'In this updated, version of this now classic volume, Patricia Coughlin, Ph.D. one of the leading practitioners of Intensive Short-Term Dynamic Psychotherapy (ISTDP) shows the reader how the psychotherapist moves from assessment to termination. At each stage of treatment case examples are provided to demonstrate the process and techniques of change. It has been my privilege to witness Dr. Coughlin's work (APA, Psychotherapy Video Series) and explore with this master clinician what makes ISTDP effective, even with some of the most challenging patient presentations. In addition to her reputation as a master psychotherapist, Dr. Coughlin is a rare clinician who is also recognized for her ability to teach and explain the complexity of this treatment in a digestible way for new and seasoned psychotherapists.'

Jeffrey J. Magnavita, Ph.D., ABPP, *CEO/Founder of Strategic Psychotherapeutics, LLC, President Elect, Society for Psychotherapy Integration (SEPI), Glastonbury, CT*

'There is no better introduction to ISTDP than Patricia Coughlin's text, a true classic, now reissued with startling follow-up data revealing the remarkable effectiveness of this treatment approach. In this book, newcomers will learn basic principles of therapy that can enhance the effectiveness of any clinician from any perspective. Her clinical vignettes make therapy come alive, and her clear explanations make complex concepts immediately understandable. I cannot recommend this book enough. There is a reason it remains a classic test after thirty years.'

Jon Frederickson, MSW, *Faculty, New Washington School of Psychiatry and author of* Co-Creating Change

'Patricia Coughlin's work has always been something of a north star for those of us practicing psychodynamic psychotherapy. Her ability to balance theoretical and technical precision with the deepest empathy for her patients has made her books sources of inspiration and edification. Here she has taken her first book—one of the definitive references in the field—and enriched it by adding new research, depth and touching follow-up data with the many patients whose lives she has transformed. As with all her books, this volume manages to communicate complex ideas in simple, immediate terms so that they provide real benefit for the practicing clinician. For anyone learning dynamic therapy, this book is a gift!'

Jonathan Entis, Ph.D.

'Consistently producing lasting, transformational change transcends theoretical differences for me, so this important update of Patricia Coughlin's influential first book on ISTDP has my endorsement. Next to her superb therapeutic results, my qualms about the psychodynamic conceptual paradigm are secondary. There can be no doubt that her work induces memory reconsolidation, the only known brain mechanism that can end symptoms permanently.'

Bruce Ecker, MA, LMFT, *co-director, Coherence Psychology Institute and co-author,* Unlocking the Emotional Brain and the Coherence Therapy Practice Manual

'This seminal work by a master clinician in dynamic psychotherapy remains essential reading for anyone serious about developing as a therapist. Long valued for its clarity, clinical richness, and vivid vignettes, the book makes a complex treatment model accessible without losing depth. Now updated with recent research and expanded content, it continues to serve as a vital and enduring guide to the practice of dynamic therapy.'

Michelle M. May, LPC, *author of* What I Couldn't Tell My Therapist
and Chair, ISTDP Program, New Washington School of Psychiatry

'The new and updated edition of Patricia Coughlin's classic *masterpiece Intensive Short-Term Dynamic Psychotherapy* is a remarkable achievement. It gives us what is exceedingly rare in the psychotherapy literature: long-term follow-up of clinical results. Once more we get to accompany Coughlin's courageous clients as they struggle, with their therapist's expert aid, to process and free themselves from deep emotional pain that had kept them stuck in life. Here we meet them again, and witness the lasting, transformative results of the collaborative work they did all those years ago.

This book is a testament to the human spirit, "blossoming once again" as pain and loss are turned toward rather than away from, in the meeting of hearts and minds that is the true therapeutic encounter.'

Tor Wennerberg, *Psychologist and Author*

INTENSIVE SHORT-TERM DYNAMIC PSYCHOTHERAPY

This long-awaited new edition of *Intensive Short-Term Dynamic Psychotherapy* is a thorough yet accessible guide for readers looking to develop their understanding of this therapeutic model and the myriad benefits it reaps as an alternative to the lengthy, and often costly, process of traditional psychoanalytic treatment.

The book is organized in a systematic fashion, analogous to the process of therapy itself, from initial contact through to termination and follow-up. Detailed clinical examples are presented throughout the text to illustrate how theory is translated into techniques of unparalleled power and effectiveness. This new edition offers a rare follow-up on nearly all of the patients included in the original, along with cutting edge research conducted over the last 30 years, to highlight the effectiveness of the method across a wide range of patients and to allow Coughlin to identify factors associated with long term change. Coughlin includes transcripts of the patients' sessions rather than a summary of her own views as a therapist, providing the reader with accurate data and allowing the patients' experience with the method to be shared in their own words.

All practicing mental health professionals, as well as students and trainees, will find this book a unique and illuminating read and an invaluable tool as they develop their own skills within the clinical space.

Patricia Coughlin is a Clinical Psychologist with over 40 years of experience as a therapist and teacher. She is the author of *Facilitating the Process of Working Through in Psychotherapy: Mastering the Middle Game* (2022), *Maximising Therapeutic Effectiveness in Dynamic Psychotherapy* (2016), and *Lives Transformed: A Revolutionary Method of Dynamic Psychotherapy* (2007).

INTENSIVE SHORT-TERM DYNAMIC PSYCHOTHERAPY

Theory and Technique

Second Edition

PATRICIA COUGHLIN

Routledge
Taylor & Francis Group
LONDON AND NEW YORK

Designed cover image: Painting by Patricia Coughlin, titled 'Evolution'

First published 2026
by Routledge
4 Park Square, Milton Park, Abingdon, Oxon OX14 4RN

and by Routledge
605 Third Avenue, New York, NY 10158

Routledge is an imprint of the Taylor & Francis Group, an informa business

British Library Cataloguing-in-Publication Data
A catalogue record for this book is available from the British Library

ISBN: 978-1-032-89307-5 (hbk)
ISBN: 978-1-032-88188-1 (pbk)
ISBN: 978-1-003-54213-1 (ebk)

DOI: 10.4324/9781003542131

Typeset in Garamond
by Apex CoVantage, LLC

To those who matter most – Megan, Katie, Anthony, James, Michael and Ben.

CONTENTS

FOREWORD XI

PREFACE XIV

PREFACE TO THE SECOND EDITION XVI

ACKNOWLEDGMENTS XVII

1 THE INTEGRATION OF THEORY AND TECHNIQUE IN DAVANLOO'S INTENSIVE SHORT-TERM DYNAMIC PSYCHOTHERAPY 1

2 THE TRIAL THERAPY 25

3 WORKING WITH DEFENSES 51

4 RESTRUCTURING REGRESSIVE DEFENSES 76

5 DEEPENING ACCESS TO AFFECT 100

6 WORKING WITH POSITIVE AND EROTIC FEELINGS 136

7 WORKING THROUGH TOWARD CHARACTER CHANGE **164**

8 TERMINATION **196**

9 FOLLOW-UP **224**

REFERENCES 247

INDEX 254

FOREWORD

Of all the factors standing in the way of therapies based on psychodynamics—which of course includes psychoanalysis—*resistance* is the most intractable. In my own practice, I recognized this many years ago, and desperation led me to try many devices for overcoming it. Most of these were derived from "alternative" psychotherapies and included using hypnosis, LSD, and Gestalt techniques, and encouraging my patients to go to encounter groups. None were of the slightest value. The attempts to shorten psychotherapy through the use of active and purely interpretive techniques, though successful, have essentially *avoided* the problem because both Balint's group in London and Sifneos's in Boston have been forced to select patients who are not resistant but highly motivated and responsive. But, in face of the kind of resistance shown by the majority of patients—perhaps 80% or 90% of the psychotherapeutic population—such methods are helpless.

In the 1970s, it became clear that Davanloo had solved the problem of resistance, without any use of alternative techniques, to an extent that would have been unbelievable if it had not been supported by videotape. In 1980, I referred to Davanloo's work as "the most important development in psychotherapy since the discovery of the unconscious"; and earlier, in 1979, I had predicted, "His work is destined to revolutionize both the practice and the scientific status of dynamic psychotherapy within the next 10 years".

I stand by the first statement, but the hope expressed in my prediction was destined to be disappointed; this simply hasn't happened. The reasons seem to include, above all, the extreme difficulty of learning Davanloo's technique, with the result that only a handful of therapists other than Davanloo himself can use it effectively. This partly stems from his use and advocacy of a highly confrontational, almost adversarial, style.

Although such an approach is extremely effective in his hands, many other therapists do not feel comfortable with it. Moreover, there has never been any textbook to facilitate the learning process.

Yet, the importance of his work cannot be overstated: he has demonstrated that a technique exists for completely overcoming the problem of resistance, resulting in a method of short-term psychotherapy with unparalleled effectiveness. The question is then whether this technique can be modified to preserve the essentials and yet permit its use by other therapists. Many professionals are attempting this task, and there are promising developments, but the results have not yet been fully documented.

That is, until the work of Dr. Coughlin described here. She has taken hold of Davanloo's technique and passed it through the furnace of her own personality, from which it has emerged softened but otherwise unchanged, and apparently equally effective—as is attested by the numerous verbatim transcripts of her interviews. There is the same persistent concentration on the defenses and the same minute attention to the transference, demonstrating that it is possible to break through lifelong defenses within the span of a single interview and thus to "unlock" the patient's unconscious. The series of observations that follow from this achievement are by now familiar, but when first made, they were equally astonishing and contradicted many pessimistic beliefs based on decades of experience with psychoanalysis: many patients can bear having the whole of their neurosis exposed within a few hours; patients rapidly reach a stage that allows direct access to the past so transference is no longer an issue; the transference neurosis can be entirely avoided; prolonged working through is not necessary; therapeutic effects can follow within a few weeks and can be *total.* Moreover, the essential therapeutic mechanism that emerges from all these therapies—as in those of Davanloo—is of extraordinary simplicity: it is the derepression and direct experience of infinitely painful feelings and memories concerned with *family relationships* throughout the whole of the patient's upbringing.

Dr. Coughlin has mastered completely both the moment-to-moment use of her technique and the theory behind it. Above all, she confronts the transference as soon as it becomes an issue; she also knows when it is necessary to back off to reduce the patient's anxiety, particularly with depressives; she understands how to judge, from physical signs, the degree to which patients are in touch with their feelings; and she is well aware of the possible danger to patients of being exposed to her powerful technique and therefore quickly detects when candidates are unsuitable and should be referred elsewhere.

It is important to say that Dr. Coughlin does not follow Davanloo's technique slavishly; she differs from him on a number of issues. She emphasizes even more than he does the importance of defenses against emotional closeness; she explicitly points out to her patients that in childhood their defenses were essential to survival; she openly acknowledges the pathology and destructiveness in other family members; she emphasizes the need to reinforce and develop the vital functions of self-care and self-protection; and she often gives the patient words of sympathy and encouragement. All these are examples of the softening that must make her technique more acceptable to other therapists and easier to use; but it in no way diminishes her toughness and determination not to let go, and therefore the effectiveness of her therapeutic work.

The book is written with exceptional clarity—the reader never has to go back and read a sentence again to understand it, but on the contrary is eager to read on.

To return to the earlier theme: in 1995, I wrote that perhaps Davanloo's most important contribution has simply been the demonstration that widely applicable brief psychotherapy is *possible*, so that other therapists are encouraged to use some of his ideas to find equally effective methods that suit their own personalities. Dr. Coughlin has unquestionably done this, and the next step will be much easier; namely, for yet other therapists to adapt her technique to suit *their* personalities—in which process the publication of this book will play an essential part. I hope the result will be a chain reaction by which the whole status of psychotherapy may ultimately be transformed.

David Malan,
Hants, England

PREFACE

My experiences as a psychodynamic psychotherapist are not unique. Like many before me, I came to believe in the power of unconscious forces in the creation and maintenance of neurotic suffering. I dedicated myself to the study and practice of psychoanalytic theory in an attempt to free patients of this suffering. Although occasionally meeting with success, nagging questions persisted. Why did treatment take so long and why were the results so sporadic and unpredictable? Was it my lack of formal analytic training, countertransference, the patient's fragility—or was I just expecting too much?

In 1987, my family and I moved to Toronto. There, in Canada, I had a chance to enroll in a psychoanalytic institute that was opened to clinical psychologists. Perhaps more study and supervision would increase my effectiveness. Several months before my analytic training was to begin, I received a notice announcing a weekend seminar in Intensive Short-Term Dynamic Psychotherapy to be given by Dr. Habib Davanloo. A vague recollection of a videotaped segment of his work, viewed in a psychotherapy course during graduate school, emerged in my mind and motivated me to attend.

That weekend was a revelation. During those 16 hours, most of them spent in a dark auditorium viewing actual therapy sessions on videotape, I witnessed something truly revolutionary.

In the past, increasing the *quantity* of therapeutic contact was the only way I had learned to intensify patient's conflicts and deepen their access to unconscious thoughts and feelings. Patients were generally seen from two to five times a week for a period of years. Dr. Davanloo presented us with unequivocal evidence that it was possible to accelerate and condense the analytic process by increasing the *quality* of therapeutic interventions. The videotaped material demonstrated a treatment protocol of unparalleled effectiveness as well as efficiency. My decision was clear. I would pursue training and supervision with Dr. Davanloo.

This book will outline what I have learned from this training. Obviously, this book reflects my understanding of Davanloo's theory and techniques. Over time I have added and integrated elements of style and substance which depart from Davanloo and these deviations are noted. Dr. Davanloo's approach remains faithful to psychoanalytic theory while radically altering standard analytic techniques. The techniques he has developed to dismantle defenses, intensify the patient's affective involvement in treatment, and identify the transference pattern of behavior result in a rapid "unlocking of the unconscious". Because these powerful techniques must be used with prudence and skill, they require a thorough understanding of the metapsychology of the unconscious in addition to careful supervision.

The book will begin from this premise, reviewing the basic concepts involved in the psychoanalytic theory of neurosis. The first chapter will outline operational definitions of dynamic concepts and strategies for developing a series of systematic interventions based on an understanding of unconscious processes.

The main body of the book will proceed in a fashion roughly parallel with the process of psychotherapy. Chapter 2 details the requirements of the initial evaluation, so crucial in determining suitability for treatment. Chapters 3 and 4 focus on techniques for working with defenses, a critical step in eliminating the resistances that prolong or disrupt treatment. Chapters 5 and 6 describe the role of affect in the creation and remediation of psychopathology, as well as techniques to intensify affective experience and facilitate its expression. Chapter 7 enumerates the various elements required to enhance and complete the process of working through. Finally, Chapter 8 discusses the process of termination and the role of follow-up in Intensive Short-Term Dynamic Psychotherapy (ISTDP).

My hope is that this introduction to the theory and technique of ISTDP will whet your appetite, increase your interest in doing effective and efficient treatment of real depth and intensity, and, in so doing, revive hope and optimism about the unique effects of dynamic psychotherapy.

Patricia Coughlin, PhD,
Albany, New York

PREFACE TO THE SECOND EDITION

When I was asked to revise and update this volume on the 30th anniversary of its original printing, I reflected upon all that has been achieved during these intervening years and decided it was worth doing.

Over the past 30 years, Intensive Short-Term Dynamic Psychotherapy (ISTDP) has accumulated increasing empirical support as both cost and clinically effective across a wide range of psychiatric disorders. Of note, it has been shown to be effective with disorders that often fail to respond to psychotherapy. These include treatment resistant depression, character disorders, chronic pain, postpartum depression, medically unexplained symptoms, and pseudo-seizures. Effect sizes are far larger than those established for medication and cognitive behavioral therapy (CBT).

Furthermore, while most medication and psychotherapeutic interventions suffer from high relapse rates, long-term follow-up studies of ISTDP have found that those who complete the treatment not only maintain therapeutic gains but continue to improve over time, with no additional intervention. In this second edition, 10- and 20-year follow-up data on many of the patients featured in the original text have been included. These verbatim transcripts reveal the depth and breadth of change that was achieved during treatment, and that continued afterward. These follow-up interviews provide clues regarding the factors associated with deep and lasting change.

ACKNOWLEDGMENTS

I feel blessed to have had the guidance and support of so many friends and colleagues through the years. I must start with my first mentor, Dr. Hal Arkes who displayed great faith in me and helped me to believe I might have something special to offer the field of clinical psychology. During my years of graduate study at Syracuse University, Drs. Jay Land and Ruth Burton stood out as models of integrity and had a profound and lasting influence on my personal and professional life.

During my years in Chicago, as a resident and a member of the faculty at Northwestern University Medical School, I was surrounded by bright, dedicated, and compassionate professionals. Drs. Edward Sheridan and Mary Dohney were most influential during my residency. Alma Rolfs, MSW, and Barbara Muday, CSW, became close personal friends as well as stimulating colleagues and models of dedicated service. Drs. Merton Gill and Ruth Westheimers were superb clinicians whose supervision proved to be an invaluable aid in my development as a therapist.

In 1987, I attended a weekend seminar offered by Dr. Davanloo, and it is no exaggeration to say that the experience changed my professional life (and undoubtedly my personal life as well). All my subsequent clinical work, teaching, and writing reflect the influence of my exposure to this brilliant man. Others who have helped immeasurably in my understanding and integration of the theories and techniques developed by Dr. Davanloo include Dr. George Glumac and the faculty at the Ontario Institute for Short-Term Dynamic Psychotherapy (STDP), Drs. Jim Schubmehl, Michael Alpert, Diana Fosha, David Malan, and Leigh McCullough Vaillant.

A deep debt of gratitude is extended to Pearl Mindell, a woman of grace and dignity, who helped me travel through the darkest night of my soul. Her influence has been deep and abiding.

My patients have granted me the rare privilege of intimate knowledge of their deepest thoughts and feelings. I have been inspired by their courage and have grown from their journeys. The generosity of spirit evident in those who have allowed their treatment to be videotaped, written about, and even viewed by professional audiences for our learning, is a gift of immeasurable value. I thank each and every one of them. Verbatim transcripts of therapy sessions are used throughout the book. Identifying information has been deleted or altered in order to preserve the patients' privacy.

Most of all, I want to thank my family for their love and support over the years, and especially during the writing of this book. I thank my mother for teaching me a love of learning and compassion for the suffering of others. To my father, who died while this manuscript was in progress, I am most grateful for his integrity of being. To my children, Megan, Katherine, and Anthony, thanks for making me happy to wake up each morning.

Finally, I want to thank Steven Sandler, MD, for his careful reading of this manuscript and my editor, Kelly Franklin. Her keen intellect and enthusiastic support were invaluable assets. This book is far better for her involvement.

1 THE INTEGRATION OF THEORY AND TECHNIQUE IN DAVANLOO'S INTENSIVE SHORT-TERM DYNAMIC PSYCHOTHERAPY

I hear a distant drumbeat
A heartbeat pulsing low
Is it coming from within
A heart beat I don't know
A troubled soul knows no peace
A dark and poisoned pool
Of liberty now lost
A pawn, the oppressor's tool.
"Breaking the silence"
Loreeao McKennitt[1]

In many ways, this songwriter has articulated the plight of neurotics, blind to their own inner world and, as such, destined to live the life of a prisoner. The discovery of such a rich and complex inner life began with Breuer and was elaborated on in great detail by Freud (Breuer & Freud, 1895).

DOI: 10.4324/9781003542131-1

Basic Tenets of Psychoanalytic Theory

Breuer's (Breuer & Freud, 1895) pioneering work with Anna O. led to the discovery of the dynamic unconscious and laid the foundation for psychoanalysis. He placed the patient under a hypnotic trance and discovered, quite by chance (Schoenewolf, 1990), that her current physical symptoms were connected to traumatic experiences from the past (caring for her sick and dying father). When he was able to get her to verbalize her feelings about these traumatic experiences, the symptoms vanished. Again and again, he found that the recall of memories and reliving of the emotions associated with the memories led to symptom removal. The original forgetting was labeled "repression", and the remembering, "catharsis" (Fisher & Greenberg, 1977). Although this cathartic treatment led to immediate relief, there were frequent relapses and no lasting cure. An additional problem arose in the treatment relationship when Anna began to have strong loving and sexual feelings toward Breuer. He became frightened and abruptly ended her treatment. In fact, he abandoned this kind of work altogether.

Freud took over where Breuer left off, making changes designed to address the problems encountered with hypnotic treatment. He decided to abandon hypnosis because this technique only provided temporary relief. He felt that the conscious ego must learn to deal directly with the trauma and integrate these memories and feelings into awareness. The task was to develop a treatment that would enable the patient to consciously tolerate what had been previously experienced as unbearable. By encouraging patients to say whatever came to mind and following their associations, Freud found that they would gradually approach previously avoided topics. The technique of free association, designed to enable patients to gradually become aware of unconscious feelings, memories, and fantasies, was the first major change in psychoanalytic technique to follow hypnosis.

As Freud began to encourage patients to say whatever came to mind, he confronted a counterforce working against remembering and reexperiencing painful and anxiety-provoking events. He labeled this force resistance and found it became the greatest obstacle to successful treatment. In many ways, all developers of subsequent technique, including the short-term dynamic psychotherapists such as Malan, Mann, Sifneos, and Davanloo, have tried to find methods for circumventing, reducing, or eliminating resistance so that patients will reach therapeutic goals. The tension between the patient's desire to get well and the desire to avoid that which is painful by resisting therapeutic intervention, is the essence of psychic conflict. How professionals deal with this conflict in the therapeutic setting is of pivotal importance and will be covered extensively in the present volume.

Another essential change in technique that followed the use of hypnosis involved using, rather than avoiding, the feelings evoked within the treatment relationship. Freud came to realize that the patient's feelings toward and perceptions of the therapist were not random but constituted a projection or transference of feelings and perceptions having to do with significant figures from the patient's past. He called this the phenomenon of transference and used it to bring the patient's inner conflicts to life in the therapeutic setting.

He combined these changes (i.e., free association, a focus on resistance and analysis of the transference) as he developed the technique of psychoanalysis. He would actively interpret the patient's defensiveness and resistance to remembering and experiencing painful experiences from the past. These interpretations were designed to release buried feelings. The process itself tended to elicit feelings toward the doctor, which were then associated to prominent figures from the patient's past. This basic technique of interpreting defense, and releasing buried feelings and memories, enabled patient and therapist to gain insight into links between the forgotten past and current behavior. This remains the essence of psychodynamic psychotherapy.

As Alexander (Alexander & French, 1946) understood it, it was not necessary for patients to remember all the events from their past that caused neurotic reactions. The essential element was the therapist's ability to reestablish the core conflictual situation in the transference relationship so that "the adult ego has the opportunity to grapple with it in a new attempt at mastery" (Alexander & French, 1946, p. 163). Being able to withstand the full impact of the previously repressed intense feelings and reactions from the past in the current relationship with the therapist, without resorting to regressive defenses, was designed in order to increase the patient's ego-adaptive capacity. Thus, the new experience in the transference would restructure the patient's defensive system. This shift in focus from emotional catharsis to conscious recall was accompanied by a shift in therapeutic goals, from that of mere symptom removal, to a permanent change in the patient's ego functioning. Dynamic psychotherapy, which had been fairly brief during Freud's early days, got increasingly protracted as the goals of treatment expanded. Following each extension of therapy came clinicians attempting to find ways to shorten the process. Contributions of the major theorists in the short-term dynamic psychotherapy movement will be reviewed in subsequent chapters.

The Importance of Theory-Guided Technique

Freud was a theorist, researcher, and clinician who wrote relatively little on technique. In the paper entitled "On the History of the Psychoanalytic Movement" (Freud, 1914), he remained vague about technique, stating that any psychotherapy which recognized the phenomena of transference and resistance as facts and made them central in the work could be considered psychoanalysis. There was little improvement in this regard over time. Analysts as a group have proven unable to agree on theory or technique. A survey of British analysts (Glover, 1958) revealed that half of the respondents reported approaching their analytic work *without* any theoretical outline in mind. A study conducted in Chicago (Henry, Sims, & Spicey, 1968) revealed that 61% of the analysts there responded in a similar fashion. Given the lack of a cohesive theoretical paradigm for understanding patient material, it should come as no surprise that other surveys were unable to find any agreement on the goals of psychoanalytic treatment (Seward, 1962–1963). In fact, the 65 analysts studied by Seward could only agree on what they *did not* expect to accomplish, including symptom relief, self-acceptance or expression, and an increase in personal responsibility. These findings have been corroborated by others (Sklansky, Isaacs, Levitor, & Haggard, 1966) who have found that analysts were "highly idiosyncratic" in their interventions.

Davanloo (1980; 1990) has attempted to correct many of these inconsistencies by having a clear grasp on the metapsychology of the unconscious, developing a systematic method of intervention based on theory, closely examining patients' responses to intervention (asking questions rather than assuming or making interpretations), and using videotapes to study the process. He has labeled this form of treatment Intensive Short-Term Dynamic Psychotherapy (ISTDP). He has repeatedly emphasized that a thorough understanding of the metapsychology of the unconscious is essential to the proper use of the techniques he has developed. Following his suggestion, this chapter will outline the metapsychological assumptions underlying Davanloo's method and then detail the technical interventions based on this theoretical understanding.

Freud's Second Theory of Anxiety

The theoretical underpinnings of Davanloo's model have been derived from Freud's second theory of anxiety. Originally, Freud viewed anxiety as a reaction to the build-up of instinctual tensions, assuming an "inherent tendency in the nervous system to reduce, or at least keep constant, the amount of excitation present in it" (Freud, 1926, p. 4). This is the essence of drive theory, which hypothesizes a motivation toward the reduction or discharge of instinctual tensions. As early as 1897 (Freud, 1950, Letter 75), Freud expressed doubts about a direct link between accumulated excitation and anxiety. Still, it was not until the publication of *Inhibitions, Symptoms and Anxiety* in 1926 that he explicitly stated his revised view: that anxiety is a danger signal to the ego, warning of the occurrence of trauma. Trauma, as he defined it, "involves separation from, or loss of, a loved object or a loss of its love" (Freud, 1926, p. 151). That such a separation or loss would constitute trauma is readily explained by the infant and child's prolonged state of mental and physical helplessness and utter dependence on caretakers for survival and well-being. As such, anxiety serves an indispensable biological function, alerting the ego to the probability of trauma.

This revision implies the central nature of human attachments and is the beginning of an object relations theory (Della Selva, 1992; 1993; Greenberg & Mitchell, 1983). Because of the child's dependence and the centrality of human attachments, any thought, feeling, or action which has led to unwanted separation from or loss of an attachment figure or their love is experienced as dangerous, evokes anxiety, and is avoided. Symptoms are considered to be compromises between the competing need to express the feeling and to defend against it. Symptoms and defenses keep the anxiety, and the feelings propelling it, out of awareness.

The following example of this theory involves a depressed woman who came for treatment. As she described a recent interaction with her father, she realized that she'd had a stubborn headache ever since the visit with him. After describing the incident, we focused on her feelings toward her father. She began to get in touch with a rage toward him that had mobilized a violent impulse. She imagined smashing his head and poking out his eyes, leaving him dead in a pool of blood. This feeling and the accompanying impulse were experienced as very dangerous and aroused considerable anxiety. There was little love lost with her father, but she imagined her mother would be furious with her. It was her mother's love and attention that she felt she couldn't afford to lose. The anxiety served as a signal to repress this feeling from her consciousness. Still, the feelings and impulses were very strong and were pushing for expression. The compromise between the impulse (smashing his head and poking his eyes) and the defense against it (displacement) was a headache. Following the experience of anger in the therapy session, the headache disappeared, providing compelling evidence that, once the patient was able to consciously tolerate the direct experience and expression affect, the need to defend against it by becoming symptomatic was no longer necessary.

Two Triangles

Menninger (1958) operationalized the notion of intrapsychic conflict by drawing a "triangle of insight" in which impulses and feelings, defenses, and anxiety each occupy one of the three corners. Malan (1979) went one step further by linking the triangle that depicts intrapsychic conflict with another triangle that represents significant others in the patient's life (called the triangle of conflict and triangle of the person, respectively). The relationship between these two triangles indicates, once again, the central importance of the interpersonal context within which psychic conflict is experienced (Figure 1.1).

Feelings do not exist in a vacuum but arise both toward and in reaction to others. There is always an interpersonal context to the arousal of emotion, even if only in fantasy. It is hypothesized that those affective states which caretakers did not tolerate will be suffused with anxiety and lead to the operation of a defense. We cannot assume that only certain feelings, such as anger, will be prohibited; for in some families nothing is experienced as more threatening and, therefore, is more heavily prohibited than the expression of tender feelings (Suttie, 1937, 1988). Careful exploration of anxiety as it arises in the dynamic interaction between patient and therapist is the most accurate way to assess this for a given patient.

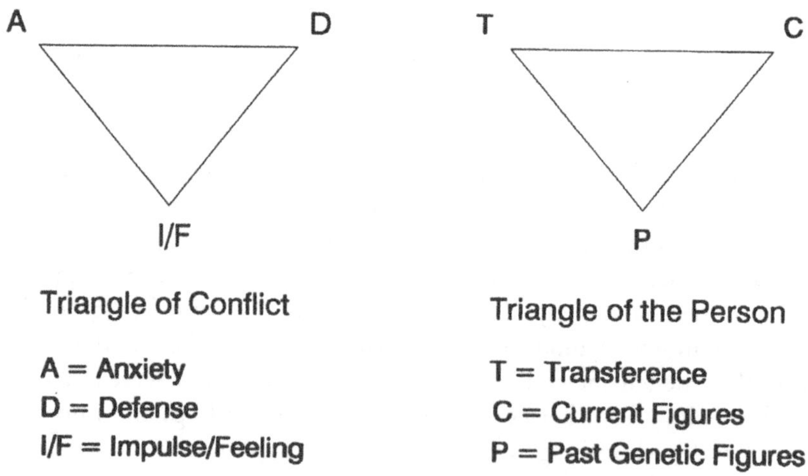

Figure 1.1 Triangle of Conflict and Triangle of the Person

Operational Definitions of Dynamic Concepts

Davanloo (1980; 1990) has made extensive use of the two triangles as a means for conceptualizing intrapsychic conflict. As such, the triangles serve as both a diagnostic tool and guide to systematic intervention. Since a full and detailed understanding of the two triangles is of such great importance in Davanloo's system, each element will be specifically and operationally defined.

Feelings and Impulses

Feelings are considered the engine of the intrapsychic system and have been placed at the bottom of the triangle. Primary feelings include joy and happiness, sexual desire and arousal, anger, and sadness or grief. Davanloo has identified three components to feeling that must be present for a patient to be considered "in touch with" the experience of affect (Laikin, Winston, & McCullough, 1991). These three components represent the cognitive, physiological, and motoric elements of emotional experience (Figure 1.2). The cognitive component involves the accurate labeling of the emotion ("I am angry"). The physiological component includes all the physical and visceral sensations that accompany the emotion ("I am feeling hot, like my temperature is up and my blood is pumping. My muscles feel strong"). Finally, the motoric element of the emotion involves mobilization of an impulse ("I feel like punching him in the face").

The absence of any one of the components of feelings indicates the operation of defense. This detailed conceptualization of feeling allows the clinician to pinpoint the specific aspect of the feeling that is being defended against and can serve as a guide to specific interventions.

For example, histrionic patients tend to experience the physiological and motoric aspects of feeling but defend against knowing *what* it is they are feeling and *toward*

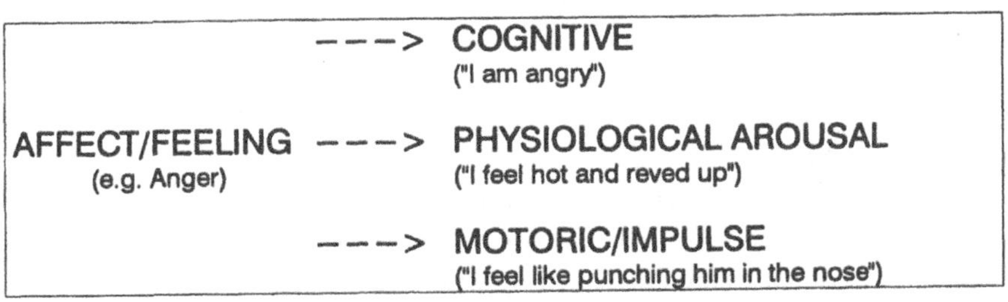

Figure 1.2 Components of an Affective Experience

FORMAL		TACTICAL	
REPRESSIVE	**REGRESSIVE**	**VERBAL**	**NON–VERBAL**
Intellectualization Rationalization Minimization Displacement Reaction Formation	Projection Somatization Denial Acting Out/ Discharge of Impulse	Vague/General Diversification Sarcasm Argumentativeness	Avoiding Eye Contact Smiling/Laughing Weepiness Arms/Legs Crossed

Figure 1.3 Defenses

whom (the cognitive element of feeling). On the other hand, obsessive patients might be able to label their feeling (cognitive) and even elaborate a fantasy of what they want to do with the feeling (motoric), but they defend against the physiological experience of the feeling, remaining emotionally detached. This brings us to the defense corner of the triangle.

Defenses

Defenses consist of cognitive, emotional, and interpersonal strategies employed by patients to keep anxiety-provoking thoughts and feelings out of awareness (Figure 1.3). Several categories of defense mechanisms will be explored here.

Formal Defenses

The formal defenses, designed to prevent conscious awareness of thoughts and feelings experienced as dangerous, can be grouped into two general categories: repressive and regressive. The repressive defenses include intellectualization, rationalization, minimization, displacement, and reaction formation. Regressive defenses include denial, projection, and somatization. Identifying the patient's characteristic defenses yields diagnostic information regarding their current level of ego functioning. For example, a reliance on regressive defenses, such as denial and projection, indicates greater impairment in ego functioning than would the characteristic use of repressive defenses, such as rationalization and displacement.

Tactical Defenses

In addition to the formal defenses, Davanloo pays strict attention to what he has labeled "tactical defenses". Whereas formal defenses are largely intrapsychic in nature, tactical defenses are employed interpersonally to prevent emotional closeness. Tactical defenses include all the verbal and nonverbal maneuvers patients use interpersonally to deflect or prevent meaningful emotional contact.

Verbal tactical defenses include vagueness and a tendency toward generalities, the use of contradictory statements, sarcasm, a high level of verbal activity making a dialogue impossible, or diversification (jumping from topic to topic). Some examples of nonverbal tactical defenses include avoidance of eye contact, smiling and giggling, weepiness, or an air of detachment. Posture is also included here, with either great stiffness and immobility or limpness indicating the presence of a defensive barrier against meaningful interpersonal contact.

Assessing Whether Defenses are Syntonic or Dystonic

Patients are sometimes aware that they are avoiding the experience of painful feelings by utilizing formal defenses. Such an awareness indicates that this particular defense is dystonic and suggests a high level of ego-adaptive capacity (specifically a good observing ego). Tactical defenses are almost always automatic and unconscious. Together, the various tactical defenses a patient employs tend to be embedded in the character and are quite syntonic ("That's just the way I am").

So, at the micro-level, the patient employs specific defenses against the experience of painful and anxiety-laden feelings, but on a macro-level, these individual defenses link together to form a barrier or wall against meaningful emotional contact with others, including the therapist (Laikin, Winston, & McCullough, 1991). To intervene effectively, the therapist must ascertain which level of defensive operation is most prominent, so that therapy can specifically address it. For example, challenging a patient on a specific defense (minimization) against a particular feeling (grief about the loss of loved one), will have very little impact if the patient has erected a massive wall against meaningful involvement with the therapist (made up of minimal eye contact, a monotone voice, and a passive, compliant stance). The therapist must proceed from the outside in, and should begin with any defenses against emotional closeness.

Defenses are employed in an effort to reduce the anxiety that accompanies "forbidden" thoughts and feelings. Understanding the nature of the patient's anxiety, the level of anxiety experienced, and the ways in which the patient typically channels anxiety is of great diagnostic significance and should be monitored throughout treatment. Davanloo has classified three primary channels of anxiety (Figure 1.4).

	-->	STRIATED MUSCLE
ANXIETY	-->	SMOOTH MUSCLE
	-->	COGNITIVE DISRUPTION/DISCHARGE

Figure 1.4 Channels of Anxiety

Anxiety

Striated Muscle

One very common channel or pathway of anxiety is into the striated or voluntary muscle. Patients who channel their anxiety into striated muscle tend to associate their physical tension with anxiety and to have a fairly accurate idea what they are anxious about, indicating some degree of integration between thoughts and feelings and suggesting a fairly high level of ego functioning. For example, a 40-year-old married man reported feeling "a little nervous" about our first meeting. When I asked how he experienced his anxiety, he said he felt physically tense (voluntary muscle). I then asked when it started and what he thought the anxiety was about. He said that his anxiety had only kicked in once he was actually in the waiting room and that, since most of his problems were of an intimate, sexual nature, he felt uncomfortable discussing them openly with "a young, attractive woman". This interchange provided evidence of a fairly high level of ego-adaptive capacity, as the anxiety was being channeled into the striated muscle and the patient was able to make a connection between his anxiety and an upsurge of feeling in the transference.

Smooth Muscle

The second channel of anxiety Davanloo has identified is into the smooth, involuntary muscle. These are patients who channel their anxiety into the soma. Frequently, they are unaware of any link between their physical state of distress (e.g., headache, or gas pains and diarrhea) and the emotional state of anxiety and nervousness. Often they will vehemently deny any such link, insisting, "It's only physical". In such cases, preparatory work is required to increase their capacity to consciously tolerate the experience of anxiety before moving on to more intense, affect-laden work. Failure to do so could lead to an exacerbation of the patient's physical ailment (e.g., headaches, irritable bowel, ulcerative colitis, asthma).

An example of a patient in this category was an older man who presented himself as "calm, cool, and collected". He reported being very interested in the process of therapy and said he looked forward to our meeting. When I asked him about any physical difficulties, he reported sleep disturbance and diarrhea, both of which had been particularly bad the day or two before our meeting. His detachment from the experience of his anxiety and failure to connect his physical symptoms with the anxiety about meeting with me indicated a lower level of ego functioning than with the man previously mentioned.

Cognitive Disruption

The third channel of anxiety is that which affects cognitive functioning. When anxious, these patients experience some sort of cognitive disruption; either losing track of their thoughts, getting weak and dizzy, dissociating, or reporting an urge to discharge their anxiety in an impulsive manner. Evidence of the use of this channel of anxiety generally signifies some fragility of the ego and is a contraindication for rapid movement into the unconscious.

For example, a young college student presented herself in a rather bubbly and effervescent manner. When asked how she felt about coming to see me, she said she was really excited about it. However, she had arrived half an hour late for our appointment. As we explored this, she revealed that she had been up all night, unable to sleep, and had lost the directions to the office. Her thinking was scattered, and she had a great deal of difficulty articulating the nature of her problems. Further inquiry revealed pervasive cognitive disruption in the face of anxiety that had significantly affected her ability to complete schoolwork. In fact, she was on academic probation. All these factors suggested that a very high level of anxiety was seriously interfering with her ability to think clearly and indicated some fragility of the ego.

Obtaining a Baseline of Anxiety

In addition to identifying the primary channel of anxiety in evidence at the time of the interview (it's not unusual to find a mix), a baseline needs to be obtained. One patient entered the evaluation with a cordless phone in hand saying, "I've brought this in case I need to dial 911. When I get anxious, I pass out". It would be easy to assume that his anxiety was exceptionally high because he was about to begin the process of psychotherapy. When asked, "How does this anxiety compare with what you experience in other situations?", he replied, "Oh, this is fairly mild. I'm least anxious when I'm alone in my apartment, and I'm also pretty good if I'm at a hospital or in a doctor's office. It's being out there with people I can't tolerate". This comparative analysis yielded valuable diagnostic data suggesting a high degree of ego fragility.

Therapeutic Implications of Theory

Psychodynamic theory suggests that all the repressed feelings and reactions to the ruptures in significant relationships lie at the root of neurotic suffering. Davanloo believes, "The vast majority of neurosis stems from the patient's conflicting feelings within family relationships . . . " (1990, p. 190).

How do these mixed and conflictual feelings develop (Figure 1.5)? At the very center of human experience, there is an innate capacity to form close emotional attachments to caretakers (Bowlby, 1973). Davanloo has clearly stated, "Only the capacity to develop warm emotional ties to caretakers is innate" (1987a; 1987b). These attachment strivings are inevitably frustrated, which causes internal pain and grief and gives rise to reactive anger toward the frustrating and depriving (if not, at times, abusive) attachment figure. At times, the pain and anger seem so great

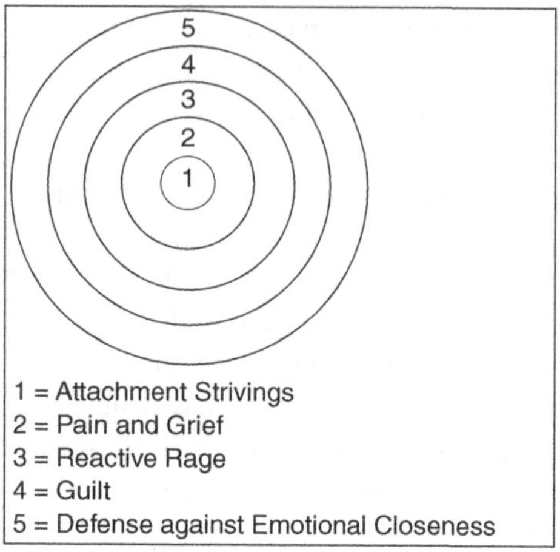
5
4
3
2
1
1 = Attachment Strivings
2 = Pain and Grief
3 = Reactive Rage
4 = Guilt
5 = Defense against Emotional Closeness

Figure 1.5 Genetic System within the Unconscious

and so unbearable that the patient unconsciously decides that no one will ever get close enough to cause such harm again. Consequently, the person builds a layer of defense around the entire intrapsychic system. This protective layer serves a dual function by fending off real or anticipated pain from both internal and external sources. Davanloo (1990–1991) refers to this as a defense against emotional closeness (DAEC). Others have called this type of defense "character armor" (Reich, 1933) or "false self" (Winnicott, 1965). What began as a layer of protection for many patients becomes an immovable barrier to satisfying human contact. These patients are often referred to as character disordered.

Traditionally, patients with a significant layer of character pathology have proven resistant to treatments of all sorts, even medication (Reitav, 1991). In all likelihood, this is the result of the therapist's failure to effectively penetrate the defensive armor of the patient.

The resistance employed by the patient has been a long-standing problem for analysts. Malan (Davanloo, 1980) has suggested that Freud took a "wrong turn" when he reacted to increasing resistance with increased passivity. Not only did this passivity on the part of the analyst prolong treatment, but it also frequently proved ineffective and patients failed to improve despite years of treatment. Reich (1933) expressed the opinion, "If one neglects such character resistances, and instead simply follows the line of the material, such resistances form a ballast which is difficult, if not impossible to remove" (p. 51).

Davanloo (1987a; 1987b) has developed a series of techniques designed to directly address, and then break through, defensive barriers that will otherwise become a resistance in treatment. He has found that clarification of defense and resistance, followed by pressure and challenge to the patient's defensive barrier, must occur from the start of treatment. This technique stirs up strong mixed feelings in the transference, followed by the patient's characteristic defenses against the same. This conflict serves as a trigger to similar conflicts from the past. Davanloo has repeatedly demonstrated that, if the defenses can be penetrated, and the feelings in the transference experienced and expressed directly, an opening into the genetic unconscious will be achieved. Theory suggests that, once patients can consciously face that which they had previously avoided, they will no longer need to rely on regressive and self-defeating defenses. The ego regains autonomy, and patients can function at their highest level of ability.

Resistance Versus Alliance

The central role of conflictual feelings in the development of neurosis makes it inevitable that patients arrive for treatment in a state of ambivalence. Patients want help from the therapist in getting to the bottom of their difficulties and achieving freedom from suffering. This part of the patient is available for the development of a therapeutic alliance. At the same time, another part of the patient operates in opposition to the therapist. This part wants to run, hide, and avoid the pain and grief the therapeutic process will entail. It is this part of the patient that fuels the resistance. Davanloo (1987a; 1987b) has found that these two variables, the therapeutic alliance and resistance, exist in inverse proportion to one another. Our job involves creating a shift within the patient from resistance to alliance. How this is achieved is a central question for all dynamic psychotherapists.

Therapeutic Stance

Many therapists have experienced occasional success in helping patients to achieve deep and long-lasting change in a brief time. The question has always been how to do so with some consistency. Alexander and French (1946), Malan (1963, 1976a, 1976b; 1978a; 1978b; 1986; Malan & Osimo, 1992), and Davanloo (1980) have all found that those most likely to make rapid and enduring changes were in some sort of acute crisis. In these cases, some external event had evoked such intense feelings and conflict that the patients' characteristic defenses were not sufficient to contain. So these patients entered treatment with little defense in operation, and strong feelings close to the surface. In addition, the pain they were already experiencing served as a potent motivator. These factors all contributed to rapid movement. Yet, this group of patients constitutes only about 20% of those seeking outpatient psychotherapy. In most cases, patients are suffering from chronic difficulties with anxiety, depression, and interpersonal relatedness, as well as character disorders. It has been assumed such patients would not be able to benefit from short-term dynamic psychotherapy. Davanloo has challenged this assumption by developing specific methods for *creating* an intrapsychic crisis in these patients. How is this accomplished?

According to Davanloo (1980; 1990), the therapist must abandon the passive stance and work actively to bring the patient's conflict into focus, intensifying the affective involvement and creating an intrapsychic crisis that makes rapid change possible. The therapist makes a direct appeal to the healthy part of the ego seeking freedom, while exerting pressure on the defenses. In this way, the ISTDP therapist is not neutral but adopts a therapeutic stance that advocates openness and honesty, even when painful. The therapist communicates a serious but dedicated approach to getting at the truth (Malan has referred to this as "the iron hand in the velvet glove"). It is clear to the patient from the outset that the therapist is working diligently and is presenting a challenge to the patient to join in and work at his or her highest level of ability.

Michael Balint (1957) has written about the element of surprise in psychotherapy and advocated presenting the patient with a counteroffer. In Freud's day, it was startling for the therapist to offer an atmosphere in which the patient could say whatever comes to mind. This was in stark contrast to the repressive attitudes of the day. In post-Freudian America, it is assumed that therapy will consist of endless talk, and it is startling for the therapist to suggest that meaningful work can occur rapidly. This counteroffer consists of the therapist placing pressure on the patient to abandon defenses while simultaneously displaying a keen interest in getting to know the patient deeply enough to be of help. Such a unique and unexpected offer evokes strong mixed feelings in the transference. In part, the patient is alarmed that the therapist wants to enter into his or her inner world, possibly closer than anyone has come before. Resistance against this is mobilized as "an inevitable consequence of the basic mechanism underlying neurosis, namely repression of feelings that are painful, anxiety-laden, and considered dangerous and unacceptable" (Davanloo, 1987).

On the other hand, there is a healthy, maturational force within the patient that yeans for the kind of emotional closeness that the therapist is offering. Davanloo (1987c) viewed this as a manifestation of "the unconscious therapeutic alliance" (UTA), which exists in tandem with the resistance. Both the conscious and unconscious alliance provide motivation for the patient to be open and honest with the therapist about her difficulties, in order to gain freedom from suffering. The conflicting desires to face and avoid one's true feelings is intensified in order to create an intrapsychic crisis within the patient. A shift from resistance to alliance results in the direct experience of all these conflicted feelings and often triggers an unlocking of the unconscious system (Davanloo, 1990).

All the techniques developed by Davanloo have been aimed at bringing buried feelings to the surface, so they can be faced directly by the patient and resolved in an adaptive manner.

Central Dynamic Sequence

The central dynamic sequence encapsulates the procedure developed by Davanloo (1988) to assess suitability for an unlocking of the unconscious and then guiding the process, should such a procedure be deemed appropriate. Malan (1980) has called Davanloo's development of this elegant and comprehensive system of intervention "the most important development in psychotherapy since the discovery of the unconscious". The central dynamic sequence involves five phases:

1. Inquiry and survey of patient's difficulties.
2. Defense analysis and triangle work.
3. Rise and breakthrough of complex mixed feelings in the C and T.
4. De-repression of significant memories and associations allowing for a meaningful exploration of the patient's developmental history.
5. Interpretation and consolidation of insights obtained in the process.

Phase 1: Inquiry

Davanloo advocated a descriptive, phenomenological approach to inquiry. This includes taking a survey of the patient's symptomatic and characterological difficulties, with an emphasis on specificity and a focus on feeling. Recent examples of the problems being reported are requested to aid in this process.

Specificity

To obtain an accurate assessment of the patient's difficulties, the therapist must make specific inquiries. For example, a patient comes in complaining of depression and inhibition at work. The therapist inquires, "What do you mean by depression? Could we look at a recent example of a time when you felt depressed? What is it that you actually experienced inside, on an emotional level, that you refer to as being depressed?"

If the patient is able to provide detailed information regarding such an experience, then a baseline and brief history of the presenting problem should be obtained before moving on to other areas of disturbance. To continue with our example, the therapist would ask, "So how long have you been depressed? Have you had other periods of depression in your life? What is the worst it has ever gotten?"

The answers to these questions suggest the nature of the underlying difficulty, as well as providing some information on the patient's ego-adaptive capacity. For example, if the patient has recently become depressed in reaction to the death of a friend and reports a history of depression following previous losses, it suggests the presence of pathological mourning. If the depression is experienced as sadness, lethargy, and pessimism about the future, but does not involve vegetative symptoms or an inability to function, the patient is likely to have fairly good ego-adaptive capacity that has been temporarily depleted and can be rapidly mobilized to deal actively with an acute grieving process.

If, on the other hand, the patient can't sleep, has lost 15 pounds in the past month, and has been calling in sick at work, the ego is so depleted that there will be little energy in the system to mobilize for the work of an uncovering psychotherapy. Either medication or supportive and restructuring work would be necessary to build the ego to the point where the patient could tolerate the repressed feelings that need to be uncovered.

Obtaining a Survey of Difficulties

Once the presenting complaints have been explored, the therapist should ask about other areas of difficulty. At times, patients will report needing help with only one circumscribed problem. The therapist might say, "So, other than this conflict with your boss, you have no other problem in your life? You are 100% satisfied in other areas?" If the patient says, "Yes, that's it", then you are sitting with one of those rare patients (5%–10% of those seeking outpatient psychotherapy) who has one circumscribed area of conflict that should be worked through in a number of hours. More often, however, patients will then volunteer several other problems.

Challenge to Lack of Clarity

The only challenge to the patient at this point in the sequence is to provide specific data necessary to delineate the areas of difficulty. In response to vagueness, the therapist might say, "It is important that you be specific so I can understand the nature of your difficulties. Could you give me an example?"

It is not uncommon for patients to externalize and either talk about problems that other people have or to say they have come at the insistence of someone else. When I asked a college student why she had come to see me, she said that her roommates were a pain in the neck, and went on to detail *their* problems. Sometimes a simple redirection will suffice to get inquiry on track. I replied, "You're telling me about some problems your roommates are having. What difficulties are you having that I could help you with?"

Securing the Patient's Will to Work

The therapist should immediately explore a patient's report that they are seeking psychotherapy at someone else's behest. It must be determined whether the patient has the inner motivation and desire to enter psychotherapy.

Another college student declared that he was in my office because his mother had told him he had to see someone. This needed to be clarified at once. I asked, "So you are here because your mother demanded it? If she had not insisted, you wouldn't be here? As far as you're concerned, you have no difficulties in your life?" If the patient were to say he had no problems of his own, there would be no point in continuing. To enter treatment under these conditions would be a farce. Conceivably, it could be quite therapeutic to refuse to engage in such a ruse. In so doing, the therapist displays respect for the patient, as we never have the right to intervene without direct permission from the patient.

In cases such as this one, the only possible intervention would be to explore the patient's compliance. "So you're telling me you have no problems and no desire to be here, but here you sit. How does that happen? Is this a unique situation or do you have a tendency to comply with others' wishes?" If the patient acknowledges this, the therapist needs to ask, "Do you see this as a problem? Is this something you would like to work on?" Patients must declare that they are in the therapist's office of their own will before the process can proceed.

Maintaining a Focus

If the patient jumps from topic to topic, the therapist must interrupt and slow that patient down. For example, "Before we go on to this other problem, let's make sure we understand the first problem you mentioned". Similarly, if the patient begins by talking about something that happened when he or she was three years old, the therapist must redirect to an inquiry of current difficulties. A statement such as "I'm sure your grandfather's death was an important event in your life and we'll be getting to that, but let's start with what brings you here now". Identifying the current precipitant of the reported difficulties is essential in establishing a context for understanding the nature of the patient's difficulties.

Phase 2: Defense Analysis

Once an adequate inquiry and survey of the patient's problems has been obtained (which shouldn't take more than 15 or 20 minutes), the therapist moves on to an examination of the patient's defenses. Recalling that the aim of the treatment is to enable the patient to experience feelings "to the maximum degree" the person can bear, all defenses against the experience of feeling must be removed. The defense work can be roughly divided into three steps or stages:

1. Identification and clarification of defenses.

2. Turning the ego against its defenses.

3. Pressure and challenge to give up the defenses.

Identification and Clarification of Defenses

While conducting the inquiry, the therapist should be noting, and filing away for future use, the kinds of defenses in operation. A patient might have erratic eye contact and have his arms folded across his chest. In response to questions about his feelings, this patient might have the tendency to smile and rationalize. The first therapeutic task in this phase is to identify and clarify the defenses in operation. "As we began to look at your feelings toward your wife, did you notice you were avoiding my eyes, you folded your arms across your chest, laughed, and then offered a rationalization?" The task here is to assess whether the patient is aware or can easily become aware of these defensive behaviors. If so, and the patient says, "Yes, I see that now", then the function of these behaviors must be made clear to the patient. "Isn't this actually a way to avoid looking at the feelings toward your wife?" If the patient can see that he *does something* to avoid feeling, it suggests that his defenses are fairly dystonic.

At other times, patients don't distinguish between what they feel (I/F) and what they do (D) to avoid it (see Figure 1.1). They may be highly identified with the defense and say, "That's just the way I am. I've always been that way", indicating a fairly high degree of syntonicity. In these cases, repeated efforts are necessary to identify and clarify the defensive avoidance of feeling in all areas of the patient's life (sometimes referred to as "working the triangles").

Turning the Ego Against Its Defenses

The second part of this phase of the work involves turning the ego against its defenses. This is done by focusing on the cost of defenses, pointing out to the patient the negative, self-defeating consequences of their use.

The following is a fairly typical intervention designed to highlight the cost of defenses and to shift the balance from resistance to alliance. "So now you see that you avoid the experience of your true feelings by laughing them off and going to a rationalization. Let's look at the consequences of maintaining this avoidant stance. First of all, if you're hiding and covering up your true feelings here with me, I can't be of any help to you. Then, you'll carry your suffering with you and be no better off. Is that what you want?" It is crucial that patients see the negative consequences of their defenses. Often, this technique is most effective if patients themselves can outline the negative consequences. If the therapist asks, "What will happen here today if you continue to rationalize, avoid the issue, and skirt around the difficult feelings?" and the patient can say, "I'll be wasting my time", then the ego is already starting to turn on the defense. The therapist is then in a good position to go on to the next step, which is to put pressure on the patient to abandon the defense.

Pressure and Challenge

Once patients can see that they are defending against feelings and, in so doing, resisting the very work they engaged the therapist to help them with, the stage is set for the phase of pressure and challenge. It is made clear to patients that insight alone is not enough. As soon as patients declare that they are defeating themselves by remaining in a defensive position, the therapist challenges them to do things differently. "So why would you want to waste your time? Let's see what you're going to do about this evasion of your true feelings?" This phase of defense work, sometimes referred to as "a head-on collision with the resistance", tends to evoke very strong feelings toward the therapist. The therapist waits for a sign, either verbal (e.g., "I'm starting to get irritated with you") or nonverbal (e.g., teeth gritting and hands clenching the arms of the chair), that the feelings are about to break through and shifts from a focus on defense to direct access of feelings.

Before moving on, it must be emphasized that it would be a grave error to proceed to the phase of pressure and challenge before the ego has been turned against its defenses. In such cases, the patient herself, rather than her defenses, will feel attacked, and a therapeutic misalliance will result.

Phase 3: Breakthrough of Feelings in the Transference

In healthy patients with low levels of resistance, facing previously avoided feelings toward current figures is often sufficient to unlock the unconscious, with links to the past emerging with speed and clarity. However, in most cases, defenses are more tenacious, requiring a phase of pressure on the patient to abandon them. This phase of pressure and challenge often stirs up intense mixed feelings toward the therapist, which the patient is motivated to avoid. These conflicting forces—to face and avoid complex mixed feelings toward the therapist—create an intrapsychic crisis. Pressure is maintained until there is a signal from the unconscious (often non-verbal) that feelings and impulses are close to the surface. The therapist must remain alert for such a sign and seize it immediately, switching focus from the defenses to the direct experience of feelings in the transference. The therapist challenges patients to be open and honest about the true nature of their feelings and impulses. Any defense against this is immediately identified:

THERAPIST: Do you notice your hand is in a fist? I sense you have a lot of feeling toward me.
PATIENT: Well, I guess I don't like what you're saying.
THERAPIST: You guess? You do like it or you don't?
PATIENT: No, I don't.
THERAPIST: Then could we look at the feeling about that? What is the feeling toward me?

Defenses and resistance increase in direct proportion to the mounting anxiety about the rise in previously forbidden feelings and impulses. In this way, the resistance is not a problem but an indication that feelings toward the therapist, the very key for unlocking the unconscious, are on the rise. It's not an indication to back off, but to proceed to a full breakthrough of feeling, provided that the patient's anxiety is at a tolerable level. During this phase of the work, persistence on the therapist's part really pays off. Backing off de-pressurizes the very conflict that these techniques are designed to intensify. Consequently, hesitance on the therapist's part will prolong treatment.

Patients who are able to declare their feelings would then be asked to describe the internal experience of those feelings. In this way, the therapist can assess the level of emotional involvement in the process and detect any remaining area of defense. For there to be a full breakthrough of feeling, all three elements (cognitive, physiological, and motoric) of the feeling must be present (see Figure 1.2).

Once patients indicate that they are experiencing the physiological components of the stated affect, the therapist asks about the impulse this feeling mobilizes. "So you are hot and feel revved up. If that energy and heat came out toward me, what would that look like?" It is made very clear to patients that the therapist is not advocating acting on the impulse (a regressive defense) but having an honest look at their feelings and impulses. Fantasy and visualization, sometimes called "portraiting the impulse" (Davanloo, 1990–1991), are techniques used to achieve full expression of the impulse.

Portraiting the Impulse

To facilitate the process of increasing the patient's access to the full experience of emotion, Davanloo advocates the use of imagery, or what he has referred to as "portraiting the impulse". Ferenczi (1924) was probably the first analyst to suggest the use of fantasy as a vehicle to enhance the experience of feelings. He felt that, until the patient's hostile feelings toward the therapist were fully experienced and expressed, no genuine positive transference could develop. He would encourage the patient to have a fantasy about the expression of rage toward the therapist.

In a similar vein, Davanloo makes sure that any sign of negative feeling in the transference is experienced and cleared away rapidly, opening the way for the development of a strong therapeutic alliance. In accordance with Freud's (1949) view that ". . . a patient never forgets again what he has experienced in the form of the transference" (p. 34), Davanloo places the experience of transference feelings at the very center of his technique.

Feelings in the Transference are Complex

In the most typical scenario, anger is the first layer of feeling experienced, followed by guilt, grief, and the emergence of tender, loving feelings (see Figure 1.5). For example, following a portrait of anger that depicted a violent impulse to rape and strangle the therapist, a patient began to weep. "I feel terrible. I just imagined doing something brutal to you and you didn't deserve it—you're just trying to help me". It is essential that *all* the mixed feelings toward the therapist be experienced and expressed; not just the anger, but also the guilt and grief which follow.

Patients are encouraged to experience each layer of feeling in a full and direct way. Davanloo (1990) suggested that we deal with grief, pain, and love in the same way that we handle anger. We challenge defenses against any and all core feelings in order to bring them to the surface. The therapist might say, "I sense a deep sadness in you and you seem to be on the verge of tears but you swallow it. Why do you want to hide the grief in your heart?" Underneath the pain and grief are love and gratitude. These feelings are also visualized.

THERAPIST: So underneath the anger is pain and deeper still, your tender loving feelings. How do you feel like expressing that?*

PATIENT: I just want to pick you up off the floor and hold you in my arms. I want you to come back.

As you may have already noted, the therapist uses highly charged, emotional language, which Davanloo (1990–1991) suggests speaks directly to the unconscious.

Phase 4: De-Repression of Unconscious Material and History-Taking

The free expression of feelings in the transference is considered the key in the unlocking of the unconscious. Meaningful memories and associations tend to flow quite readily following the breakthrough of affect in the transference. Sometimes patients will make spontaneous links with the past. For example, a man who imagined raping me went on to say, "This is just how I felt with my mother. She was such a difficult woman, always on my case about everything. I just wanted to kill her. But since she died, I am miserable. I miss her. When I was young, we were very close. I was her favorite".

On occasion, there is no spontaneous outpouring of supporting material. In these cases, a brief review of what has just occurred within the transference relationship and a question about who else comes to mind is typically sufficient to facilitate the de-repression of significant memories.

Therapeutic Value

The experience of intense affect has three major functions:

1. It desensitizes the ego to the experience of previously toxic affects;

2. It leads to a loosening in the intrapsychic system with a de-repression of meaningful memories, dreams, and associations revealing the nature of the core conflicts underlying the neurosis; and

3. It allows patient and therapist to make meaningful links between the triangle of conflict and the triangle of the person (Been & Sklar, 1985).

Developmental History

Now that defense and resistance have been removed and there is direct access to the unconscious, the stage is set for a meaningful exploration of the patient's developmental history. Davanloo warns that if history is obtained before defenses have been cleared away, the material obtained may well be skewed and inaccurate.

Phase 5: Interpretation

Once there has been a breakdown in defense and resistance, followed by an intense experience of affect in the transference, with an outpouring of unconscious material, meaningful interpretations are possible. Nearly all Davanloo's innovations have been in the pre-interpretive phase of therapy and pave the way for making accurate and effective interpretations (Malan, 1986).

Interpretations consist of links between the triangle of conflict and the triangle of the person (see Figure 1.1). An example would be, "So now we can see that your smiling—the submissive, compliant attitude you initially displayed with me—was a cover for all the angry feelings you came in with. When you faced that directly, there was an outpouring of grief-laden feeling and, deeper still, we saw the positive feelings and craving for closeness. It then became clear that this was almost identical to all the mixed feelings you have regarding your mother. It sounds like this gets played out in virtually all your relationships with women". This re-analysis of the therapeutic process is essential to drive home the insights obtained and consolidate the process of change. In addition, once these T-C-P links have been made, distinctions between people become clearer. To continue with our example, this patient was able to say, "When you were pressing me, I felt angry and thought you were just like my mother. But my mother was never interested in my real feelings and I feel like you are".

Making a Therapeutic Contract

Once this process has been completed, a meaningful therapeutic contract can be made. The therapist emphasizes to the patient that this initial work is only the beginning of the process and that therapy will involve hard work. The sense of relief and revival of hope that frequently accompany this initial work is a powerful motivating force for the patient. It is within this hopeful and collaborative atmosphere that a meaningful therapeutic contract can be made. Often the therapist will roughly estimate the expected duration of treatment while emphasizing that the achievement of the stated therapeutic goals will be the decisive factor, and not a prescribed time limit.

Therapeutic Tone

Throughout this procedure, the therapist should be gentle but firm. The therapist should never argue with a patient but remain mindful to step out of any such interpersonal struggle by redirecting the patient to the internal struggle being experienced. Patients often identify with only one aspect of their conflict and tend to project the other aspect of the conflict onto the therapist, thereby avoiding the tension and discomfort of containing both aspects of the struggle. In ISTDP, we seek to intensify the patient's internal conflict. The following type of intervention is designed to achieve this goal: "Now you want to argue with me. It's not up to me to decide. Only you can say whether you are hiding and covering up your feelings with intellectualization and rationalization. What do you think—is that happening here with me or not?" Again, the therapist is firm but not harsh and must be ready "to extend the hand of warmth and closeness the moment the patient is ready" (Malan, 1963, p. 76).

Summary

While adhering quite strictly to psychoanalytic theory, Dr. Davanloo has developed ISTDP, which is designed to make rapid entry into the unconscious. This is achieved by breaking through barriers of defense and resistance and focusing on the patient's experience of painful and conflicting feelings, especially in the transference. This chapter has outlined the metapsychology of the unconscious, defined dynamic concepts in operational terms, and detailed the method for "unlocking the unconscious" developed by Dr. Davanloo.

Note

1. From "Breaking the Silence". Music and lyrics by Loreena McKennitt. "Parallel Dreams" Quinlan Road 1989.

2 THE TRIAL THERAPY

> You need that rite of passage
> before you can continue on,
> That great self understanding
> you can lean your dreams upon.
> *"Right of Passage"*
> *Dougie MacLean, 1991*[1]

This chapter will outline the process of the trial therapy, as developed by Dr. Davanloo (1990). The development of this elegant system for assessing suitability for treatment and, when indicated, rapidly entering the unconscious, is surely one of Davanloo's greatest contributions to the field of dynamic psychotherapy. Three cases from my own practice will be used to illustrate some typical responses to the trial therapy. While these patients had nearly identical presenting complaints, the trial therapy revealed different origins to the symptoms as well as varying capacities for the work at hand. Consequently, each had distinct requirements for treatment.

The trial therapy is a complex and systematic method for assessing the patient's symptomatic and characterological difficulties, determining the unconscious forces behind these difficulties, and evaluating the patient's current ego-adaptive capacity. This extended (2–4 hour) evaluation is, indeed, a rite of passage for both patient and therapist, providing an opportunity for a deep understanding of the unconscious forces responsible for the patient's suffering.

DOI: 10.4324/9781003542131-2

Assessing Suitability for Treatment

Patient as Evaluator

Although the therapist assumes a great deal of responsibility for the pace and direction of the initial evaluation, patients must understand from the outset that the process is a two-way street, creating the kind of collaboration associated with successful outcomes in psychotherapy. Patients are informed that the purpose of the evaluation is threefold: 1) to get to the bottom of their difficulties; 2) to understand the driving forces responsible for their problems; and 3) to ascertain whether this particular form of treatment will be useful to them. The therapist must determine patients' suitability for treatment, whereas patients must weigh their willingness to do the work at hand. In this sense, it is a two-way evaluation. We encourage patients to be active participants from the start. Vagueness, passivity, and compliance with the therapist are targeted from the inception of treatment.

Selection Criteria

In the field of dynamic psychotherapy, professionals have paid little attention to developing therapeutic techniques tailored to the specific requirements of the opening phase of treatment. The initial evaluation serves a dual purpose: (a) to determine the factors responsible for the patient's suffering; and (b) to assess the patient's ability to benefit from intensive short-term dynamic psychotherapy. Because of the abbreviated nature of this form of dynamic psychotherapy, pioneers in the field (Davanloo, 1978; 1980; Malan, 1976; 1979; Sifneos, 1972) have focused much effort on the development and application of reliable criteria for patient selection.

Some, like Sifneos (1972; 1979), were very demanding in the characteristics they required of a patient to be considered suitable for treatment. These characteristics include above-average intelligence, motivation for change, an ability to make meaningful contact with the evaluator, ready access to feelings, and the ability to articulate a chief complaint. In addition, candidates must evidence a willingness to endure hardship and frustration in order to obtain help. So few patients fit these rigid criteria, that the short-term treatment developed by Sifneos has had very little applicability.

Malan (1963) and Balint (1957) began their studies on the effectiveness of short-term dynamic psychotherapy with the assumption that only patients with recent, mild, and circumscribed difficulties would be suitable for this type of brief treatment. When they were unable to find a large enough group of patients to fit their criteria in the outpatient population of their clinic, they reluctantly expanded their parameters for selection and, much to their surprise, found that the majority of those who made substantial and long-lasting gains in brief (up to 40 sessions) psychotherapy suffered from chronic and debilitating symptoms.

These studies (Malan, 1976a; 1976b; Malan & Osimo, 1992) indicated that the patient's ability to develop a focus within the first four sessions and to respond positively to trial interpretations provided the most accurate predictors of outcome. In this context, "focus" referred to the demarcation of a central theme or conflict that had precipitated the patient's current distress and was linked with similar conflicts from the past. The kind of response to interpretation they were looking for was one in which genuine and deeply-felt affect was experienced, leading to new insights. The insight felt to be most crucial involved an understanding of the relationship between the triangle of conflict and the triangle of the person (see Figure 1.1). Follow-up studies (Malan, 1976a; 1976b; 1979) have confirmed that a successful outcome is significantly related to the frequency of a positive response to these very interpretations.

Davanloo (1980), expanding on Malan's notions regarding the importance of the patient's response to trial interpretations, has stated, "No one can tell anything about the patient's likely response without exposing him to some of the important ingredients of the therapy he will receive" (p. 99). Therefore, "The major part of the interview contains exactly the same interventions as are used in the main body of therapy" (Davanloo, 1980, p. 100). In fact, Davanloo asserted that exposure to the vital ingredients involved in short-term dynamic psychotherapy, along with a vigilant monitoring of the patient's responses, is the only reliable way to assess whether they can withstand the impact of their own unconscious material. This is what the trial therapy was designed to accomplish. In addition to, and, in fact, preceding, the use of interpretation, Davanloo has developed a series of pre-interpretive interventions designed to assess a patient's current ego-adaptive capacity and to break through defensive barriers, making previously inaccessible patients open to intervention. He referred to these series of interventions as the "central dynamic sequence (outlined in chapter 1)".

Recent research suggests that the trial therapy is a powerful therapeutic tool, as well as a vehicle for an accurate assessment of patient functioning. Abbass, Joffres, and Ogrondniczuk (2008 compared an Intense Short-Term Dynamic Psychotherapy (ISTDP) trial therapy with a standard intake interview and discovered significant differences. Fully one third of those patients receiving the trial therapy, when evaluated six weeks later, required no further treatment. Seven of the 30 patients in the trial therapy condition stopped all psychotropic medications following this one session and two went back to work, having been on disability. None of these results were noted in the traditional intake condition.

Additional studies on the effectiveness of the trial therapy have confirmed these findings and expanded upon this initial data. Aafjes-vanDoorn, et al. (2014) and Abbass, et al. (2018) studied 500 patients with mixed diagnoses who were offered a trial therapy. These subjects evidenced significant reductions on both the Brief Symptom Inventory (BSI) and Interpersonal Problems Inventory (IIP) following this single session. Of note, Abbas, et al. (2018) found that those patients experiencing a breakthrough into the unconscious during this initial contact had the most striking reduction in symptoms and presenting problems. Abbass, Kisley, and Town (2018) were able to demonstrate significant cost savings, as well as therapeutic effectiveness, for those receiving the trial therapy. At intake, the patients investigated had significantly higher medical expenses than the average Canadian. Yet, after only one trial therapy, their medical costs plummeted. Three years post intervention, the average savings per patient was more than $10,000 Canadian dollars, far exceeding the cost spent on this single session. This research provides compelling evidence for the effectiveness of this extended and intensive initial evaluation.

Spectrum of Psychopathology

The first goal of the trial therapy is to obtain a dynamic diagnosis and place the patient on the spectrum of psychopathology (Figure 2.1). On the left side of the spectrum are those rare patients who come for help with one narrowly defined problem. Their anxiety is relatively low and generally channeled into the striated (voluntary) muscle. Their defenses are repressive (intellectualizing) in nature and are often dystonic. These patients erect no barriers to emotional closeness and tend to perceive the therapist as helpful. They utilize this help, participate actively in

NEUROTIC	CHARACTER DISORDER	FRAGILE EGO
<------------	------------	------------>
Single Focus	Multi-Focus	Multi-Focus
Anxiety in Striated Muscle	Anxiety in Smooth Muscle	Anxiety with Cogniti Disruption
Repressive Defenses	Mix of Repressive and Regressive Defenses	Regressive Defenses
No Defenses against Emotional Closeness	Moderate level of Defense against Closeness	Significant Defenses against Closeness
Defenses Dystonic	Defenses Syntonic	Defenses Syntonic
Highly Functional	Impaired Social & Occupational Functioning	Impairment in Self-Care
Highly Motivated	Ambivalent about Treatment Process	Motivation Severely Compromised

Figure 2.1 Spectrum of Psychopathology

treatment, and respond rapidly to intervention. The central dynamic sequence moves with ease from inquiry to a breakthrough of feeling, usually toward a significant other in their current life, with meaningful links made to figures from the past.

Most often, however, patients come for treatment complaining of several symptomatic disturbances and significant impairment in their social and occupational functioning. These patients, who fall in the middle of the spectrum, are the most frequently encountered in daily practice. For these patients, anxiety is likely to be of sufficient intensity that repressive defenses alone cannot contain it. Consequently, as anxiety rises, it may be channeled into the smooth muscle or even temporary cognitive perceptual disruption. In addition, when highly anxious, patients can resort to regressive defenses, such as acting out or somatization. Characterological defenses, such as helplessness or defiance, are common in this group of patients and create a barrier to meaningful communication. These defenses become an obstacle in treatment if not addressed immediately. Although the range of symptoms and presenting problems may be plentiful and severe in this group, they tend to cause significant distress and undermine effective functioning, providing a real incentive to work that milder forms of psychic disturbance may not. This distress, along with the concomitant desire to heal, are the therapist's allies.

On the right side of the spectrum are patients with ego fragility, who tend to display cognitive/perceptual impairment when anxious and resort to highly regressive defenses, such as dissociation, splitting, and projection. These patients have difficulty distinguishing between their genuine feelings, the anxiety they generate, and the defenses they employ to avoid them. For these individuals, the triangle of conflict is more like a circle of conflict (Celentano, personal communication, 1992) in which anxiety, feelings, and defenses are fused and lack definition. These patients often require a gradual and titrated approach to their unconscious feelings and impulses. Treatment efforts must be directed toward building ego structures that are more resilient and adaptive than those currently at their disposal. Once they can distinguish between the corners of the triangle, and can experience anxiety in their striated muscles, approaching their anxiety-provoking feelings is indicated.

Contra-Indications

It must be emphasized that no one sign or symptom obtained in the trial therapy should be evaluated out of context or be, in and of itself, a reason for determining suitability or lack thereof. Patients can have episodes of dissociation or severe depression in their history, but display a high degree of motivation, and prove very responsive to intervention. Contra-indications that are readily obtained through inquiry include evidence of psychosis, untreated major affective disorder, severe impulse control disorder, or active alcohol or substance abuse.

Response to Intervention

To assess suitability for treatment, the patient must be subjected to the vital ingredients of the treatment itself. The central dynamic sequence and the triangles of conflict and person serve as guides in this process. Each therapeutic intervention is met with a response from the patient that provides data regarding their current ego-adaptive capacity and suitability for ISTDP. The therapist assumes an active stance, focusing on the patient's inner life and challenging defenses as they arise. Patients are not assumed to be fragile but are challenged to work at their highest level of ability.

In general, there are three categories of response to this intense and focused approach. In the most responsive patients, focusing on symptom generating situations leads to the production of affect-laden unconscious communications that readily shed light on the genesis of their neurotic conflict. Another frequently encountered response to this approach is increased defensiveness, particularly in the form of transference resistance. Individuals falling into this category are often openly defiant and consciously resistant ("I am not going to answer any more of your questions"). In between these two extremes are those patients who respond with a mix of feelings and defensive attempts to avoid them.

These responses to intervention indicate the patient's current level of ego functioning and serve as a guide to further intervention. In the first case, the therapist can simply proceed from the experience of feeling a breakthrough of unconscious material shedding light on the origin of the patient's symptoms. In the second case, there is a fortification of defenses, along with a mobilization of resistance in the transference, requiring the application of pressure and challenge to the resistance. The third case requires a mix of challenge to defenses, while encouraging the direct experience of emerging feelings.

Three clinical examples, each representing one of the three categories of response just outlined, will be presented. Various technical interventions and a theoretical understanding of the emerging clinical data will be interspersed throughout the case material.

Clinical Example

The Manic-Depressive's Daughter

In the following case, the patient proved highly responsive to a focused approach. There were virtually no defenses against meaningful emotional contact with the therapist. Little more than clarification and interpretation were necessary to render defenses against anxiety-provoking thoughts and feelings dystonic and to shift the balance from repression to a full experience of previously warded-off affect. The result was a rapid de-repression of memories and associations that made sense of her current difficulties.

THERAPIST: So, tell me what brings you.

PATIENT: What brings me is the fact that I often have difficulty coping with my oldest son, who is six. He is, by all accounts, a very difficult child. About a year and a half ago, we took him to see a child psychiatrist.

THERAPIST: Difficult? How do you mean?

PATIENT: Temperamentally. He throws tantrums, is mercurial—a difficult person to live with. He's extraordinarily bright but labile and a behavior problem. He's not of a piece. He's very developed intellectually but emotionally and socially underdeveloped. He was thrown out of preschool for aggressive behavior and then we took him for treatment.

THERAPIST: Is there a diagnosable disorder?

PATIENT: The doctor has had to reassure me about that on any number of occasions because there's a history of mental illness in my family. My mother was a manic-depressive and my husband's father is just a depressive. In many ways, he reminds me of my mother and that's, I think, part of why I have such trouble dealing with him. She was very unpredictable. I never knew what I'd be facing when I came home, and it's the same with my son. When I wake up in the morning, I don't know whether he'll say "Hi, Mommy" or "I hate you". I find that kind of unpredictability very hard to deal with (the patient is becoming tearful).

So far, this woman proved quite capable of articulating her plight in relation to her son, and demonstrated considerable insight by linking this current difficulty to unresolved feelings toward her mother. The patient was emotionally activated and made excellent contact with the therapist, sitting forward in her chair, maintaining eye contact, and speaking with clarity and specificity. The treatment moved rapidly to an exploration of the feelings toward these two key figures, along with an assessment of the defenses that would inevitably come into operation as these feelings got aroused.

THERAPIST: What do you mean difficult? As soon as you make the link to your mother and what it was like for you growing up, you get tearful.

PATIENT: Yeah.

THERAPIST: What's the feeling?

PATIENT: Well, it's hard to be precise—it's painful.

THERAPIST: Can you describe how you feel that pain inside?

PATIENT: Well, it's almost physical. It feels like a tightness (points to her heart) and I feel like crying. It's a reminder of what was a very painful childhood—one I've done my best to put to bed so I can go on. And I was pretty successful at it (the patient got a scholarship to college, went on to postgraduate study, is highly successful in her career, and is married to "a very good man"). Then having a child like this has set me back and prevented me from leaving the past alone.

The patient was clearly in touch with the pain she was feeling. She was able to label the feeling, experiences it viscerally, and knew about who the feelings involved. The recent upsurge of symptoms (anxiety and depression) occurred because her characteristic defenses had failed her. As long as she was able to "forget about the past", she could avoid all the painful feelings associated with that period in her life. The birth of her son, who had physical and temperamental difficulties reminiscent of those of her very disturbed mother, evoked intensely painful feelings that could no longer be repressed in her typical fashion. Putting these thoughts and feelings out of her mind no longer worked and she resorted to less adaptive defenses, such as isolation and withdrawal. These defenses were highly dystonic, since they were in direct conflict with her desire to be a good mother. This conflict led to symptom formation and motivated her to seek treatment for the first time in her life.

C-P Link

THERAPIST: So these current experiences trigger deep pain from your childhood that you've long been avoiding.

PATIENT: Yes, and my moods are totally dependent on his mood and behavior, which is no good. I want to maintain some equanimity and deal with him more effectively and to do that I can't be so emotionally at one with him.

THERAPIST: The question is how to get there. It sounds like the way you've dealt with trauma in the past, and all the painful feelings that evokes, is to suppress them and try to go on by distancing yourself. You were able to do that as long as there was no external trigger. To detach from feelings you detached from people. To do that now means detaching from your son. You don't seem to want to do that, so instead of detaching and avoiding the feeling, you will have to go through it.

PATIENT: I want to be free so I can go forward (becoming tearful). I want to be a good mother, but it gets so hard. I want to run away or send him away. I've said to my husband, "I can't live with him, I feel like he's killing me" (crying very hard now).

The genesis of the intrapsychic conflict this woman was struggling with became crystal clear in response to the cost–benefit analysis regarding the defense of emotional detachment. To avoid facing the anger toward her son, and the part of her that wished she was rid of him altogether, the patient had to detach from him. The emerging grief about the cost of such a defensive strategy was a direct indication that this defense was becoming highly dystonic. This painful feeling proved a powerful ally to the therapeutic process. In addition to the painful cost of this defense, there was a genuine desire to attach to her son and to be a good mother to him. This was another factor in her strong motivation to face what has been avoided.

Her psychological mindedness, intense emotional involvement in the process, lack of resistance, and genuine desire to change indicated that the process was able to move rapidly to the most painful and anxiety-laden area of the conflict in an effort to resolve her conflicts as quickly as possible

Focus on Anger and Defenses against It

THERAPIST: Could we look at one of those times when you felt like you wanted to be rid of him?

PATIENT: When I had a three-month-old, was moving into a new house, and he got thrown out of preschool.

THERAPIST: Do you notice you smile as you tell me about this? (Patient smiles again.) I wonder if that's a cover because, obviously, that wasn't funny.

PATIENT: I don't think I'm angry (denial).

THERAPIST: What about the smile?

PATIENT: It's only recently that I've felt like I can't take it anymore.

THERAPIST: It looks like these feelings toward your son are hard to face; you smile, sigh, look away.

PATIENT: I don't remember.

The patient became increasingly defensive as the anger toward her son was approached directly. The "slippage" in her memory was especially noticeable, as she was initially able to give a very specific example of a time when she wanted to get rid of him. Yet, to experience this rage directly was so threatening that the ego resorted to regressive defenses such as denial and forgetting. The strength of the defenses was in direct proportion to the strength of the anxiety regarding the underlying feelings and impulses. Therefore, the increase in defensiveness is "to be welcomed as an indicator that painful conflicts are not merely being approached but can be brought to the surface and resolved" (Davanloo, 1990, p. 3). Because there were no contra-indications for this intensive approach, the conflictual feelings toward her son were brought to the surface rather than avoided. An attempt to avert her "forgetting" by focusing on her current feelings toward her son was attempted.

THERAPIST: What about now? How do you feel toward him when you go back to that time?

PATIENT: I don't blame him (rationalization). The school was inept in their handling of him (displacement).

THERAPIST: You see, what gets passed over are the feelings toward your son. Isn't that why you are here—to deal with those feelings?

PATIENT: It's a fear of losing control. I feel like I'm close to beating the crap out of him.

In the foregoing interchange, the therapist called on the therapeutic alliance to tip the balance from avoidance to facing the feelings of rage toward her son. The pressure to have an honest look at these feelings paid off, as the patient revealed her fear (and wish) of losing control and acting on her rage. The basis of such a fear must always be explored in detail.

Fear of Loss of Control

It is not unusual for patients to report a fear of losing control when strong affect is approached. The basis for this fear must always be explored. If there is a history of impulsive discharge of affect, then the fear is considered "realistic" and the therapist would avoid any intensification of feeling until the patient was able to exhibit good impulse control.

If, on the other hand, there is no history of acting on impulses, the fear is considered "neurotic". The patient fears the feelings associated with forbidden action and has failed to make a clear distinction between the two. Gradual exposure to the feared stimulus, the experience of anger in this case, is required to de-toxify the affect. In essence, the feeling of anger and the anxiety it generates get separated. Consequently, the patient can experience the anger without getting so anxious that she has to defend against it. Then, the affect is available as a source of information and energy to the patient, who can deal with it in a conscious and deliberate fashion. This process increases ego strength, freedom, and adaptability.

In this case, I decided that the direct experience of rage toward her son was too threatening so early in the therapeutic process. I summarized the information already gathered, making a link between the triangle of conflict in the current situation with her son and that in the past with her mother. We returned to the phase of inquiry to see what other conflicts might emerge. The therapeutic alliance was very strong, revealed in the next vignette, when she raised the issue of anger toward her husband. On some level, she is aware that there is a link between these two important figures in her life.

Return to Inquiry

THERAPIST: Any other problems you want help with?

PATIENT: The conflict with my son is primary, but I have some conflict with my husband too. He procrastinates and I get angry.

THERAPIST: Could we look at this anger toward your husband?

PATIENT: With my son, I'm afraid I'll lose control and do harm. With my husband, I couldn't because he can defend himself, but I'm afraid I'll do something I will regret, like smack him.

The same conflict the patient has with her son, over control of her violent impulses and the consequences of same, emerged in relation to her husband. Examining the rage toward him seemed less threatening than that with a small child, so it was a good place to begin.

THERAPIST: There is a physical impulse to lash out. How do you imagine that? (It is important to make clear we are talking about fantasy and imagination and not advocating that the patient act on impulse.)

PATIENT: Smacking him on the face.

THERAPIST: What else?

PATIENT: Pounding on him. (Patient is waving her hands and shaking her fists, indicating that the impulses have been activated and are being directly experienced.)

THERAPIST: Where?

PATIENT: On his chest. To smack him and punch him.

THERAPIST: That's the full extent of it? You said you were afraid you'd do something you regret.

PATIENT: Do I imagine going down to the kitchen, taking out a knife, and stabbing him? No, I don't.

That this last response was a thinly disguised expression of the exact impulse she feared was quite clear. Because the patient had been highly involved and very responsive, a touch of humor was used to see if the defensive disavowal of the impulse could be lifted readily.

THERAPIST: Well, where did that come from? It's pretty specific!

PATIENT: Gee, I don't know. I did lose it once, and I slapped him in the face. We were dating for years, and he kept dragging his feet about getting married. One night I got so angry and upset, I hit him. He just held me, like we do with our son when he gets out of control. So, I know what that's like.

THERAPIST: It sounds like there's some real anger toward him, but it seems to tap into a reservoir of rage from the past. Who else comes to your mind?

PATIENT: My mother. She was the one who made my life miserable. But, you know, I adored her (Patient starts to sob). She died 20 years ago, and I still can't talk about her without crying. I feel very much like a motherless child.

Now the full picture of all the intense and conflicting feelings toward her mother emerged and helped us to make sense of the patient's turmoil over similar conflicts with her husband and son. In fact, it was only in the closest relationships, where these feelings got evoked so strongly, that the patient experienced such intense conflict. Memories of tremendous closeness with her mother emerged. She was an only child, and her parents were divorced when she was seven, leaving her alone with her mother almost all the time. They spent many happy hours together talking, playing, and laughing. Then, her mother would sink into an intractable depression and have to be hospitalized, or would become manic and bring men into the home for sexual encounters. She also frequently embarrass the patient with wildly inappropriate behavior on the street.

As a child, the patient could not reconcile the intense love and hate she felt toward her mother and withdrew to avoid the anxiety this conflict would precipitate. In the relationship with her son, she felt a similar desire for closeness alongside the same pain, rage, and frustration at not being able to achieve and maintain that closeness with an erratic, unpredictable family member. Facing these mixed feelings directly led to an outpouring of crucial developmental material, making a meaningful exploration of the past possible. Interpretations followed quite effortlessly.

This patient was successfully treated in 20 sessions and reported, in our final session, that she was not only getting along better than ever with both her husband and her son, but that she felt free and truly happy for the first time in her life. She said she felt as though a tremendous weight had been lifted off her shoulders, allowing her to move forward in her life now, rather than running from the past.

The case of the Manic-Depressive's Daughter illustrates a fairly smooth evaluation with a highly motivated and responsive patient. Such cases are the exception rather than the rule in practice. Typically, patients arrive in a highly anxious and defensive state or rapidly become so in response to the therapist's focus on painful feelings. In such cases, much more time and effort must be spent on the phase of defense work to turn the patient's ego against the self-defeating defenses that are interfering with the therapeutic goal. Working the triangles and focusing on the central dynamic sequence are guides in this process.

Use of the Two Triangles in the Trial Therapy

Davanloo (personal communication, 1989–1991) has exhorted us not to make assumptions, but to test out our hypotheses in real time, basing our diagnostic assessment on the patient's response to intervention. Once a detailed account of the patient's symptomatic difficulties has been obtained, the therapist begins the inquiry into the feelings involved in the situations where symptoms erupted. During this phase of the evaluation, the triangles of conflict and person are used as models for understanding the intrapsychic workings of the patient. In addition, this model provides a structure for assessing the ego's resources and weaknesses and, when followed properly, gives order and coherence to the process of therapeutic intervention.

During the trial therapy, the therapist conducts a three-step analysis of the triangle of conflict. This involves:

1 Assessing each corner of the triangle (anxiety [A], defense [D], and impulse/feeling [I/F]).

2 Determining the extent of clarification and differentiation within the triangle of conflict.

3 Linking the three elements within the triangle of conflict to the elements of the triangle of the person (transference [T], current figures [C], and past genetic figures [P]).

Step 1: Assessing the Corners of the Triangle

Anxiety

In most cases, anxiety is the first dynamic factor to be assessed. Exploration of the patient's experience of anxiety should provide the answers to several crucial diagnostic questions. How is anxiety being channeled within the system? Is the patient aware of being anxious and does he have an accurate idea about the source of the anxiety (facing difficult feelings or opening up to someone new)? Does the patient seem to have a reasonable amount of tolerance for the conscious experience of anxiety? The response to each question indicates something about the patient's level of current ego-adaptive capacity and will guide the process. For example, very high levels of anxiety channeled into the smooth muscle would indicate the need for a stepwise approach to feelings, lest this lead of an exacerbation of symptoms.

Defenses

The second aspect of the conflict to be examined is the defensive system. Because anxiety mobilizes defenses, the examination of anxiety usually leads quite naturally into the area of the patient's characteristic defenses. What are the patient's typical defenses? Do they seem to be directed internally against the awareness of threatening thoughts and feelings (defenses against impulse/feeling) or externally against emotional contact with others (defenses against emotional closeness)? How varied and flexible are the defenses observed and reported? Of particular importance is the assessment of how syntonic or dystonic the defenses are to the patient.

Impulses and Feelings

Finally, an exploration of the patient's access to affect is conducted. Assessment of the three elements considered necessary for a full experience of feeling (cognitive, physiological, and motoric) needs to be conducted to evaluate the patient's current capacity for emotional involvement in the process. The range and depth of the patient's emotional involvement should also be noted. How freely can the patient access the affective reactions toward and in response to others? What is the balance between the two?

Patients are often aware of some feeling toward others—say love and appreciation—but can't seem to tolerate having mixed feelings, including anger toward this same individual. For example, a particular patient might experience an internal feeling of sadness regarding a separation in a free and unencumbered fashion but seem heavily defended against the awareness of the reactive feelings of anger toward the person who left. This type of constellation of feeling and defense is typical in depressives. There are also cases in which the opposite configuration is apparent. In narcissistic characters, there is ready access to anger toward others who hurt or disappoint them, but significant defenses against the internal experience of pain and grief.

The assessment of the three corners of the triangle of conflict yields rich diagnostic data, helps place the patient on the spectrum of psychopathology, and guides the therapeutic process by pinpointing critical areas of conflict or ego weakness.

Step 2: Differentiating the Corners of the Triangle

Once each element involved in the triangle of conflict has been labeled and evaluated, the therapist must determine whether the patient can distinguish between them. Can the individual distinguish between the experience of a feeling (say, grief), the anxiety it arouses (butterflies and heart palpitations), and the defenses that come into play (intellectualization and isolation of affect) in order to avoid them? In particular, the clinician should look for any area of fusion between feelings and anxiety, feelings and defense, or anxiety and defense.

For example, if the therapist inquires about the internal experience of anger, and the individual describes the physiological experience of anxiety, then some fusion between these internal states is in operation. Clarification is required to help facilitate the distinction between the two. Failure to make these distinctions can result in an unanticipated and undesirable exacerbation of anxiety when the patient is pressed for the experience of feeling.

Can the patient differentiate between anxiety and the defenses the anxiety calls into play? If a patient tells you about defenses (distancing) when asked about the experience of anxiety, some fusion is suspect. Again, a process of clarification and distinction between anxiety and defense is required until the patient can see (cognitive clarity) and then indicate the ability to experience (emotional) the difference between the two.

Evidence of fusion between feelings and defenses is quite common and is essential to detect early on in the process. Spending some time clarifying the difference between the experience of a feeling like anger, and the defense against it (criticizing and blaming the self), pays off in the end. The process leads to clarity and increases ego functioning. Failure to systematically assess and clarify areas of fusion before proceeding to a breakthrough of feeling can lead to an increase in anxiety, symptoms, or defensiveness, any of which can inhibit a swift and smooth therapeutic process.

Step 3: Linking the Corners of the Triangles

The third step in the process of assessing the triangle of conflict is to determine whether the patient can both distinguish between feelings, anxiety, and defense, and link them in a meaningful way (e.g., he was angry with his boss, which mobilized anxiety that he dealt with by withdrawing and rationalizing). In addition to linking together the three elements within the triangle of conflict, links between the triangle of conflict and the triangle of the person also need to be made. Can the patient see that the constellation feelings, anxiety, and defenses evident in the current situation are related to unresolved conflicts from the past? Further, can this patient see the same dynamic forces in operation with the therapist?

In the following two cases, a good deal of defense work is necessary for the therapeutic work to begin. Heavy use is made of the triangles (see Figure 1.1) to acquaint the patients with their defenses and render them dystonic.

Clinical Examples

A Gentleman Scorned

The following transcript provides an example of a type of response frequently encountered in the trial therapy. The patient entered the session expressing a conscious desire to participate and obtain help from the therapist yet resisted exploring painful feelings. Such patients typically provide adequate factual responses to inquiry and are quite "cooperative" as long as you "stick to the facts". However, defensive efforts increase markedly as the therapist began to focus on the patient's feelings about the people and events being reported. Emphasizing the conflict between the part of the person that wants help, and the part that wants to run and hide from the pain entailed in the process, precipitates the sort of internal crisis and disequilibrium necessary to enable a rapid entry into the unconscious. Often, when patients enter treatment in a state of crisis, this intrapsychic disequilibrium may already exist. In contrast, patients who are chronically disturbed and highly identified with their character defenses require therapeutic intervention to tip the balance between motivation and resistance.

THERAPIST: What brings you?

PATIENT: An agreement with my wife to remain married but live apart for six months, then we'll decide.

THERAPIST: Who instigated the separation?

PATIENT: Mutually agreed, but my wife instigated it.

THERAPIST: She wanted you to see someone as part of the agreement?

PATIENT: I've been in therapy three times. I went to see a friend, who's a therapist, two years ago. I spent eight hours with him to find out if there was a problem. He asked me, "What do you want?" I realized I had never asked myself that question. To understand that you have to understand my background (begins to rattle off his history with rapid-fire speech) . . .

It is important not to get embroiled in past history or to let the patient diversify before the current difficulties have been adequately explored. Again, the only pressure at this stage of the trial therapy is to maintain focus and be specific.

THERAPIST: I'm sure that's important but let's start with what you're here for now. What are the problems you want help with?

PATIENT: Confirmation of my own health and well-being. I've been exploring what I want and am making changes.

THERAPIST: Like what?

PATIENT: Like a career change.

THERAPIST: So you've made changes in your career, but what have you come here for?

PATIENT: There's a sense of loss regarding the relationship ending.

Exploring the Patient's Feelings in the C

THERAPIST: So you have a lot of feeling about the separation.

PATIENT: Well, when you're married for 25 years and this woman you've loved all along says she doesn't love you anymore (uses sarcastic tone and smiles, to avoid any painful feeling) . . .

THERAPIST: You smile. What is your feeling about this?

PATIENT: Initially, it was devastating, very painful. Now I'm confused and ambivalent. I'm living alone for the first time in my life, and there's a sense of newness and excitement. I've come to terms with the fact that I've held on for ten years even though it's been very difficult. I was depressed.

THERAPIST: Clinically depressed?

PATIENT: No physical signs, but emotionally down. I didn't care—flat affect.

THERAPIST: You were very detached.

PATIENT: Very detached and just didn't care.

Examining Resistance in the T

THERAPIST: This detachment still seems to be present. We don't get to see what feelings you have. This is what you avoid.

PATIENT: You're assuming. (Resistance in the transference is becoming evident. Now the patient contradicts himself and becomes defiant.)

THERAPIST: Isn't this the problem, that . . .

PATIENT: I don't know if there is a problem.

THERAPIST: You are happy and satisfied with your life?

PATIENT: No.

THERAPIST: It is important for us to look at this. Either you have problems you consider psychological in nature and that's why you've consulted a psychologist, or you are here to appease your wife.

PATIENT: No. If she wanted me to, I wouldn't come. I'm unhappy with the way my personal life has turned out. I invested a lot in a marriage that isn't functional, and I held on for a long time. No one else was surprised.

THERAPIST: Are you saying you have a blind spot? You didn't see it coming when others did?

PATIENT: Yeah. I knew it was bad but didn't . . . chose to ignore it and was very passive.

THERAPIST: You tend to be passive and avoidant and you're concerned about how you let this happen.

PATIENT: Yeah, but since we've decided to separate, all the intellectual pieces are in place. I'm feeling liberated. I'm at ease, at peace.

This pattern of identifying and then denying areas of conflict or difficulty continued for 20 minutes. It became increasingly clear that the primary resistance was in the transference. It seemed he would rather be damned than agree with me.

This defiance was undermining therapeutic efforts and had to be eliminated for the process to proceed. Despite the high level of defensiveness in evidence, some important information was revealed. The patient reported a lifetime of self-defeating behavior that had affected both his career and home life. At the age of 25, unemployed with three children and a wife to support, he had contemplated suicide. The tendency toward self-defeat was already in operation within the therapy and became the focus of intervention.

Exploration of Self-Defeat in the C and the T

THERAPIST: Let's look at this. Is there a pattern of self-defeat in your life? You keep yourself from being happy and sabotage your own goals?

PATIENT: Until recently I have, and it's all based on being responsible. I got married right out of college and then had three children by the time I was 25. I was so overwhelmed, I seriously contemplated suicide.

THERAPIST: So, how did you get yourself into such a situation?

PATIENT: I could tell you the jokes I lay on others but between then and now I've also had two disastrous business failures in which friends betrayed me. (Now the patient admits a long history of self-defeat which, in fact, continues to the present.) The problem was I trusted people I shouldn't have trusted. Now, for the first time I can say "I want . . . " and if you don't like it, too bad.

THERAPIST: You're better at knowing what you want and declaring it, but for some reason you're having difficulty with that here—to declare what kind of help you want from me. Do you notice?

PATIENT: You're acting very much like my wife and I find this approach very annoying.

THERAPIST: So you're feeling angry with me.

PATIENT: It's the emotion I have the most trouble with.

THERAPIST: Could we look at this?

PATIENT: I was really looking forward to coming here. The experience intrigued me, the three-hour intensive session, the short-term approach . . .

THERAPIST: So there was a part of you looking forward to it, specifically being focused, intensive, and short-term but obviously there is another part of you in operation because you interfere with that very approach. The element of self-defeat is already in operation here.

PATIENT: Maybe just a self-fulfilling prophesy because I don't see an intensity of problems or emotional distress.

This vignette speaks to the intensity of the conflict this man was experiencing about the prospect of opening up to the therapist. The patient was mired in ambivalence. He said he wanted to get to work and have an honest look at the feelings being evoked, but remained evasive. Pointing out the two opposing parts of him was necessary in order to create an intrapsychic crisis. The work had to take place in the transference, where the majority of the defenses were being directed.

Anger in the T

THERAPIST: You say that, as we go to look at your difficulties, you feel angry with me. How do you experience this anger?

PATIENT: I don't know what the problem is, I feel inadequate (D).

THERAPIST: That's not your anger, could we look at the anger?

PATIENT: The problem is I'm not clicking with you, and I find your approach offensive.

These comments suggested that the patient could not distinguish between his feeling of anger and the defenses against it (feeling inadequate or finding fault with the approach). This needed be clarified before any pressure was brought to bear on the defense. Failure to make such a distinction will lead to a misalliance, as the patient himself, rather than his defeating defenses, would feel attacked or criticized.

THERAPIST: When I ask you about your feelings, you go to your head. Do you notice, from the beginning, when I ask you how you feel, you tell me what you think and give an explanation? You stay emotionally detached, so we don't know what you're feeling inside. Now you say you're angry with me. So, we have a choice, we can have an honest look at your emotional reaction toward me or you can stay detached.

This man's characteristic defenses of sarcasm, defiance, and self-contradiction were very provocative. It was essential not to get caught in an interpersonal struggle with him, as this was another way for the patient to avoid dealing with his own intrapsychic conflicts. At this point, I decided to make his options clear and leave the decision up to him. The decision to do the work must be his alone.

Triangle of Conflict in the T

PATIENT: I want to look at it.

THERAPIST: You say you're angry. How do you feel this anger inside?

PATIENT: Just backing off (D). I don't need this.

THERAPIST: That's not the anger, that's the position you take to avoid the experience of the anger—you distance and withdraw. Haven't you been distant and withdrawn this whole time? You stay in your head, are vague and general, you don't look at me when you speak—you erect a massive wall.

PATIENT: I just met you half an hour ago.

THERAPIST: Why do you want to waste more time? You told me you wait passively and hang onto dead relationships. You somehow think you are protecting yourself, but we have to look at whether you actually end up wasting opportunities. You don't let me get to know you.

PATIENT: Um . . . (Patient shifts in his chair to face the therapist directly, rubs his chin, and looks the therapist in the eye.) I spend a lot of time letting people get to know me and they hurt me a great deal.

THERAPIST: You've been very hurt, and the way you've dealt with that is to withdraw and detach. Now you're hiding behind a wall.

PATIENT: Most people don't notice because I can seem very engaging.

THERAPIST: But if I'm going to be of help, I have to get to know you in a deep and honest way. That's what you avoid.

PATIENT: Right.

THERAPIST: This is a massive conflict.

PATIENT: I don't trust you.

THERAPIST: And, in a sense, why should you? But we also have to ask, why shouldn't you? You have no evidence either way.

PATIENT: I used to blindly trust people and I was a trusting fool.

THERAPIST: Who are you thinking of?

PATIENT: The business partner that stole $25,000 from me.

THERAPIST: So people you trusted have violated that trust. Obviously, you have feelings about that, but it sounds like you've gone to the opposite extreme and won't trust anyone. You seem to be saying, "I won't let anyone in".

PATIENT: Oh, I have. It's been a very hard week. I had to tell my sons about the separation, and they were very harsh and rejecting, yelling at me.

T-C-P Interpretation

Focusing on the cost and benefit of keeping the therapist at arm's length finally paid off, with increased emotional involvement and meaningful communications regarding the genesis of the patient's difficulties. The recently evoked feelings of grief and anger experienced toward his sons reminded the patient of a similar mix of feeling toward his parents in the past. Upon return from their honeymoon, the patient and his wife revealed that the bride was already three months pregnant. His parents berated and "disowned" him. This was how his sons behaved when they heard of their parents' separation. So now, as then, he was criticized and rejected by his family at a time when he needed their support. Making these connections and having the opportunity to experience the feelings associated with these events, increased the therapeutic alliance and his motivation to do the work. As a result, there was marked reduction in defense and resistance. In addition to linking the present conflict with a core conflict from the past, the patient was able to understand his readiness to view me in the same way, as someone who would criticize rather than help in a time of need. This all-important T-C-P link was made by the patient toward the end of the trial therapy, boding well for success. In fact, his treatment was completed in only ten sessions.

The Woman with Two Failed Marriages

The third example of a response to the trial therapy illustrates what occurs when a patient arrives in a state of resistance that prevents a factual inquiry from being completed. In such cases, the initial phases of the central dynamic sequence must be abandoned. The process must proceed rapidly to the phase of clarification, while applying pressure on the defenses, which serve as resistance to any meaningful contact with the therapist.

In the following case, the patient entered the trial therapy with a ready-made transference based on past experiences with other therapists. If feelings toward the therapist are not brought directly to the fore in a speedy fashion, the defenses against these feelings will greatly distort the process. Consequently, an examination of the defenses and the underlying transference feelings must precede inquiry.

Inquiry

THERAPIST: Why don't you start by telling me about the problems you're having right now.

PATIENT: I'm in a major transition in my life and it hasn't been easy. I'm going through a second divorce from a guy who's not unlike my first husband—actually, a carbon copy (smiles broadly). I saw it coming so I left after six months.

It should be noted that, although the patient was obviously in a crisis, she was speaking as if recounting an amusing story about a day at the beach. Her affect was not congruent with the content being reported. I noted this to myself but proceeded with inquiry before addressing the character defenses.

THERAPIST: So it was a very brief marriage.

PATIENT: Extremely brief, and it had a lot of false starts. I know I didn't want to go through this again, the first was so bad. I just wanted to get out quickly. Well, he didn't agree, you know how that is, and it was an extreme case.

THERAPIST: What do you mean?

PATIENT: He's gotten very angry and so when I call, even just to say, "Gee, I can't believe this is happening", and just wishing maybe it could have worked out, or at least we could be amicable, he would go and say I am unbalanced. He'd use a threatening tone.

THERAPIST: Has he actually threatened you?

PATIENT: He was physically abusive, so it wasn't a very happy situation (smiles). I just moved back home, and I'm not really very excited about therapy, by the way (another big smile), because I've been through a lot of therapy with my husband and it was always about how they could make me change, so I'm having a lot of negative feeling about being here.

The patient was not able to provide basic, factual information in response to inquiry. She was vague and overly general in her responses to specific questions and tended to diversify, jumping from topic to topic. Her affect was inappropriate to both the content being discussed and the feelings she reported having about being in the therapist's office. Exploration of the negative feelings being reported needed to take precedence over the factual inquiry.

Exploration of the Ready-Made Negative Transference

THERAPIST: So you have a lot of negative feelings about being here. Could we look at that?

PATIENT: Yes. I feel a bit defeated (D). I'm put on antidepressants.

THERAPIST: Who prescribed those?

PATIENT: The marital therapist. He said, "Oh, you're depressed, you should go on antidepressants". That was OK because, given the situation a person can become sad or depressed.

THERAPIST: What are you taking?

PATIENT: I don't know. Xanex? Elavil?

THERAPIST: You don't know?

PATIENT: I'm at the point where I don't even care anymore.

THERAPIST: We need to look at this. You complain about how poorly you're treated. Your husbands mistreat you and the doctors mistreat you. You have negative feelings about being here, but here you sit. How do you understand this? Somehow you allow yourself to be used and abused. Do you see that?

PATIENT: It sounds, on the surface, like I allow myself to be taken advantage of but, in a sense, I don't have a choice.

THERAPIST: You don't have a choice about going to a therapist? You are here under coercion or you came of your own will?

PATIENT: No one is forcing me. I came of my own will. But, like with a husband, you don't have a choice. My husband, in his usual state, looks wonderful, he's well-dressed and has a wonderful education, a good job. Then you go into the house and suddenly there's World War III. Do you see what I mean?

Clarification of Defenses

Each attempt at clarification of the patient's current situation results in more defensiveness and confusion. The first issue to be clarified involved the issue of the patient's will to be in therapy. Since she declared that she was seeking help of her own accord, the next step was to assess whether an intrapsychic focus could be obtained. If the patient considered all her difficulties to be externally imposed, then insight-oriented psychotherapy was not what she was looking for. However, if she was able to view her tendency to externalize and assume a helpless, victimized stance as a problem within her that significantly contributed to her recurrent interpersonal difficulties, then we could proceed with an analytic focus. This is the central issue at this juncture in the process.

THERAPIST: So you see yourself as helpless.

PATIENT: No, I see myself as out of control. I had to leave, even though I have to come home (she had just returned to her parent's home) and I feel very dependent. If you ever saw me at work, you'd never think I'm helpless.

THERAPIST: No, it's not how *I* see you, it's how you present yourself and you don't seem to be aware of it. I'm sure there is some truth to what you say. Your husbands have mistreated you and therapists are certainly capable of that, but that's not what we're here to look at. We're here to look at how you handle this. We can see, even with the issue of medication, that you take a passive, submissive stance and then feel victimized and taken advantage of. There is a way in which you give up control and allow others to take over. This looks like a pattern, and the question is, do you want to know what is going on inside of you that you should repeatedly let yourself be treated in this way? This is the central issue, do you want to examine what is going on inside of you and get to the bottom of your difficulties?

This last intervention was aimed at clarifying the character defenses of passivity and helplessness evident in the patient's interactions with both the therapist and other significant figures in her current life orbit. The way in which these defenses cost her, by allowing others to use and abuse her, was outlined to bolster her observing ego and encourage an intrapsychic focus.

As this transcript illustrates, these character defenses were highly syntonic and formed a massive resistance to meaningful communication and therapeutic progress. If the patient's tendency to externalize blame and assume a passive, victimized stance in relation to others was not clarified, the therapist would become another abuser in the patient's eyes, and the unconscious would remain inaccessible. Therefore, assessing the patient's ability to distinguish between feelings and defenses was essential in determining suitability for treatment.

PATIENT: I thought I should come since I'm at the point of taking medication. I felt so sick I just thought, "Give me something".

THERAPIST: You got sick?

PATIENT: People can get physically ill, you know, physically exhausted (reported with increased sarcasm).

THERAPIST: People? You mean *you* got sick? How?

PATIENT: I haven't been sleeping well, I'm exhausted, I have pains in my chest, pain down my arm, migraines. I'm not doing well. (These complaints were listed in a rapid-fire manner with a decidedly hostile edge to her voice.) So, when a person says, "Here, take this, it'll make you feel better", you take it.

The patient's seemingly intractable defensiveness and list of physical symptoms suggested some ego fragility. Still, until the defenses and resistance in the transference were clarified, one can't be certain. The increase in defensiveness could be driven by a rise in negative feelings toward the therapist. These feelings became the focus.

Mix of Feeling and Defense in the Transference

THERAPIST: Let me ask you how you're feeling right now.

PATIENT: I'm sorry, I'm being very belligerent toward you right now.

THERAPIST: And why is that? There is some feeling toward me.

PATIENT: Yes, there is. It's not you personally (D)—it's easy for a person to say (patient becoming tearful) . . .

THERAPIST: What is your feeling toward me?

PATIENT: You can say, "Take control of your life" (D).

THERAPIST: That's a thought, what's the feeling?

PATIENT: The problem is, I sit here in a therapist's office (more weepiness) and people tell me (D) . . .

THERAPIST: Did I tell you to do anything? We are here to look at your difficulties, and as I inquire into that, you say you get "belligerent". Obviously, you have a lot of feeling toward me.

PATIENT: No feeling toward you personally (D).

THERAPIST: Sure you do, you said you have a lot of negative feelings about being here, and then you realized you were becoming belligerent. That's a behavior. What's the feeling underneath?

PATIENT: (looks therapist in the eye and speaks calmly) Resentment.

THERAPIST: You feel resentment. We should look at this because you didn't declare that to me. First you denied it, then put it into the behavior of belligerence and sarcasm. Then, when I asked you about the feelings directly, you became weepy. The same thing happens here as you say happens with your husband (T-C link). This could be a really crippling problem. Is this a problem in your life, for you to become aware of your feelings and to be able to declare them directly?

PATIENT: Oh, angry feelings get me into big trouble.

This patient presented herself as a passive victim in life, indicating that her character defenses were highly syntonic. In accordance with this view, she identified the source of her problems as external. Such a belief prevents the delineation of an intrapsychic focus and, if intractable, would constitute a contra-indication for ISTDP. A focus on the feelings in the transference, along with an examination of the defenses against them, was an essential step in assessing whether the patient would be able to develop an observing stance. When the angry feelings toward the therapist were finally revealed, the patient changed noticeably. She calmed down, made direct eye contact, and began to give detailed information regarding both her history and current difficulties. Then an accurate assessment of her ability to use this type of treatment became possible. The patient reported a history of psychotic depression with two previous hospitalizations. This information, along with that gathered through the dynamic interaction between patient and therapist, confirmed the diagnosis of ego fragility, a clear contra-indication to further uncovering. Medication and supportive treatment were recommended.

Summary

The transcripts from three trial therapies have been used to illustrate some typical responses to the trial therapy. Of note, all three patients presented with similar complaints. Each was experiencing anxiety and depression in response to conflicts in their close personal relationships. The systematic evaluation involved in the trial therapy revealed very different levels of ego functioning in each case. The Manic-Depressive's Daughter proved highly motivated and responsive. The patient arrived with an intrapsychic focus, indicating a high level of ego-adaptive capacity. This assessment was further substantiated as the evaluation continued. The standard technique of pressure and challenge to the defenses with the goal of unlocking the unconscious via a breakthrough of feeling was indicated.

For the Gentleman Scorned, the current problems being described were only the most recent manifestation of lifelong difficulties resulting from the patient's character pathology. His character defenses created a barrier to meaningful communication with the therapist and, left unchecked, would have prevented an intrapsychic focus. Techniques designed to create an intrapsychic crisis were employed, as no signs of ego fragility were obtained during inquiry. His response to this challenge was a mixture of increased defensiveness and mounting anger at the therapist. Once this anger was directly expressed there was a decrease in defensiveness, followed by direct and emotionally meaningful communications with the therapist, along with increased motivation. All these factors suggested suitability for treatment.

The trial therapy of the Woman with Two Failed Marriages revealed significant ego fragility, which served as a clear contraindication for dynamic psychotherapy. The patient's defensiveness could have easily masked this fact. She was well-dressed and groomed and reported a high level of education and a responsible, professional career. Failure to address the defenses could have led to an assumption of greater capacity than the patient possessed. In fact, two weeks after the patient was referred to a psychiatrist for medication and supportive therapy, she was hospitalized once more, after threatening her mother with a knife. The obvious advantage to this method of assessment is the rapidity with which suitability can be determined, preventing the experience of finding out, well into treatment, that the patient cannot make use of dynamic psychotherapy, or, as in this case, that there is an underlying psychotic illness.

Note

1. From "Rite of Passage". Music and lyrics by Dougie MacLean. "Indigenous" Dunkeld, 1990.

3 WORKING WITH DEFENSES

Slip sliding away
Slip sliding away
You know the nearer your destination
The more you're slip sliding away

Slip Slidin" Away,
Paul Simon, 1977[1]

Many (Abbass, 2015; Frederickson, 2013) consider Davanloo's (1980; 1990) technical innovations for handling defense and resistance to be his greatest contribution to the practice of dynamic psychotherapy. The tight focus on defenses from the inception of treatment is also the most controversial aspect of his work. This chapter will review the concepts involved in the mechanisms of defense, will provide a working definition of defense and resistance, and will outline a detailed schema for the conceptualization and handling of these dynamic forces within the treatment setting. The work of those clinicians most directly affecting the development of Intensive Short-Term Dynamic Psychotherapy (ISTDP) will be highlighted.

Key Concepts in Defense Theory

It was during his early work with hysterics that Freud (1894; 1895) first outlined the concepts involved in the notion of intrapsychic conflict— that patients mobilize forces (D) to prevent awareness of painful and anxiety-provoking (A) thoughts

DOI: 10.4324/9781003542131-3

and feelings (I/F). He went on to say that the mobilization of these forces, which he called defenses, was a function carried out by the ego.

The Ego

The ego refers to that aspect of psychic functioning responsible for the observation of and mediation between internal wishes, feelings, and impulses clamoring for expression and the need to control the expression of these "instincts" in accordance with external constraints.

Defenses

Defenses are not psychic entities, and cannot be understood in isolation, but only by the functions they serve. Brenner (1976) contended that the entire range of ego functions can potentially be used in a defensive manner. Consequently, no list of defenses can ever be exhaustive. In addition to identifying typical defenses, we need to understand their function within the context of the intrapsychic conflict of which they are a part. In particular, defenses cannot be understood without addressing the anxiety that calls them into action. Freud's second theory of anxiety (Freud, 1926) shifted the focus of psychoanalytic inquiry and therapeutic efforts from the realm of id impulses to the functioning of the ego. It is the ego that perceives anxiety and then mobilizes forces to defend against the anticipated danger presented by the uprising of threatening feelings, impulses, and wishes. This theoretical revision places a greater emphasis on the role of the environment than that focused primarily on innate instincts. Given this, the ego is strapped with double duty, controlling internally generated feelings and impulses, and modulating external demands.

Resistance

Frequently, the terms defense and resistance are used interchangeably. In *Interpretation of Dreams*, Freud (1900) stated, "Whatever interrupts the progress of analytic work is resistance" (p. 517). He noted that such resistances often proved stubborn and required specific technical interventions. He came to feel that the "overcoming of resistances is the part of our work that requires the most time and the greatest trouble". Despite Freud's awareness of the central importance of helping the patient overcome resistance, he developed no specific techniques to accomplish that goal. Instead, he advocated patience, and the slow, judicious use of interpretation. This involved letting patients get acquainted with and experiencing their impact. Eventually patients would be encouraged to discover the feelings that were driving these avoidant behaviors.

Most analytically oriented therapists have followed Freud's lead, developing a whole rationale for continuing in this, a gentle manner based on assumptions about the inflexibility of defenses and the fragility of most patients. This has become a self-perpetuating system. The lack of activity on the part of the therapist and the paucity of specific techniques for overcoming the resistance leads to protracted treatments of dubious value, reinforcing the notion that resistances are intractable. It also leads to pessimism about our effectiveness in overcoming these counterforces. In fact, near the end of his life, Freud went so far as to say we must "bow to the superiority of the superego's resistance, which has our efforts come to nothing". As the reader will note, Davanloo turned this around, returning to Freud's initial sense that resistance is to be welcome as a sign that forbidden feelings and impulses are close to the surface. Therefore, we must move forward, rather than retreat, as resistance intensifies.

Advances in Defense Analysis

Anna Freud (1937/1966) was a pioneer in the study of defenses. She was the first to outline a range of *formal defenses* designed to "avoid painful or unendurable ideas or affects" (p. 42). In addition to repression, she discussed the defenses of denial, displacement, projection, and reaction formation. She also advanced the theory that defenses could be directed toward environmental influences, as well as against instincts and their vicissitudes. "Identification with the aggressor" and "defense against reality situations" (such as dissociation) are examples of behaviors aimed at modifying the traumatic effects of external conditions.

The success with which a given individual navigates between external demands and internal pressures came to define the ego's adaptive capacity. For this reason, Ms. Freud (1937/1966) advocated examining the defensive system to assess the functioning of the ego. These two theoretical advances—(a) an appreciation that defenses can be directed outward toward anxiety-arousing situations; and (b) that an examination of the defensive system can provide a vehicle for assessing a patient's current ego functioning—have been incorporated into Davanloo's thinking and have influenced the development of his technique.

Ferenczi and Rank (1925), and Reich (1933) were other clinical theorists whose work on defense and resistance influenced Davanloo. Their findings converged on a number of theoretical issues and technical maneuvers. Each felt that analysis had become a sterile intellectual exercise, requiring a shift in focus to the patient's emotions. Furthermore, they suggested that defenses needed to be confronted and eliminated in order to increase the kind of affective involvement in the treatment process necessary for deep and permanent change to occur. To accomplish this goal, they advocated an active approach on the part of the therapist, focusing on an understanding of the contemporary meaning of behavior. References to the distant past were only made once defenses had been eradicated and an affective involvement in the process was palpable.

Although there is a wide area of agreement among these clinicians, each has made individual contributions worth noting. Ferenczi (1924) encouraged the use of fantasy to break through resistance and activate feeling. He also encouraged his patients to openly express their feelings toward the therapist, especially negative and aggressive feelings. These techniques have clearly been incorporated into Davanloo's technqiue.

Reich (1933) agreed with Ferenczi that resistances must be attacked from the inception of treatment. He focused on what he called "character resistance" or "character armor"; those mannerisms and attitudes that permeate every aspect of patients' functioning, including their posture, gait, and tone of voice. He noted that these characteristic defenses formed a "ballast" around the patient and, unless penetrated, would prevent any interpretation from having a mutative effect. He insisted that it was not enough for patients to remember; they had to *experience* what was remembered. Hence, he was not as concerned with *what* the patient was reporting (content) as with *how* he or she reported it (process). For example, if a patient is remembering a painful and humiliating scene from her schooldays but reporting it in a light and humorous way, the focus would be on the smile and the purpose it serves in the current interaction with the therapist. In this case, the patient is avoiding the experience of the pain and outrage associated with the memory *and* hiding these feelings from the therapist.

Like Ferenczi, Reich felt that the direct expression of resentment, rage, hurt, and longing toward the therapist was an essential step in breaking through a patient's defensive armor. He also felt that negative transference feelings had to be cleared up before any genuine positive feelings could develop. If the negative feelings have not been experienced and expressed, then what might look like cooperation and a positive transference would be more likely to represent a defensive compliance on the patient's part. His (Reich, 1933; 1987) clinical experience with this technique confirmed what seemed to have been forgotten by most analysts; "that the neurosis itself is contained in the resistance, and that, in dissolving a resistance, we also dissolve a part of the neurosis" (1987, p. 81).

Davanloo's Approach to Defense Work

Davanloo (1978; 1979; 1980; 1990) incorporated all the preceding strategies and techniques into his system of ISTDP, while adhering strictly to three fundamental psychoanalytic principles: "releasing hidden feelings by actively working on and interpreting resistance or defenses; paying strict attention to the transference relationship; and actively making links between the transference and significant people in the patient's current life and in the past" (1978, p. 45). In so doing, he came to find that "unconscious conflicts emerged in an unmistakable way" (1978, p. 45). Davanloo's work has been built upon the foundation laid by Anna Freud, Ferenczi, and Reich.

Specific Techniques for Working with Defenses

The real question for most practicing clinicians is, "How can defenses be rendered inoperable, making treatment more rapid and effective?" According to Davanloo (1986a; 1986b), defense work involves three separate but frequently overlapping parts:

1 Acquainting patients with their defenses.

2 Elucidating their function.

3 Examining the cost of defenses that perpetuate his suffering and undermine treatment efforts.

Each aspect of this phase of treatment will be detailed and illustrated.

Part 1: Acquainting Patients with Their Defenses

In conducting the initial inquiry into a patient's difficulties, the therapist is alert to any signs of defense against clarity, emotional activation, or meaningful contact with the evaluator. In particular, as the therapist probes for feeling, it is important to monitor the balance between defense and resistance on the one hand, and motivation and therapeutic alliance on the other. In this vein, it is important not only to render the resistance inoperable but to release the force toward health buried beneath it. This is what Coughlin calls "the one two punch", simultaneously speaking to the alliance while challenging defenses that undermine progress.

During this phase of the evaluation, the therapist will begin to make use of the information gathered during inquiry by pointing out the operation of defenses against feelings as they arise. This is a three-step process involving the identification, clarification, and examination of the consequences of those defenses in operation. In particular, it is crucial to note how reliance on defenses creates and perpeatuates the patient's presenting problems.

Identification

First, the therapist needs to identify defenses as they arise in response to an inquiry about the patient's true feelings. An example of this would be, "Do you notice that, when I ask you about your feelings toward your girlfriend, you smile, make a joke, and change the subject?" The patient's response will yield diagnostic information and direct the next intervention. If the patient is able to acknowledge that he was smiling and joking, the therapist can proceed to the stage of clarification of the function. If the patient says, "No, I didn't notice that", further examples must be obtained and utilized to increase the observing function of the ego. "It happened again, just now, as you talked about being annoyed with your boss—that smile reappears. Did you notice?" The patient must be aware of the behavior before an exploration of its function will be of any therapeutic value.

Responses generated by the process of defense identification yield preliminary information about the observing function of the ego, particularly regarding the syntonicity of defenses. As such, this exploration quickly alerts the therapist to the direction the work will take.

Clarification

Once a defense has been identified, its function must be clarified and made explicit. "The smile and the joke are not your feelings toward your girlfriend but a way you avoid those feelings. Do you see that?" Once again, the patient's response to this clarification will yield important diagnostic information.

The therapist is assessing whether the patient is capable of distinguishing between the defense and impulse/feeling corners of the triangle of conflict. If the patient can make such a distinction, and, furthermore, can see how defenses are employed to avoid feelings, we would consider them "dystonic". To assess whether the patient can actually distinguish between feelings and defenses, the therapist would ask, "Now we see the laugh was a cover for your feeling, not the feeling itself. So, what was your feeling toward her?" If he can now say, "I was angry", a contrast between the current experience of the anger and the initial report, in which the experience was warded off with the smile, will consolidate this important insight. This type of interaction between patient and therapist highlights how this technique is employed to test out the patient's abilities in the here and now. It is not enough for the patient to agree with the therapist. Some actual demonstration of the ability in question is necessary before moving on to the next phase of work.

So far, the focus has been on highlighting the distinction between feelings and defenses. To complete the phase of clarification, all three corners of the triangle must be assessed and made explicit. Patients will either volunteer or be made aware that, as the therapist begins to probe for feeling and remark on defensive efforts to avoid it, they become increasingly anxious. In many cases, the patient will volunteer that information. For example, the patient may say, "I dread feeling that sadness". If the anxiety does not emerge spontaneously, the therapist might ask, "We have to wonder why you run from these feelings", or might venture, "You seem terrified to experience your anger". Because it is anxiety about the "danger" involved in the experience of the feelings being targeted that propels the defenses into operation, understanding the role of anxiety in the intrapsychic system is an essential element in the phase of clarification. Davanloo (1990) believes, "The patient needs to be given insight into the ways in which he has been defending himself against his underlying feelings and the anxieties that have led him to do so" (p. 8). Once this understanding has been outlined, and it is clear the patient can see how the defenses operate, an examination of the consequences can occur.

Examining the Consequences of Defenses

Once the above-mentioned information is obtained, a summary of what has been learned about the patient's characteristic defenses, as well as the feelings and anxieties that they are designed to avoid, can proceed. Assuming that the patient has indicated a similar understanding of these dynamic forces within him- or herself, the focus can shift to an examination of the consequences of these defenses in both the patient's life and in the therapy itself. Looking at the consequences of defenses, and helping the patient appreciate the cost involved in their utilization, has great therapeutic value. For example, the patient would be asked, "What effect will it have on your goal if you this mask of good humor?" The ways in which the defenses defeat the patient must be identified. As always it is best to ask, so the patient can elucidate the costs themselves.

Responses to Defense Analysis

There are several predictable responses to defense work. Cases in which patients are deeply involved in the process and appreciate the terrific cost of their defenses, often experience grief over these consequences. This grief becomes a powerful incentive to abandon defenses in favor of approaching previously avoided feelings. Such patients demonstrate a low level of resistance. Treatment, in these cases, proceeds quite rapidly to uncovering.

At times, a patient might acknowledge the operation of self-defeating defenses, but adopt a helpless position in the face of them, with comments such as, "I don't know what else to do". They might even say, "Yes I know I'm covering up, but I don't' like to cry in front of people". These comments suggest a moderate level of resistance. Additional pressure and challenge are typically required to turn them on defenses.

Another common response to defense analysis is an intensification of defensive efforts, creating resistance in the transference. This dynamic suggest that the patient's conflicts are becoming crystalized in the transference. Anger and irritation with the therapist for challenging his defenses exist alongside a high-level resistance against experiencing and sharing them. Patients can become overtly resistant, saying, "I am not going to open up to you. I hardly know you". Or "Maybe this whole therapeutic procedure is just a pile of horseshit". In these cases, a combination of pressure to honestly face his feelings toward the therapist, along with a challenge to defense and resistance (culminating in a head-on collision with resistance) are required to precipitate a breakthrough of feelings, leading to an unlocking of the unconscious. While this type of interaction can be quite challenging for therapists to manage, they can also create the deepest breakthroughs and most dramatic change, as there is a direct relationship between the strength of the resistance and the intensity of the complex feelings they are designed to repress.

We will begin with the first type of response to defense analysis, in which grief over the cost of defenses emerges.

Clinical Example

A Grief Response: The Lonely Businessman

THERAPIST: Tell me why you're here.

PATIENT: I've been seeing a marital therapist on and off for two years because my marriage has not been good for three or four years. He helped me with that, but I want to stress I'm not here for the same reason I went there. My own position now is that I expect we'll separate. We have four kids which is why we've stayed together. To all intents and purposes, we're separated but living at the same address.

THERAPIST: But you come now for your own reasons.

PATIENT: One reason we haven't separated is because I've been reluctant to make a change. Some of these are practical reasons, but at least 50% are reasons I have for not wanting to be alone. I've discovered this since separation became a real possibility.

This opening interchange contains a great deal of valuable information. The patient arrived with an intrapsychic focus and made it clear he had come for treatment of his own accord. He also proved quite insightful regarding the core of his difficulties—the fear of being alone and the painful feelings that would evoke. Intellectually, he was involved and insightful. As he relayed this information to the therapist, he appeared to be choked up. An exploration of his feelings was indicated.

THERAPIST: It looks like you're fighting a lot of feeling.

PATIENT: Yes I am. I've felt this way for four to five years now, since the marriage started to decline.

THERAPIST: So, once separation became a possibility, you began to confront fears about being alone and a lot of pain inside.

PATIENT: Yes, and I realized that played a large part in staying together and getting together in the first place.

THERAPIST: Any idea what that's about—why you're so afraid to be alone?

PATIENT: No I don't. I'm an intellectualizer by nature and seek isolation. I'm not a socializer, so it's a surprise to me to find this. I was remembering an event when I was 20 or so (patient is now in his 40s). Before going to college, I traveled for six months. I remembered looking forward to traveling and being alone. But then I suddenly realized, midtrip, that I was really depressed and didn't want to go on alone. I beat a hasty path to the airport and went home to stay with my older brother. I only remembered that in the context of the feelings evoked in this situation.

When patients are this insightful, sometimes all that is required is inquiry to unveil the causes of pain and anxiety. After initially saying he did not understand this, he was able to recall an earlier time in his life when he achieved the solitude he thought he wanted, only to become depressed. He seemed well acquainted with both his formal (intellectualizing) and tactical (isolation) defenses.

Examination of the Triangle of Conflict

THERAPIST: So there's a combination of anxiety and depression that comes when you're alone, and then you want to be reunited with a loved one. Was that the first time, at age 20?

PATIENT: It was the first time I got the isolation I thought I wanted. Many memories before that of looking to escape from people, all very tied up with experiences at boarding school. I thought if I just made it through there and got out, I'd be all right.

THERAPIST: How old were you when you went to boarding school?
PATIENT: Seven.
THERAPIST: Obviously that was traumatic.
PATIENT: Very.
THERAPIST: The way you dealt with that was to go to withdrawal and isolation. Now you find you can physically escape from people, but it doesn't solve the problem. Then you confront the feelings inside.
PATIENT: Precisely. I'm fairly sure that's why I got married, to prevent those feelings about being alone.

Here the therapist ventures the first interpretation of the triangle of conflict—that the anxiety (A) was a response to an upsurge of painful feelings, (I/F) which he attempted to avoid with emotional detachment and social isolation (D). The therapist added that the avoidance of feelings hadn't provided a solution, as the painful emotions associated with being left alone were still pressing for expression. The patient's response to these interpretations provided further evidence that he was well acquainted with his defenses, as well as suggesting that they are becoming dystonic.

Exploration of Anxiety

THERAPIST: So let's look at this anxiety. Are you aware of feeling that now?
PATIENT: Yes.
THERAPIST: Where do you feel it?
PATIENT: Emotionally, I suppose I have enough defense mechanisms in place that I don't particularly relish dismantling them.
THERAPIST: We'll get to that, but how do you experience the anxiety?
PATIENT: Some tension but mostly inner guardedness.
THERAPIST: Guarded is a way you avoid these feelings you dread and a way you keep me away from them. But, physically, you feel tense?
PATIENT: Mostly it's a raised heartbeat, stomach tension, and sort of bodily rigidity.

The preceding vignette indicates some fusion between anxiety and defenses. His defenses worked quite well in containing the anxiety but came at a considerable cost. As the process of clarification continued, the patient was able to describe the physical experience of anxiety, which was being channeled into the striated muscle. These responses indicated that the patient's ego-adaptive capacity was quite high, suggesting that he would be able to tolerate a rapid unlocking of the unconscious.

Anxiety in the Transference

PATIENT: When it's at its height and I'm in an "on the spot" situation, there's an overall feeling of nervousness.

THERAPIST: Like here—being on the spot. You smile.
PATIENT: I've put myself on the spot. I did this intentionally.
THERAPIST: But it makes you anxious. What about coming here to see me today makes you anxious?
PATIENT: I've never been in a situation where someone has put me on the spot and been there, and I don't intend to take refuge in those usual devices (defenses).
THERAPIST: So you've decided to come here and get to the bottom of your problems, but you're terrified to face it and to let me close to you. It raises the issue of intimacy and closeness.
PATIENT: Yes, without question.

The exploration of the patient's anxiety with the therapist leads unquestionably to his fear of closeness. Therefore, the following interventions are aimed in that direction.

Focus on Defenses against Emotional Closeness

THERAPIST: So the question is, will you let me close enough to be of help?
PATIENT: No one has ever been there. I've never really been there.
THERAPIST: You want help but you're running. Are you aware of how you're avoiding me right now?
PATIENT: How I would prevent someone from coming close? I rationalize a lot, but at the same time, I have a distinct feeling people can get there. They get in touch with those things underneath. I actually can't stop them. I'm thinking of boarding school. It was easy, because they were superiors and had authority, to simply invade that space and waste it.
THERAPIST: What do you think brought that to mind?
PATIENT: The feeling that we're already below levels I'm comfortable letting people in.

It is extraordinarily important to clarify at this point whether the patient is beginning to experience an upsurge of feeling about the past or is actually experiencing the therapist as invasive in the here and now.

Cost–Benefit Analysis of Defenses

Whereas Davanloo advocated a focus on the cost of defenses, I believe it is also crucial to acknowledge the benefit and the attempt at adaptation involved in defensive efforts. A good deal of developmental and longitudinal research (Stern, 1985; Vaillant, 1993) suggests that human beings are continually striving to adapt to the environment to the best of their ability. Although outmoded strategies developed in childhood certainly have self-defeating consequences in adulthood, there is no solid evidence that self-defeat is the motive behind the use of defenses. If the focus remains solely on the cost of defenses, without an acknowledgment of the attempt at adaptation, the patient can feel deeply misunderstood, creating the possibility for a misalliance. Making it clear to patients that their defenses worked at one time, or in a particular situation, while inviting them to examine whether they work now prevents any iatrogenic resistance from developing and increases the therapeutic alliance.

Grief Regarding the Cost of Defenses

THERAPIST: It reminds you of being invaded. Let's make sure I'm not invading where I don't have permission to go.

PATIENT: You're not. I am inviting you there but also unnerved.

THERAPIST: You keep a safe distance. I'm sure that served you well in boarding school, but here with me, if you stay distant and detached, what impact will that have?

PATIENT: It would have the impact which would be to waste my time and yours, which is why I don't plan to do it, but it's not to say it's going to be easy.

THERAPIST: It's a central conflict. Are you aware you avoid my eyes?

PATIENT: It takes a lot of effort to talk, to verbalize and communicate, to let someone in.

THERAPIST: You're terrified of closeness.

PATIENT: I've always been frightened and so . . .

THERAPIST: I'm sure you have reasons. Initially, it was for protection but now it traps you. It must be terribly lonely.

PATIENT: Yes, I always have been, as long as I can remember. I don't remember ever having anyone there (starts to cry).

Examining the cost of these distancing defenses revealed how they had perpetuated the painful loneliness this man hoped to avoid. Not only did he understand this intellectually, he experienced the cost with an outpouring of grief-laden affect. This indicated that he was turning on this previously entrenched defense. With the initial breakthrough of grief, the genesis of his difficulties became quite clear. The patient had been cared for by servants in his early childhood and was sent to boarding school at the tender age of seven. All his attempts to connect with his parents were met with rejection. They were described as both demanding and critical.

Following the work on defenses against emotional closeness, the deep pain about feeling so alone in the world was easily accessed. However, the reactive anger toward those who abandoned him was still being defended against. Until these defenses were removed, there would continue to be resistance in the transference and possible distortion of the material being reported.

Anger in the Transference

THERAPIST: It sounds like you are making a connection between your mother and me. You're saying that, without ever having established a warm, close relationship with you, she would barge in and demand a response. It sounds like you're saying to me, "Listen lady, I don't know you. You haven't paid your dues. I'll be damned if I'm going to let you in".

PATIENT: That's right.

THERAPIST: So there must be a lot of feeling toward me. Are you aware of feeling angry with me?

PATIENT: Oh yes. I've felt angry for about an hour now.

THERAPIST: How do you experience this anger?

PATIENT: Tension and defensiveness.

THERAPIST: That's not the anger, but a way to avoid it. What happens to the anger?

PATIENT: It says inside, unexpressed.

THERAPIST: Who suffers with it then?

PATIENT: I do, but I don't know what else to do with it.

This last interchange, regarding the experience of anger toward the therapist, and the mobilization of the patient's characteristic defenses against it, was very important. It became clear that he habitually internalized his rage and became depressed. Insight into the link between the repressed rage and the symptom of depression was necessary to turn the ego against this defense.

Turning the Ego against Its Defenses

THERAPIST: So, it stays inside and you suffer. It also creates a barrier. To avoid the experience of the anger you have to keep a distance from me.

PATIENT: Right.

THERAPIST: And then I can't help you. That's self-defeating.

PATIENT: Yes, yes it is.

THERAPIST: Why do you want to do that?

PATIENT: I don't.

The patient clearly indicated that he was aware of how defending against anger toward the therapist had a substantial cost. Furthermore, he declared his will to give up the defense in favor of facing and experiencing his anger directly. As pressure to feeling was initiated, the therapist monitored the patient for signs that aggressive impulses were getting mobilized in the body.

THERAPIST: So let's look at how you experience this anger toward me.

PATIENT: I don't know how to work it.

THERAPIST: The questions is, how do you experience the anger? Do you notice your hands are moving (referring to significant movement in the patient's hands that has just become evident)?

PATIENT: Yes, that's right. I just feel like shaking and strangling you.

Following the breakthrough of the anger toward the therapist, along with the aggressive impulses that accompanied it, the patient made spontaneous links to similar feelings and impulses toward both his wife and mother.

T-P Link

PATIENT: I wanted to shake and strangle my mother too, but not to kill her, to wake her up and get a response. Why was she never there for me? The anger is easy compared to the pain underneath. (The patient is crying and clearly in touch with the deep emotional pain he has run from all his life.)

THERAPIST: What is it like to experience this now?

PATIENT: It's a place I've tried to remove as far as possible. There were times I've felt my heart break, and I can't handle it (sobs). Nobody cared. It felt like death, in a way.

THERAPIST: It sounds like something died inside. It's as if hope died the night you were sent to boarding school. How could you bear it? It sounds like you killed off the longing to deal with the pain. While you couldn't bear it as a child, you can now. You're able to share it. What is that like?

PATIENT: For the first time, I feel reasonably safe feeling it.

THERAPIST: So as painful as it is, facing it directly and sharing it provides the very kind of emotional connection you've always longed for.

PATIENT: Yes, it's hopeful. It's the only hope. The entrance in was so hard, but now I want to stay there. I get the mental image of a three-year-old, sitting in a cave. Somewhere, back there, this connection exists.

THERAPIST: There was a real, live, feeling little boy back there.

PATIENT: There's a sense of hope and abandonment at the same time. Loneliness and hope, together. It's painful but not terrifying anymore.

Experiencing and expressing all the complex feelings of longing, pain, and rage with a concerned and engaged therapist provided a "corrective emotional experience" (Alexander & French, 1946). As central as this experience is in the process of healing, a deep understanding of the process is required to drive home the insights obtained. Initially there was a connection between the therapist and the patient's mother. As the feelings from the past were faced and shared with the therapist, the contrast between them became vivified. Instead of feeling violated he felt "reasonably safe" in sharing his true feelings for the first time in his life.

Another important change tends to occur subsequent to the direct experience of previously avoided feelings. Once feelings are faced, shared, and accepted, the anxiety that had accompanied them gets stripped away. In this case, anxiety was replaced by deep relief and the dawning of hope. Not only had the symptoms of anxiety and depression been lifted, but they were replaced by a sense of calm and reasonable hope that greatly enhanced the alliance, strengthened motivation, and accelerated the process of change. These changes were evident in the follow-up session, three days later. The patient entered the session ready to work, taking an active role in the process, and reporting a flood of memories from his early life, helping him to make sense of his current difficulties.

Part 2: Turning the Ego against Its Defenses

For highly responsive patients, such as "The Lonely Businessman", clarification and gentle challenge to the defenses is usually sufficient for the patient to abandon them in favor of experiencing previously avoided thoughts and feelings. In most cases, however, things do not progress so smoothly.

Syntonic character defenses are, by definition, deeply ingrained and tightly held, even when patients acknowledge how self-defeating they are. Reich (1933), one of the most "radical" analysts in his relentless attention to defense and resistance, declared, "We leave it up to him whether or not he wants to make use of his knowledge to change his character" (p. 52). Freud felt a strong lever against the resistance was required to tip the balance. He suggested that defenses had to be deprived of their value or even replaced by more powerful ones, though he never elaborated on the means to accomplish this end. This is exactly what the techniques of pressure and challenge, designed by Davnaloo (1990) were designed to do. A good deal of ego strength is required (by patient and therapist alike!) to endure the anxiety and intensely conflictual feelings toward the therapist that this technique evokes. In many cases, the restructuring of the defenses, which significantly increases ego strength, is a necessary prerequisite to this work. This process will be outlined in detail in the following chapter.

Part 3: Pressure and Challenge

The technique of "pressure and challenge" was designed to create an intrapsychic crisis, leading to psychic disequilibrium in patients with rigid character pathology. Pressure to experience his true feelings by abandoning his ultimately self-defeating defenses can create an internal crisis. This series of interventions often lead to the intensification of complex transference feelings, as well as crystallization of the defenses against them. The patient becomes affectively mobilized "within an atmosphere in which he senses, both consciously and unconsciously, that the therapist is directing him toward his most painful buried feelings out of a genuine and compassionate concern, a determination not to spare him pain but to face it, with the sole purpose of freeing him from the self-defeating patterns that have spoiled his life for so many years" (Davanloo, 1990, p. 7).

Pressure and challenge (exerting pressure on feelings while challenging the healthy part of the ego to abandon defenses) are the technical elements necessary for creating an intrapsychic crisis. Once the treatment has reached this stage, the clinician must proceed in a determined fashion. This involves relentless attention to each defense as it comes into operation, as each defense is like a brick in the wall of resistance which will prevent healing. Interventions must occur in a rapid-fire manner in order to interrupt defenses as they arise. At the same time, the therapist must remain alert to any signal that underlying feelings are ready to break through into conscious awareness. Once observed, a shift in focus to a full and direct experience of the complex transference feelings can occur. The phase of pressure and challenge has been referred to as a "head-on collision" with resistance in the transference. This is considered the most difficult intervention for most therapists to master. Yet, pressure and challenge can be a "do or die" procedure when dealing with patients enmeshed in rigid character pathology. Anything less tends to bounce right off the wall of resistance. A detailed example of the phase of pressure and challenge, culminating in a head-on collision with the resistance, will be provided.

Goals of Defense Work

The goals of this phase of the treatment, whether achieved through clarification and interpretation in highly responsive patients, or pressure and challenge in the case of more resistant patients, are threefold:

1. De-sensitization of the ego to previously toxic affects.
2. De-repression of memories and associations pertaining to the genesis of the patient's intrapsychic conflicts.
3. Use of this affective and cognitive information to make meaningful T-C-P interpretations and consolidate insight.

Anger in Response to Defense Analysis

It is not unusual for a patient to respond to defense analysis with anger and irritation toward the therapist. Some compromise between the feeling of anger and defenses against it is frequently observed. Although the anger toward the therapist must eventually be dealt with, it is up to the therapist to maintain a focus on ·the cost of defenses before proceeding to the experience of the anger. At this stage of defense work, anger toward the therapist is most often a diversion from the pain and grief patients have caused themselves by relying on these defenses. Only when patients can see their contribution to the problems they've been experiencing should the transference feelings be explored. Failure to stick with the task of clarification of the defense can distort the transference, such that the therapist is viewed as just another insensitive and demanding individual.

Clinical Example

The Detached Observer

The following vignettes illustrate the techniques of pressure and challenge to the patient's character defenses, which had become a major resistance to emotional involvement in the treatment. These interventions were designed to break through the defensive barrier and gain access to the patient's inner life. This young man exhibited the same kind of massive emotional detachment in the treatment setting that had characterized his entire life. To continue in this manner would result in the same sort of sterility and disappointment in the treatment that marked all his other relationships. The self-defeat in operation needed to be addressed directly. As the patient's defenses were repeatedly brought into focus, there was a rise in complex transference feelings.

The patient came for help with the symptoms of anxiety and depression, as well as social isolation and withdrawal. He was 27 at the time he entered treatment and, although intelligent and attractive, was functioning far below his capacity in both social and occupational realms. He repeatedly failed to take advantage of opportunities that came his way, due to his tendency to withdraw in the face of anxiety around contact with others. In fact, he had rarely left the house since a catastrophic car accident left him a quadriplegic. His core conflict, between the desire to connect authentically with others and the habitual avoidance of such contact, became evident in the therapeutic relationship.

The patient entered this, the sixth session, reporting anxiety about coming for his appointment. Previous sessions were spent on defense analysis and tracing the triangles of conflict and person. He was increasingly able to distinguish between feelings, anxiety, and defenses and was motivated, but anxious, about proceeding. He claimed that he wanted to open up but was nervous about doing so. The increased anxiety in the transference he reported suggested an intensification of complex transference feelings. In order to move forward, all his defensive attempts to avoid the experience of his feelings toward the therapist needed to be rendered inoperable. Pressure and challenge to the defenses was required to achieve the goal of emotional activation and access to the unconscious.

Exploration of Anxiety in the Transference

PATIENT: I'm really nervous about being here. I was thinking about it, and I really want to open up, but I get anxious.

THERAPIST: What are you experiencing with the anxiety?

PATIENT: Fidgety.

THERAPIST: Inside?

PATIENT: Tense in my chest and my arms. I'm kind of braced.

THERAPIST: There's lots of muscle tension. Anything else?

PATIENT: I get more quiet.

THERAPIST: That's not the anxiety, is it? You're getting quiet is a retreat in the face of anxiety.

PATIENT: I get the wandering mind too. If I'm with people, especially. That doesn't happen when I'm alone, I notice.

THERAPIST: So the anxiety has to do with being with other people, like being here with me. When did that anxiety start?

PATIENT: A few days ago when I realized I wanted to come here and open up to you.

THERAPIST: So there's something about opening up to me that makes you very anxious, and in the face of the anxiety you go to emotional distance—by avoiding eye contact, keeping constricted, even your voice is low and controlled, no emotion, and your mind wanders, you tend to be vague. Are you aware of that?

PATIENT: Yes, pretty much. It comes very automatically.

The last intervention involved an interpretation of the triangle of conflict in the transference with particular attention paid to the types of defenses the patient was using to erect a wall and remain detached. His response indicated that he was able to see that he was backing off in the face of anxiety about close emotional contact but felt as if it was automatic and against his conscious will. This indicated that these defenses were still syntonic. As such, some pressure was required to turn the ego against them and render them dystonic.

Examining the Consequences of Detachment

THERAPIST: Right. It's automatic and pervasive. It's not just here with me but you get anxious and then distance yourself from everyone, which has had a devastating effect on your relationships. You end up leading an isolated, constricted life. So, if you establish the same kind of detached relationship here with me, we are at an impasse.

This intervention constituted an attempt to examine the consequences of the patient's characteristic defenses, particularly in the transference, and to tie that to the devastating consequences of this stance in his entire life.

PATIENT: Right.
THERAPIST: Is that what you want?
PATIENT: No.

Now that the patient has declared his will to give up the defenses that have perpetuated the pain in his life, the process proceeded to the phase of pressure and challenge. The patient was challenged to follow through on his declaration of will.

Challenge to the Defense of Detachment

THERAPIST: So then we have to see what you are going to do about the detachment here with me.
PATIENT: (stays silent and looks to the floor).
THERAPIST: You stay silent, look away, sigh—you maintain the distance.
PATIENT: (throws up his hands).
THERAPIST: Now you go to a helpless, defeated position. Do you see the barrier this creates here between you and me?
PATIENT: Yes.
THERAPIST: If you maintain the barrier, what will happen to your goal of getting to the bottom of your difficulties so you can be free of your suffering?
PATIENT: It won't happen.
THERAPIST: More self-defeat. This will be another failure. Is that what you want?
PATIENT: No.
THERAPIST: Then what are you going to do about the detachment that kills off your potential for a helpful relationship here?
PATIENT: (returns to silence and withdrawal).

As pressure was exerted on the patient to take responsibility for acting on his stated intention to open up, defenses and resistance in the transference increased. One line of defense after another came to the fore in rapid succession. The patient started with emotional detachment, retreating to silence and stubborn withholding, then resorted to helplessness. The resistance was a sign that underlying complex transference feelings were rising. Therefore, a relentless focus on the defense, with an appeal to the part of the patient that wants to be free to directly express himself, had to be maintained until the defenses were exhausted and the feelings broke through the repressive barrier.

Pressure and Challenge

THERAPIST: You look away, sigh, and remain silent.

PATIENT: I don't know what to do.

THERAPIST: That's helplessness. You say you see that you erect a wall of emotional detachment.

PATIENT: Yeah. I know it's there.

THERAPIST: You put it there, and you're the one who can keep it there or take it down. If it stays?

PATIENT: Nothing will get done.

THERAPIST: So it becomes another part of the self-defeat in your life. You come here of your own will to get help but end up sabotaging that by remaining uninvolved—a detached observer. The problem here between us is the same problem that spoils your life—detachment. So the question is, what are you going to do about that?

PATIENT: I don't know.

THERAPIST: You don't know. Now we're in limbo.

PATIENT: Yeah. (There's a decided edge to his voice and a defiant quality to this sequence of the interaction.)

THERAPIST: Where does that get you?

PATIENT: Nowhere.

The "Head-On Collision" with the Resistance

The following sequence demonstrates a combination of interventions refered to as "a head-on collision with the resistance" (Davanloo, 1990). This focused attempt to help the patient confront the strength of his tendency to hold onto self-defeating defenses, while challenging the healthy ego to assume control, takes place in the transference in the here and now. The therapist places responsibility in the patient's lap and refuses to let the patient off the hook or to do the work for him. The therapist makes it clear that they are on the side of openness and honesty, no matter how painful, and will not collude with the part of the patient that wants to skirt the experience of painful feelings and memories. The therapist must be ready to detect and then withstand the full storm of complex transference feelings once they surface. Facing the fact that therapy will fail if the patient continues to resist is an essential element of the head-on collision.

THERAPIST: Isn't this the problem in your life? Why should we continue in this "nowhere"? Let's have an honest look and you decide—it's up to you.

Because, if there is a part of you that has decided, "There is no way I'm going to let this woman into my life", we might as well say our good-byes, because to continue in this way is to perpetuate the misery. Maybe we could have a nice chat but that is not going to help you with your problems. Which is it going to be?

PATIENT: I want to, but I don't know if I can change it.

THERAPIST: You want to change, though?

PATIENT: Yes.

THERAPIST: You're not content to remain an observer in life—detached and alone?

PATIENT: No. No.

Again, his conscious will to change was solidified while pressure to experience his true feelings was intensified.

Anger in the Transference

THERAPIST: So what are you going to do about the detachment here with me?

PATIENT: (The patient is silent but physically charged, moving around in his chair and breathing deeply, a sign that transference feelings are close to the surface and can now be tapped.)

THERAPIST: Is there some feeling toward me?

PATIENT: Yeah.

THERAPIST: Which is what, if you don't avoid it?

PATIENT: I can't let it out.

THERAPIST: Could you declare what the feeling is toward me?

PATIENT: It's real anger.

THERAPIST: How do you experience this anger toward me?

The patient was able to declare anger toward the therapist, indicating a breakdown of the defense against cognitive awareness of his feeling toward the therapist. Now the physiological and motoric elements of the anger needed to be assessed, and any remaining defenses removed, so that the patient could achieve a full experience of the complex transference feelings.

Breakthrough of Sadistic Impulses

PATIENT: I want to but . . .

THERAPIST: But there's another part that fights you, keeps it inside, and the attack is on you. You become more depressed, more isolated, constricted in your life.

PATIENT: Yeah.
THERAPIST: Is that what you want, to let that part rule? Or are you going to decide and take the risk to face this anger with me directly right now.
PATIENT: (retreats to silence).
THERAPIST: This is more avoidance, which is a decision not to let me close to these feelings.
PATIENT: That's because they're almost murderous.
THERAPIST: Very powerful, huh? So, there's a murderous rage toward me?
PATIENT: Toward more than just you.
THERAPIST: But, first toward me.
PATIENT: Yeah.
THERAPIST: And if that were to come out, in your imagination, how would you murder me, what is the impulse?
PATIENT: The impulse is to swear at you.
THERAPIST: But that is not to murder me. How would you murder me? Your hands start to move.
PATIENT: Just to strangle you. I'd squeeze your neck with such force, it would come right off. I'd sever your head from your body, take it by the hair, and just smash it against a brick wall.

At long last, the patient became deeply immersed in the experience of his angry feelings toward the therapist. To get there, all the defenses he had erected against emotional contact had to be systematically identified and challenged until they were exhausted. The last-ditch efforts to avoid the direct experience of the rage toward the therapist, including diversifying ("Toward more than just you") and minimizing ("The impulse is to swear at you"), were pushed aside. In a sense, the patient was testing the therapist to see if they would take an easy out or would settle for a half truth.

It is crucial to access all the feelings in the transference before moving on to the other figures with whom the therapist is associated. If the feelings toward the therapist are not directly experienced, they are, by definition, being defended against and will contribute to ongoing resistance. In addition, an opportunity for a powerful corrective emotional experience would be lost. As Freud (1917; 1920) reminded us, what is learned directly through the transference relationship is never forgotten. Experiencing and expressing the very feelings the patient has dreaded, without encountering any of the anticipated damaging consequences, is a potent corrective experience. So, the resistance is substantially decreased and the therapeutic alliance bolstered by facing these feelings directly. Once the feelings in the transference have been experienced, the genetic figure the therapist has come to represent will become clear. This transfer of images, in which the picture of the therapist morphs into the face of an attachment figure, is the hallmark of the unlocking of the unconscious. No interpretations are necessary, as the crucial figure from the patient's past emerges in an unmistakable fashion.

T-P Link

THERAPIST: So what happens to me? My head is a bloody pulp and my body?

PATIENT: I throw your head down and take your body and break it over my knee. Then I raise it over my head and the blood drenches over me. (The patient is motorically, as well as emotionally involved, going through the physical motions he's describing.) Now I see my mother, only it's more gruesome.

THERAPIST: So as you get in touch with this massive rage toward me and the impulses that come with that, you get a picture of your mother?

PATIENT: Yeah. Only it's worse with her. I break every bone in her body. I target her fingers and break them one by one. It was those fingers, all that twitching and crazy shit she did with her hands, I target that. The sounds are deafening. (Patient begins to tear up.)

THERAPIST: As you face this rage toward her, other feelings seem to come. This is a horrendous scene.

PATIENT: I don't think it's horrendous.

The patient was very involved in the experience of anger but did not seem ready to move to the underlying guilt and grief. As our time was up, I summarized what had occurred in the session, linking the triangle of conflict in the transference with that in the past with his mother. He entered the next session noticeably changed. There were no signs of anxiety, and rather than being quiet or hesitant, he started speaking right away, declaring that he still felt angry. This provided evidence of character change.

De-Repression of Memories

PATIENT: I'm still really pissed about the last session.

THERAPIST: I think it's very important that we examine what happened and what your reactions are.

PATIENT: I'll tell you what I've been thinking. I thought I'd come in here and lay it on you but then it got transferred—you were my mother, you were her. Because I felt like it was an attack and it felt unprovoked, it was similar to what I got with my mother. It had nothing to do with what I did, she would just come at me.

THERAPIST: So, as you began to face the feelings toward me for what felt like an unprovoked attack . . .

PATIENT: It went right to my mother. I said, "For 17 years (she died when he was 17) I was right in front of you, and you basically ignored me". The only attention I got was "You're a lazy bum", "Why don't you go out and make friends?", shit like that. And then she bought a dog. It was for her, because she felt lonely . . . (getting choked up with emotion) . . . and I was right there. I hated that fucking dog. I know, when she died, we kept that dog. I'd open up the door and it would fucking growl at me. That dog was just like her. The only person it cared about was her—wouldn't let anyone next to it. I used to beat that fucking dog sometimes. And I wanted to beat her.

THERAPIST: The rage toward her is a reaction to all your needs to love and be loved being repeatedly thwarted.

PATIENT: I don't understand it because, you know, I tried to be the best I could, I was good, I don't cause trouble. (In fact, the patient was an A student and star athlete while his mother was alive.) So what was it? It was her.

THERAPIST: But that doesn't make it any less painful. You tried to be so good, but she still couldn't respond and would sometimes lash out in an unprovoked way?

PATIENT: That leads to another thought I had. We're in a padded room and I'd just keep slapping her, to stop this ranting and raving (his mother appeared to have a serious mental illness, with tics, phobias, and paranoid ideation), just keep slapping her (arms waving) until she'd stop all this wild talk and these crazy body movements and she'd just look at me—just see that I need her, I need her love (begins to cry and is clearly grief-stricken).

Now the full range of intense feelings toward his mother, which had been precipitated by the uprising of complex transference feelings, came pouring out. This was followed by the de-repression of significant memories shedding light on the very real trauma this man experienced in relation to his very disturbed mother. This material also provided an example of the direct relationship between the extent of the trauma to the early attachments, the intensity of the reactive anger and sadism, and the strength and tenacity of the defenses erected against them. When the full intensity of this man's rage, and the horrendous trauma that gave rise to this rage became apparent, it was fairly easy to see why such massive defenses were required to contain it all. Once the feelings were experienced directly, the patient's adult ego had another chance to put it all in perspective. Although initially there was a direct connection between the feelings and perceptions of the therapist and the patient's mother, by the end of this session, clear distinctions were made. Even though I had, in fact, put pressure on him and repeatedly pointed out the ways in which he was avoiding me and rendering me useless to him, I did not attack him personally as his mother had. In addition, my motive was to help him, not berate him. He made these distinctions spontaneously, and they were accompanied by a feeling of gratitude toward me for going through all this with him. The direct experience of anger toward the therapist did not result in feared death and destruction, but actually led to relief, a greater understanding of himself, and a genuine feeling of closeness with and gratitude toward the therapist. This is the essence of a corrective emotional experience.

Summary

In most cases, patients arrive for treatment in an ambivalent state and tend to become increasingly defensive as painful areas of their life are explored in depth. Because defenses, when left undisturbed, create resistance to the treatment, they must be eradicated as quickly as possible if treatment is to be efficient and effective. In rare cases, a focus on the high cost of the patient's defenses evokes deep grief, which is sufficient to shift the preexisting psychic equilibrium. Such was the case with the Lonely Businessman.

To deal with more intransigent defenses, Davanloo developed a whole series of interventions designed to break through the barrier of resistance, rendering patients who have been poorly motivated to collaborate more accessible to intervention. In the case of the Detached Observer, a heavy dose of unrelenting pressure and challenge was required to shift the balance from resistance to engagement.

Note

1. From "Slip Sliding Away". Music and lyrics by Paul Simon. Warner Bros. Music, 1982.

4 RESTRUCTURING REGRESSIVE DEFENSES

Tell me and I forget
Teach me and I remember
Involve me and I learn
Xun Kuang, translated by
H. H. Dubs, 1928

As has already been demonstrated in Chapter 3, many of Davanloo's techniques are employed pre-interpretively, to prepare the patient to withstand and then effectively utilize material from the unconscious. Intensive Short-Term Dynamic Psychotherapy (ISTDP) is quite demanding on both cognitive and affective levels and can only be successful if both patient and therapist are deeply involved in the process. In rare cases, patients come for the initial evaluation with the motivation and ability to become freely involved and make use of this focused and intensive approach. More often than not, however, patients arrive in a state of ambivalence—wanting help but resisting the process of opening up and experiencing anxiety-provoking and guilt-laden feelings. This resistance prevents the kind of emotional involvement necessary for a successful outcome. Davanloo (1980) has developed a standard technique for handling highly resistant patients, in which "pressure and challenge to the resistance are steadily increased and are not relaxed until the patient directly experiences the complex transference feelings" (Davanloo, 1987a, p. 77). Following this experience, there is an outpouring of unconscious material that not only provides a deep understanding of the genesis of the patient's difficulties but dramatically increases the unconscious therapeutic alliance. This process

DOI: 10.4324/9781003542131-4

was illustrated in the case of the Detached Observer (see Chapter 3). The patient's resistance was massive and prevented any meaningful contact between patient and therapist, as he was keeping the innermost part of himself sealed off from view. Because all the initial interventions indicated a strong ego, the standard technique of applying unremitting pressure and challenge to the defenses was employed. The outpouring of memories and associations following the breakthrough of complex transference feelings confirmed this assessment.

Restructuring

Indications for Restructuring

The standard technique involving pressure and challenge to the patient's defenses is contra-indicated in those cases where patients suffer from depression, functional disorders (e.g., headaches, irritable bowel syndrome), panic, or impulsive discharge. Common to all these disorders is a deep-rooted inability to distinguish between the elements involved in the triangle of conflict. Most often, various defenses are mistaken for the impulse itself. With this type of fusion, challenge to the defenses, with pressure to experience the underlying impulses, can result in an exacerbation of symptoms and/or unmanageable anxiety. Modifications to the standard technique are required in these cases. The technical requirements involved in restructuring and clinical examples of this process will be detailed in this chapter.

The Technique of Defense Restructuring

The technique of restructuring defenses involves the systematic and repetitive reworking of the triangle of conflict in both the transference and the patient's current relationships. Restructuring involves the following elements:

1. Clarification and differentiation within the triangle of conflict.
2. Gradual exposure to the direct experience of feelings and impulses, keeping anxiety in the optimal range.
3. Cognitive re-analysis of the process.

The goals of this phase of therapeutic intervention are directed toward an increase in the adaptability, flexibility, and strength of the ego. This is achieved by:

1. Increasing insight into the link between repressed impulses and anxiety or other symptoms.

2 Decreasing the patient's reliance on regressive defenses.

3 Reducing the intensity of anxiety that accompanies the direct experience of affect.

4 Increasing motivation and capacity to face one's feelings honestly.

All this work must occur before attempting any access to unconscious impulses and feelings toward central figures from the patient's past.

Working the Triangle of Conflict in Current Relationships

During the phase of inquiry, special attention is devoted to the examination of recent episodes preceding depression, panic, or exacerbations of psychosomatic complaints. As these episodes are explored, slow and repetitive work on the triangle of conflict begins.

It is essential that patients become aware of the mechanisms by which they have avoided particularly painful impulses and feelings. Since these patients are typically very identified with their defenses and don't distinguish defenses from feelings, repeated clarification is required to achieve this insight. A clinical example will be used to illustrate this process.

Restructuring with Depressives

Patients who are currently experiencing depression require a phase of defense restructuring that follows inquiry and must precede any pressure or challenge to experience the feelings they typically avoid. A detailed inquiry should cover all areas of symptomatic disturbance, history of previous episodes of depression, including severity and duration, examination of past treatments, and assessment of current ego functioning and character structure. When depression is severe or is deeply embedded in a patient's character, patients cannot participate actively in the treatment process. Their slowness, passivity, and helplessness form a barrier of resistance in the transference that must be addressed from the outset. Clarification of the self-defeating nature of this resistance in interactions with the evaluator, as well as in other areas of the patient's life, is necessary to turn the ego against these ego-syntonic character defenses.

Davanloo's (1987a; 1987b) work with depressives has demonstrated that a reliance on the defenses of repression and internalization is a central and overriding feature of this disorder. Fosha (1988) has stated:

> Thus, Davanloo conceptualizes the phenomenological hallmarks of depression—the withdrawal, the self-reproaches, the passivity, the helplessness,

> the sense of inferiority and inadequacy—as the result of regressive mechanisms used not only to defend against sadistic impulses but also to avoid the experience of the associated painful feelings, such as guilt and grief.
> (Fosha, 1988, p. 189)

This last point is very important. Depressives are defending against guilt and grief as well as aggressive impulses. The following clinical example will illustrate several of these crucial factors.

Clinical Example

Woman on an Emotional Roller Coaster

THERAPIST: Why don't you start by telling me about the problems you came for help with.

PATIENT: First of all, I got cancer. My marriage is falling apart and I'm about to leave. I have one child still living at home who doesn't know yet. One older child has known since last year. I have been disconnected from my parents for three years, so they don't know. I have a boyfriend, lover . . .

THERAPIST: You're telling me about events but . . .

PATIENT: You want feelings.

THERAPIST: Well, how is this causing you a problem?

PATIENT: Pain, I'm on an emotional roller coaster.

Exploration of Anxiety

The patient began by presenting a list of highly traumatic events in a rather businesslike fashion. Before the therapist could complete her first intervention, the patient took over, indicating a strong tendency to be compliant with what she imagined was expected of her (in this case, a focus on feeling). At this opening stage, what needed to be delineated were the problems in her current life. The patient reported the onset of anxiety attacks and depression nine months prior to our meeting. An exploration of the phenomenological experience of the symptoms and exploration of the precipitating events follows.

Exploration of Depression

THERAPIST: So let's look at how you experience this anxiety and then we'll look at the depression.

PATIENT: It's like hot flashes, but they're emotionally precipitated. So I become flushed and sweaty and feel anxious in the pit of my stomach.

THERAPIST: And this started?

PATIENT: After my husband left and my older daughter went back to college.

THERAPIST: So you realize the anxiety is a reaction to emotion.
PATIENT: When I contemplated leaving or talked about the separation.
THERAPIST: The anxiety was a reaction to the feelings about separation.

The patient was able to give a good account of the physical experience of anxiety and indicated an awareness that anxiety was a response to an emotional trigger. Her ability to distinguish, yet meaningfully link, anxiety and a rise in unpleasant feelings indicates a fairly high level of insight into her own inner workings.

PATIENT: Separation anxiety, yeah. Depression was about ambivalence. I want to break loose, but there's a loss. In part I want to re-do adolescence; drive a motorcycle, have sex; but I also want to be secure with my family around.
THERAPIST: Clearly, the cancer diagnosis created an internal crisis and you began to reevaluate your life.
PATIENT: That, and midlife, and the kids taking off with their own lives. Even the youngest doesn't need me as much, so the loss of the role of mother. And I lost my mother too, and when you're in pain, you want to call "Mommy".
THERAPIST: What's that about?
PATIENT: I disconnected from my parents. I was an abused child and had a difficult childhood. I always tried to be good, to work hard to try and please them, and, on a very erratic schedule, I'd manage to do that. So, I kept trying, but just as often I'd get slapped down and I became very rebellious and I began to believe what they said about me.

C-P Link

THERAPIST: So this recent separation, and the ambivalence about that, brought all these unresolved feelings from the past close to the surface. On the one hand, wanting to be good and pleasing to secure the attachment but then enraged about having to win their love, which goes into rebellious behavior. You say, "To hell with you". So there's a sense in which this emotional roller coaster is not just about now, which is traumatic enough, but stirs up unresolved feelings from the past. How do you understand it?
PATIENT: I was trying to be tough and independent to survive it on my own, but cracks in the armor that covered the pain started to show. I think there is tremendous anger (getting weepy) because I spent 25 years of marriage being a good girl, good wife and mother, and he was conditionally loving.

Both the precipitant to the recent crisis and a meaningful link between that and an unresolved conflict from the past emerged rapidly, making sense of the patient's intense struggle. To work the triangle of conflict, the process moved to an examination of the current conflictual relationship. While the relationship between anxiety and affect had been established, the exploration of defenses was just beginning and needed to be solidified by a repetitive process of examination.

Triangle of Conflict in the C

THERAPIST: You were angry with your husband and how did you deal with that?

PATIENT: By leaving.

THERAPIST: So you run (D) in the face of your anger (I/F).

PATIENT: And the other is to go into manic behavior (D)—exercising, buying and spending, like $2,000 on clothes, having an affair.

THERAPIST: Characteristically, you don't let yourself experience what you're feeling. You suppress it, are compliant, the good girl, then get angry and fed up and channel the anger into rebellious behavior. The anger goes directly into behavior.

PATIENT: Yeah, I went to this tough stance and shut down my feeling, went to being self-sufficient. I'm not sure what triggered the actual breakdown, but when my husband left, I felt I didn't want to get up anymore. I had been rebellious, the bad girl, and then went to helplessness. I liked being rebellious better.

THERAPIST: You go to various positions, rebellious or helpless, but these are not the feelings themselves.

PATIENT: Yeah, I was running away.

THERAPIST: Right. It was a way to avoid feeling.

This work provided evidence of some fusion between feelings and defenses. The internal experience of angry feelings was avoided by acting on the feelings in some external way, either passivity and compliance or rebellious behavior. Such acting out would trigger guilt, and she punished herself by becoming depressed, helpless, withdrawn, and fairly nonfunctional. Her responses to this phase of the work indicated that she now had a cognitive understanding of how feelings were being avoided. She spontaneously commented that she had dealt with her anger toward her parents in the same way—by cutting them off. However, in that situation, it was more accurate to say she provoked a rejection. This interaction was explored to re-work the triangle of conflict and increase her capacity to experience the feelings themselves in a direct manner.

Triangle of Conflict in Relation to Her Father

PATIENT: I wrote to my parents to ask for a "hearing" in which I could tell them what I really thought about them. I knew they would put me down, but I thought that surviving it and telling them what I really thought would be cathartic.

THERAPIST: You thought that this action—telling your parents what you really thought—would lead to a resolution of your own conflicted feelings toward them?

PATIENT: Yes, but my father said, "No, it'll be two adults against a child whose memories are warped". He was furious and wanted to know why I had to cause trouble. So, I sent them a letter. It wasn't a poisoned pen letter but it was accusatory. They each wrote me separately saying nasty things and that they wanted nothing to do with me. That was it. I got really manic in my behavior. I was furious.

THERAPIST: So you were furious (I/F) with them but channeled it into manic behavior (D).

PATIENT: I didn't know what to do with it.

THERAPIST: You immediately want to do something with it but the first question is, how do you experience this fury toward your parents? When was it most acute?

PATIENT: When my father called and said he didn't like the idea.

THERAPIST: How did you experience this anger toward him?

PATIENT: I started crying (patient gets tearful).

Restructuring the Depressive Mechanism

THERAPIST: But crying isn't your anger. It's just like what's happening now. You get tearful as we look at your anger.

PATIENT: If I have a good crying jag I feel relieved.

THERAPIST: Is this the anger or the way you avoid it?

PATIENT: That's how I get angry. (This response indicates fusion of feeling and defense.) If I have a good crying jag, I feel better.

THERAPIST: For the moment, but what happens to the anger?

PATIENT: I act on it.

THERAPIST: How adaptive is that?

PATIENT: But I'm scared of it (getting weepy). I don't know what else to do or how to feel it, because my mother is an extremely angry, hostile person, and when I feel that kind of rage and fury toward someone, that she so easily expressed, it scares the hell out of me, and I don't want to be like her, so I try to do something else.

THERAPIST: You are terrified (A) of your own anger (I/F). We can see it here. There's some rise in your anger (I/F) but that mobilizes a lot of anxiety (A) and you go to weepiness (D).

PATIENT: But then it gets back under control.

THERAPIST: But at what price? Does this work for you, or is it a very self-defeating way of dealing with your anger?

PATIENT: I suppose, but I'm not convinced. I'm ambivalent. I like to go into high gear. I just don't like getting depressed.

Turning the Ego against Character Defenses

The preceding work was designed to turn the patient's ego against these regressive and self-defeating defenses. They are quite syntonic, and the patient openly expresses her hesitance to give them up. The manic behavior, in particular, was hard to relinquish, as it provided some immediate sense of satisfaction. These defenses work by fending off depressive affect and by providing revenge on those she was feeling angry with. These defenses needed to be rendered dystonic before any more anger was evoked, otherwise the acting out could accelerate.

THERAPIST: They are flip sides of the same coin. You either swallow it or spit it out, but in neither case do you really let yourself experience the anger, know who it's toward, and decide the best way to deal with it. But you're saying maybe you don't want to because it's very gratifying to feel pumped up. It's gratifying in a direct way to act on these feelings and indirectly by getting back at others.

PATIENT: It's also the way I punish myself for feeling something bad. I'm my own judge, jury, and executioner. I make myself suffer.

This was an extraordinarily important communication from the patient, signaling the turning of the ego, the easing of the resistance, and an increase in the unconscious therapeutic alliance. She went on to solidify her determination to do things differently.

THERAPIST: How?

PATIENT: By embarrassing myself, wearing myself out.

THERAPIST: So it is self-defeating and you end up suffering. You don't want to . . .

PATIENT: I really don't. I want to be an autonomous person.

THERAPIST: So do you want to take this opportunity to have an honest look at your feelings, to get to the bottom of what drives you?

PATIENT: Yeah, I really do. I don't have a chance to be happy if I don't. Otherwise, I'm on this roller coaster, always mildly manic-depressive.

Cognitive Re-Analysis of the Process

To consolidate the insights obtained by clarifying and differentiating the triangle of conflict, a period of cognitive re-analysis should follow each gradual increment toward a full experience of affect. This phase of the work is aimed at strengthening the observing function of the ego.

Two rounds of this work have been conducted thus far. The patient's responses indicated that she was gaining clarity about the distinctions between feelings, anxiety, and defenses. Further, she was beginning to acknowledge just how self-defeating her defenses have been, motivating her to approach directly the feelings behind the defense. A third round of work was required to highlight these distinctions and prepare the way for a direct experience of her mixed feelings toward others. We proceeded to examine her feelings and reactions to the doctor who gave her the cancer diagnosis.

Triangle of Conflict in a Current Relationship

PATIENT: It took two weeks to get an appointment with the OB-GYN. Halfway through the exam, my doctor, a female, was called out on an emergency C-section. They asked if I wanted to reschedule or have another doctor finish the exam. I didn't want to wait, so I said, "Send in another doctor". In came this Oriental male who, without introducing himself, just said, "Lie down, I'm going to do a pelvic". I thought to myself, "I'm here for a breast exam but he must just want to do a Pap smear". So, I laid down, but by the time he was through, I felt as if I had been raped (patient is tearful). I was already really angry with him, and then I started crying right there on the table. Then he asked if the Nurse Midwife could come in and have a look. I thought, "Why should she come in? Oh, maybe it's just a lactating cyst". So, I said it was OK. Then he said to her, without ever speaking to me, "You wanted to feel a tumor, right?" She was so patronizing! She said, "Did you find this yourself? Aren't you good to do your self-exam and aren't you brave to come to the doctor". I really felt like smacking her! I just wanted to punch her out, so I started crying.

There are several important points to be noted regarding this last segment of the transcript. The patient was describing an incident in which she was, in fact, treated very poorly. While this must be acknowledged, the therapist should guard against getting caught up in personal feelings about such incidents and stay focused on the task, which was to point out the operation of regressive defenses against feelings that interfered with the patient's optimal functioning. This can be a tricky task. When patients are highly identified with the victim role, they are likely to respond defensively to any attempt at exploring their own role in their victimization. Tact and precision are absolute requirements to achieve this end. The following interventions will illustrate the therapist's attempt to direct the patient's attention toward an examination of the self-defeating nature of her characteristic defenses against anger.

THERAPIST: Just like now. You cry, but what was the feeling inside? Already you have waited a long time for the appointment. Then your doctor is called out. You're quick to be understanding, she has an emergency, OK, but it doesn't mean you don't have feelings about it. Then this man comes in who treats you in a highly impersonal, even cold, manner. What was your feeling toward him?

PATIENT: Why couldn't he . . .

THERAPIST: That's a question. Your feeling?

PATIENT: Helpless.

THERAPIST: That's a position you take but the feeling?

PATIENT: Angry.

THERAPIST: You were angry. You don't like to be treated this way, so how did you deal with that?

PATIENT: It was quiet resentment.

THERAPIST: You kept it inside, stayed quiet, and behaved in a compliant manner. This is for you to look at. Somehow you allow this, like you did for the first 25 years of your marriage. You were the good girl— quiet and subservient—but all the anger and resentment were building until you explode.

PATIENT: I don't think I was even in touch with those feelings. It all happened so fast.

THERAPIST: And that's the problem. It's not the interaction that happened so fast but these automatic mechanisms you employ to stuff your feelings. Because you do not allow yourself to know what you're feeling and to use that information in your own behalf, you make yourself vulnerable to mistreatment. Do you see what I mean?

PATIENT: Yes, but in general, I'm not passive.

THERAPIST: I don't know about in general, but in this situation.

PATIENT: It's with anger.

THERAPIST: And what's the purpose of anger? It has a self-protective function. If you don't have access to it, you can't protect yourself. (Patient nods.) So, you can see that, with the doctor, you were angry but went to tears and took a victimized stance. Then you look foolish, and no one pays attention to your outburst. Pretty self-defeating.

PATIENT: I agree with that. It is a way I defeat myself. Still, I don't like to hear it.

THERAPIST: So this is what you want help with? (Patient nods.) The problem is clear then, but you don't like to look at it. You must have a certain feeling toward me, as I point it out to you.

Graded Pressure and Challenge

As defenses are identified, clarified, and rendered dystonic, graduated pressure is placed on patients to experience their feelings directly. The initial aim of this intervention is to increase insight into the mechanism by which patients turn feelings and impulses into anxiety, depression, or symptomatic disturbances. In the case at hand, the patient turned her anger into tears and adopted a helpless stance in the face of her violent rage ("I just wanted to punch her out, so I started crying").

As soon as patients indicate a clear cognitive understanding of the link between the repressed impulse and the symptom being targeted, the focus shifts to the experience of the feeling itself. Patients are encouraged to face their feeling without resorting to defense and to compare this new experience with that which they had previously mistaken for the feeling.

This step-by-step approach is more horizontal than vertical. The process moves from example to example in the patient's current life orbit and then expands to include the therapist. There is no attempt to break through to the unconscious and expose the genetic links at this juncture, as there would be in the standard technique. Each small breakthrough of feeling into conscious awareness is highlighted and compared with past examples. This process is one of consolidation in which these distinctions become increasingly clear to the patient. The therapist continually looks for direct evidence that the patient can now experience anxiety-provoking affects without resorting to regressive defenses.

Similarities to Systematic Desensitization

This carefully graded approach to the experience of affects that have been avoided in the past is quite similar to the kind of graded exposure used in the process of systematic desensitization. The difference lies in the stimuli that are being targeted. In behavioral treatment, feared external stimuli are gradually approached. Here, the focus is on the gradual exposure to the internal experience of internal feelings. Such exposure is designed to reduce the anxiety that's been associated with these emotions, thus reducing the tendency to automatically avoid or defend against them. Once the feared stimulus—in this case the experience of angry feelings or impulses—is approached and experienced without the feared consequences coming to pass, the patient's perceptions change. In fact, the direct experience of feelings that had previously been avoided constitutes an experience of mastery. This is typically followed by a deep sense of relief, a new understanding of oneself, and a feeling of closeness with the therapist, all of which are profoundly reinforcing.

Goals of Restructuring

To summarize, the goals of restructuring include:

1 Undoing regressive defenses.

2 Re-directing the pathway of impulse and feeling into consciousness.

3 Building the patient's ego-adaptive capacity so that these feelings and impulses can be experienced directly.

To achieve this, a phase of cognitive re-analysis of the process must precede the breakthrough of feeling. This incremental process begins with a low level of intensity that is steadily increased until the patient indicates a tolerance for the direct experience of affect. Each round of work is followed by systematic re-analysis, leading to consolidation of insight within the session. Ultimately, direct experience of the complex transference feelings is achieved.

To return to the present clinical example, this repetitive work on the triangle of conflict in the current situation with the Gynecologist was required to consolidate the insights already obtained. This phase of the work was perused until the patient provided clear evidence that she understood the link between repressed impulses and symptoms and indicated a desire to give up these defenses. The statement that she now sees her defenses as self-defeating was followed by several other examples which indicated real insight on the patient's part and not mere compliance. She also signaled that she was ready to approach the feelings being evoked in the transference by saying that she "doesn't like to hear it".

Triangle of Conflict in the Transference

THERAPIST: What is your feeling toward me, as I point this out to you?

PATIENT: I know the answer should be "I don't like you" but . . .

THERAPIST: "I don't like you" isn't a feeling.

PATIENT: Anger. I guess I feel annoyed.

THERAPIST: How do you feel that inside?

PATIENT: Kind of a tightening—wanting to rip tissues.

THERAPIST: There's a mix of anger and anxiety. You want to discharge it by ripping the tissue, but the feeling is toward me.

PATIENT: Right.

THERAPIST: What's going to happen if we skip over this?

PATIENT: I'll stuff the feelings, I won't trust you, I'll cry a lot and be manipulative.

THERAPIST: So what effect would that have?

PATIENT: But people don't like the anger.

THERAPIST: You have a terrific problem with your anger, and you come to me for help with that. Don't you want to see if I'm capable of helping you with it?

PATIENT: I don't think we should avoid it, but it won't be easy.

THERAPIST: Who said it would be easy? How do you feel this anger toward me, if you don't look away?

PATIENT: Feels like a growing pressure pushing up (motions with her hands).

THERAPIST: And if that came out toward me, in your mind, what would that be like?

PATIENT: It would be ugly and show all this bad stuff I have inside.

THERAPIST: What do you feel like doing?

PATIENT: Be sarcastic, imitate you, be prissy, just be mean.

THERAPIST: To be mean is to put it into behavior. How would you declare this anger?

PATIENT: (voice raised) Stop pigeon-holing me.

THERAPIST: You're pleading. That isn't declaring your anger toward me. Do you see that your arms and legs are going?

PATIENT: A lot of power.

THERAPIST: What's the impulse in your hands?

PATIENT: It's growing. Like strangulation, if I let it go. Get off your high horse, leave me alone, let me be. You don't know me. (The patient is deeply involved in the emotion and is motorically activated, making strangling motions as she speaks.)

THERAPIST: With this anger is an impulse to strangle me and shut me up. What happens to me?

PATIENT: ou'd go "Ahhhhhh" and faint.

THERAPIST: Faint?

PATIENT: Or pass out and then I'd get scared and try to revive you. I'm getting dizzy; it's like it's happening to me.

Techniques to Lower Anxiety

Every attempt is made to engage patients in the process of treatment at their highest level of capacity. If no anxiety is being experienced, there will be no therapeutic movement. On the other hand, if the anxiety getting aroused by a focus on affect becomes too high, patients cannot process what is being experienced. In fact, if patients become overwhelmed by anxiety, they may resort to highly regressive defenses such as projection, which will have a corrosive effect on the treatment process. Therefore, it is essential to be familiar with fairly simple and direct techniques to rapidly reduce anxiety and prevent the mobilization of regressive defenses.

There are three direct methods for lowering anxiety: (a) switch the focus to an exploration of the physiological manifestations of anxiety; (b) return to phenomenological inquiry; or (c) switch focus on the triangle of person; for example, from the transference to a figure in the patient's current life. Once the patient's anxiety has been lowered to a tolerable degree, a cognitive re-analysis of what has occurred is necessary before returning to the feeling in question.

This is a crucial point in the therapeutic interaction. The patient in our example was beginning to experience directly the intense rage she had always avoided. When the impulse to strangle the therapist began to break through the repressive barrier, there was a sudden and intense spike in anxiety with an instantaneous internalization of the impulse. This had to be analyzed immediately, in order to interrupt the defense and consolidate the insight into the link between the repressed impulse and the symptoms. In this case, the link between the repressed impulse and the symptom was very specific; she did to herself what she wanted to do to me. Once this crucial insight had been achieved, it was essential to return to the moment of the surge in anxiety to see clearly what was previously too frightening to comprehend.

T-P Link

THERAPIST: Exactly. This is it, right here. You do to yourself what you want to do to me. (Patient nods.) You barely let yourself experience this impulse to strangle me before you internalize it, and then you're the one who is dizzy.

PATIENT: And I feel all choked up (puts her hands to her throat).

THERAPIST: What happened is, you've been working really hard, and you begin to let yourself free to experience this anger toward me. You got further than you've probably ever gotten before (patient says "yes") and got to the point of getting in touch with an impulse to strangle me, but there's something about that which is so threatening, so terrifying, that you get flooded with anxiety. In an instant, that impulse is redirected from me to you—you get dizzy and choked up. It makes me wonder what happened at that moment when you got in touch with the impulse. I wonder if someone else came to your mind?

PATIENT: Yeah, my mother.

Several rounds of work on the triangle of conflict in a number of current relationships have resulted in an increase in the patient's capacity to face her true feelings without resorting to regressive weepiness and helplessness. This done, feelings in the transference were approached. There was a sudden surge of anxiety as the repressed impulse came into consciousness. After lowering the patient's anxiety to a tolerable level, cognitive re-analysis of the process solidified the insight into the link between the repressed impulse and the self-attack. Following the breakthrough of sadistic rage toward the therapist, a direct link was made with the generic figure that she had come to represent. Then, feelings of guilt, grief, and longing emerged.

De-Repression of Feelings and Memories from the Past

PATIENT: Yes, my mother (starts to cry), when she was younger and prettier. She choked me and I felt helpless. Anytime I'd express anger . . .

THERAPIST: Do you have a memory?

PATIENT: Being enraged and wanting to choke her when she was choking me.

THERAPIST: This actually happened?

PATIENT: I was 12 and she was 36 and pretty but she was livid, enraged, with hate-filled eyes, like she wanted to kill me. And I wanted to kill her, but I couldn't raise a hand—father was outside the door. She had me by the throat and was knocking my head against the tiles.

THERAPIST: She did literally?

PATIENT: Yeah, and calling me names and saying I was bad, ruining her life and driving her crazy.

THERAPIST: So your mother would completely lose control.

PATIENT: Usually she would tell my father and he would take out his belt, but sometimes she would be physically abusive herself.

THERAPIST: Here's a situation where she's out of control. You are feeling both terrified and enraged. If that rage came out?

PATIENT: I'd be punished, get it four-fold.

THERAPIST: But even now, you punish yourself. The feeling is toward her. Can we look at that or are you dizzy?

PATIENT: No, I'm OK.

THERAPIST: In your mind, if you had taken over?

PATIENT: I would have smashed her against the medicine cabinet window and watch her bleed.

THERAPIST: Her head smashes on the glass?

PATIENT: Glass shatters, her head bleeds.

THERAPIST: That kills her?

PATIENT: No, it wouldn't. I'd take a piece of glass and drive it into her heart (makes stabbing motion).

THERAPIST: In her heart?

PATIENT: Make her bleed. In a pool of blood on the floor.

THERAPIST: What do you feel toward her when you see her dead on the floor?

PATIENT: OK—still feel hatred and some relief.

The patient was able to experience rage toward her mother directly, but avoided the complex feelings of guilt and grief. It is essential that all of the complex, mixed feelings toward others be directly experienced, lest the defenses against them, and their attendant symptoms, return. The therapist must be persistent in order to achieve this goal. Here, it was accomplished by returning to the scene and intensifying emotional involvement by looking closely at her mother's face (use of visualization).

THERAPIST: Initially relief. What does her face look like?
PATIENT: It's soft, soft and blank, her eyes are rolled up, she's powerless (becomes teary).
THERAPIST: It looks like there's feeling there.
PATIENT: All the anger had gone out of her, drained. Then I'd want her back some other way (deep sobbing) . . . See, being brutalized by my mother, it didn't start that way. I loved her so much when I was little. She was gorgeous and had a beautiful voice. She would sing me lullabies and read me stories. I want her back that way—soft and cuddly and warm.
THERAPIST: So beneath the anger toward her, there is tremendous grief about the loss of closeness with her. There's also tremendous love for her.
PATIENT: Yes, I thought she must be good, and I was bad.
THERAPIST: How did this happen?
PATIENT: My sister was born when I was three-and-a-half.

The origins of the patient's core conflict were revealed following the experience of complex, mixed feelings toward her mother. The patient's mother was not always an angry, hostile person, as the patient had initially described her. It was only once she got in touch with the rageful feelings and murderous impulses toward her mother that the underlying pain and grief about love lost could be experienced. While the patient initially described her mother in wholly negative terms, a more complex and nuanced picture emerged following the breakthrough. This underscores the importance of waiting until this junction to obtain an accurate developmental history.

The restructuring in this case was largely completed within the three-hour initial evaluation. Because we were able to achieve a breakthrough of feeling in the transference, with an outpouring of memories from the past, the patient's core neurotic structure was readily exposed. She proved highly responsive to these interventions and left the evaluation feeling tired, but relieved and hopeful. Treatment was completed in two 12-session blocks. The first segment of treatment focused on the current crisis. After a six-month break, the patient came back to therapy to work on the relationships with her parents and children. Of significance, she re-engaged with her estranged parents, and was both surprised and delighted by their responses to the changes in her. The rupture between them was repaired and healing took place.

Restructuring with Patients Suffering from Functional Disorders

As in the case of depressives, patients who suffer from functional disorders display a marked inability to distinguish between the three corners of the triangle of conflict. Physical symptoms function as a defense against the awareness and experiences of anxiety-laden feelings. There is frequently a direct, one-to-one correspondence between the repressed sadistic impulse and the specific symptom the patient experiences. As such, the symptom contains both expressive and defensive elements. The symptom expresses the impulse while simultaneously disguising the aim through displacement. In addition, suffering what was wished on the other serves as a punishment for the disguised act of sadism. Great economy is involved in such symptom formation.

Clinical Example

The Woman with Headaches

This single woman in her mid-30s entered treatment because she was unable to decide whether to marry her current beau. Inquiry revealed a history of anxiety, depression, and headaches going back to childhood. The patient's mother was seriously ill throughout her childhood, was frequently hospitalized, and almost died on several occasions. Her father was a brutal man who beat both his wife and children. The patient and her older brother seemed to bear the brunt of her father's uncontrollable rage.

Course of Treatment

The patient presented a whole host of intellectualizing defenses. Isolation of affect was especially prominent. She was intelligent and insightful, but almost completely shut down on an emotional level, which contributed significantly to the difficulties with her boyfriend. In fact, at times of extreme stress she fell into fugue states that lasted days. She also reported a history of severe migraine headaches that started when she was eight years old and required hospitalization on a number of occasions. Both her headaches and severe, systemic shut down were the result of instant repression of rage, which required restructuring to reverse. In the following session, the patient came in complaining of a headache that, as she described it, "is killing me".

Exploration of the Symptom and Its Trigger

PATIENT: I don't know what to talk about today. It's been a non-week. I've had a headache all week which is killing me right now.

THERAPIST: You mentioned the last time that you haven't had headaches for some time now (since therapy had begun, some two months earlier).

PATIENT: But this one has been for two weeks now. I'm not sure why.

THERAPIST: Could you describe what it feels like?

PATIENT: Behind my eyes. I've been diagnosed with ocular migraines, although the Neurologist couldn't confirm that. There's throbbing from my eyes to temples, a pounding that even wakes me up at night. It can even hit my stomach with vomiting (the patient is squinting and appears to be in considerable pain).

THERAPIST: When did it start?

PATIENT: I've had headaches since I was a child.

THERAPIST: But this particular one?

PATIENT: About two weeks.

THERAPIST: What was going on then?

PATIENT: I went home to visit, and I had it when I came back.

THERAPIST: So you got it when you were down there, visiting your family?

PATIENT: I didn't really want to go. I was there to see my mother but I was really angry with my father. He was tense. I was too. I had to run around and visit all the relatives (sighs). I couldn't relax. And my big brother, at dinnertime (smiles)—I could just smack their heads together. I think I've told you how my mother turns on the radio at dinner so she doesn't have to listen to silence. Then my brother or father starts to complain about it. I turned it off. There was tremendous tension. My father is glaring at my brother with complete hatred because he's eating too much and my father resents him living at home.

THERAPIST: You're telling me this story, but you seem very emotionally detached. What was it like for you sitting at the table?

PATIENT: I was angry (I/F), I get tense (A). It's like an automatic response when I go back there—angry and tense.

Inquiry Into the Situation Surrounding the Symptom

The patient entered the session complaining about a painful and intransigent headache. Exploration of the precipitant to this symptom provided clear clues regarding the underlying feelings and impulses involved. The patient recalled going to her childhood home for a recent visit, in which vicious anger toward her father was triggered. However, there was no indication that she was actually in touch with the experience of the anger. In fact, responses to intervention suggested a clear pattern in which her rage toward him was instantly turned back upon the self. It was also clear from the previous vignette that she was not able to differentiate between the experience of anger and that of the anxiety it induced. The patient described increasing tension as her anger mounted, which culminated in a massive tension headache. This lack of differentiation within the triangle of conflict required clarification.

THERAPIST: So there's a tremendous anger and then tension. Do you think the tension is from trying to keep the anger in check?

PATIENT: Yeah, because I just want to flail my arms and send the plates flying.

The distinction between the anger and the tension, with an emphasis on how the tension is designed to rein in the anger, had the effect of loosening its grip and the patient became animated and involved in the process. Her voice, which had been very soft and slow up until this point, became suffused with energy. However, there was still evidence of defensive displacement, as the patient talked about wanting to throw plates, when she had already declared she wanted to smash heads.

THERAPIST: But you had said, "Smash their heads together". Whose?

PATIENT: My brother—he's manipulative—and my father. My father hates him but I blame my father.

THERAPIST: So let's look at it, what's the impulse as you sat at the table, viewing all this?

PATIENT: I want to push the table away and them away. I feel trapped by the table.

Linking the Symptoms with Repressed Feelings

It is essential that all three components of affective experience (cognitive, physiological, and motoric) be clearly in evidence before proceeding to pressure and challenge. At the start of the session, the patient was able to cognitively label her feeling toward her father (anger), but she was completely detached from the physiological and motoric aspects of the feeling. These elements were instantly internalized, with a headache and depression the result. As she began to get in touch with the physiological experience of anger and the aggressive impulses they mobilized, she started to lose the cognitive focus—in that the anger was getting displaced from her father onto inanimate objects. She was clearer about *what* she felt and *how* she felt it but lost sight of *who* she felt this rage toward. All three elements needed to be present simultaneously for the patient to be considered in touch with the experience of her feelings. In addition, evidence of all three elements of feeling is a pre-requisite to moving onto the phase of increased pressure and challenge.

Internalization is really just one aspect of displacement in which the rage toward another is displaced onto the self. Given depressives' reliance on the defense of displacement, it is not unusual to find that they also have episodes of explosive temper tantrums in which they displace rage from the actual target to an inanimate object or less threatening figure. All elements of displacement must be removed so that the patient can have a full and direct experience of their rage.

THERAPIST: So you want to push the table away and then?

PATIENT: My father is glaring at my brother. His table manners are horrible and he eats like a baby, but so what? Big deal. My father is glaring at him . . .

THERAPIST: And the feeling inside you?

PATIENT: Hatred toward my father and disgust with my brother.

THERAPIST: How do you feel that inside?

PATIENT: With my father, it's just this cold . . . I'm so disgusted I just want to push him and smack him.

THERAPIST: But you go cold?

PATIENT: It feels like a cold hatred. If icicles could come out of my eyes and pierce, I would give it to him that way.

THERAPIST: How?

PATIENT: I would send daggers out to pierce him, make puncture wounds.

THERAPIST: Where?

PATIENT: I don't know, now my eyes hurt (patient hangs her head and rubs her eyes).

Reemergence of the Symptom

Throughout the process of restructuring, the therapist must vigilantly monitor for any signs of undue anxiety or an increase in symptoms will result. In the previous sequence, the use of the word "cold" to describe her intense hatred toward her father, and the slow quiet manner in which she was relating to me, suggested that she was detached from the actual experience of anger. The crucial question here is, where does that go? Since the patient had experienced several episodes in which she was curled up in a fetal position and unable to get out of bed for days, it was of the utmost importance to block the mechanism in which her red-hot rage turned to cold, frozen immobility.

In this case, having the symptoms of head and eye pain appear during the session was both good news and bad news. The re-emergence of the symptom at that moment suggested that the impulse had intensified and was threatening to break through into consciousness. That was the good news. The upsurge of feeling was experienced as dangerous, so the defenses which were driving the symptoms came marching back with a vengeance. Left unchecked, that would certainly be the bad news. The mechanism of internalization had to be undone to prevent any further exacerbation in symptoms. Reducing the patient's reliance on this defense would also increase the functioning of the ego so that she would be able to tolerate the direct experience of rage. To accomplish this, insight into the link between the repressed impulse (to pierce and wound her father) and her symptoms (piercing pain in her eyes) had to be reinforced.

THERAPIST: See, isn't that what happens? Do you see this connection? Inside, there is this terrific rage toward your father with an impulse to pierce him and wound him, but you keep it inside and you get it—you suffer the very thing you wished on him—the piercing in your eyes. There is a one-to-one connection. You want to smash their heads, but you get the headache. You want to pierce and puncture him, but you get the stabbing pain in your eyes.

PATIENT: I didn't even think of that.

THERAPIST: Do you see it now?

PATIENT: Yeah. We're talking about heads and eyes and that's what's hurting.

THERAPIST: So you end up experiencing the pain you wanted him to feel.

PATIENT: But I don't know why.

The patient's attention, curiosity, and desire to understand herself were evident. She was making direct eye contact with the therapist, and the alliance felt strong. Rather than respond directly to her query about why she would internalize this pain or make an interpretation about it, I continued to explore with her what would happen if she directly expressed the impulse. The information to emerge would allow the patient to answer her own question.

THERAPIST: Let's look at what you imagine would happen if it came out toward *him*.

PATIENT: I'd smash him. I'd go for my father, smash him in the face.

THERAPIST: Do you feel the anger inside or are you still cold?

PATIENT: Inside, I feel my muscles tense. This is funny, this always happens, I go cold.

THERAPIST: At one time, it was all you could do; you were a child.

PATIENT: I was trying to survive.

THERAPIST: But now, shutting down and going cold doesn't help you survive, it leads to suffering. Now the enemy is inside. You keep yourself trapped in the suffering.

PATIENT: I keep trying to picture it, but it doesn't go anywhere.

THERAPIST: The feelings drive the picture, and you don't let yourself feel it. This has been inside you for 35 years. As much as it costs you, you're terrified to experience this rage.

Cost–Benefit Analysis of the Defense of Internalization

The preceding interventions were aimed at turning the patient's ego against these highly syntonic character defenses. It was acknowledged that these defenses may have helped her at one time but were presently outmoded and self-destructive. Focusing on the cost of the defenses will help turn her against them.

PATIENT: To really face it, I'd have to let it go. Maybe I could if I felt better.

THERAPIST: But the two are intimately connected. Only by feeling it emotionally will the symptoms be relieved, because you turn an emotional pain into a physical one.

PATIENT: I used to scream at the top of my lungs. Last week, I beat up the car because I was so angry. It was a rage.

Again, there is evidence of both an increase in the patient's ability to get in touch with the experience of her rage (as evidenced by a rise in her voice, sitting up in her chair, and an angry look in her face) and of displacement from her father onto the car. Now that the feelings and impulses were mobilized, the therapist continued to proceed with a pressure to connect with the experience of her rage.

THERAPIST: The rage was toward your father?

PATIENT: Yes. I wanted to kill him, wanted to kill him.

THERAPIST: Now you feel it *and* can imagine it? It was *him* you wanted to beat and kill?

PATIENT: Yes. I want to face the rage toward him, but there's a loop inside my head and it keeps derailing and I run in a circle. I can almost see it in my head, getting away.

The cyclical process involved in restructuring is quite evident in this transcript. We were making incremental steps toward the full experience of the warded-off feelings and impulses. The loop was getting progressively smaller and the diversions fewer and fewer as we progressed in the hour.

THERAPIST: What would happen if you let out toward him all that rage that came out toward the car?

PATIENT: I would lose. He's stronger than me. When I was 14, I started to fight back but he would overpower me, then lock me in the bathroom. If my mother was around, I felt I had to protect her because if she tried to intervene, he would go after her. As a child, it was unbearable. I would rather be beat up, otherwise I would feel it was my fault, that I caused her to get hurt.

Although the emergence of this new material certainly shed light on the very real predicament she had faced as a child, at that moment in the session it served as a diversion from the anxiety she was feeling about facing her own rage now. Rather than getting caught up in a discussion about the past, focus was maintained on the current feeling welling up in her and the defenses against it.

THERAPIST: So you wouldn't just want to provoke him. You said you'd kill him.

PATIENT: What entered my mind was a knife. I can't watch movies with knives, anything entering people.

THERAPIST: Like the daggers.

PATIENT: I never thought of that, but yeah. I'm seeing it in the kitchen again, there are knives in the kitchen. I could plunge it into him, in his chest, over and over, in a frenzy, with lots of strength. It would even get stuck sometimes (making stabbing motions), it's that deep. It's my Tazmanian devil, I'd go berserk. Then he can't fight back. He's on the floor, white as a ghost, blood all over. I'm sweaty, that's how much energy, like running 30 miles. I can see him on the floor, all bloody, but I don't care. I almost want to see him get up again so I could do it again.

THERAPIST: You don't want him to die so soon.

PATIENT: Yeah, I want to torture him.

THERAPIST: Let him see what it was like.

PATIENT: Well, he knows because his father tried to kill him a few times. He was an alcoholic. He set the house on fire once with all the little kids inside. He tried to throw him out an apartment window when he was 18 and had joined the service. My father won't talk about it, but once I said to him, "You're doing what Grandpa did to you".

Davanloo (personal communication, August 1990) has suggested that there is a direct relationship between the severity of the suffering involved in the symptom and the severity of the sadistic impulse being repressed. In this case, the sadistic rage the patient has felt toward her father was enormous and was a direct response to his brutal attacks on the patient herself, her siblings, and her mother. Killing him didn't seem like enough. Very often, in cases where patients have been severely abused, their reactive rage takes on the form of an impulse to torture. There is often a desire to respond in kind with the same mal-treatment they suffered.

In this case, when the impulses came into consciousness, a deep feeling of sadness over all the damage done emerged. Although there was relief in facing the reactive sadism, there was no satisfaction in it. In fact, the patient began to experience some empathy for her father's pain. This empathy should not be confused with forgiveness. The patient still has a great deal of anger toward her father for the very real pain and damage he inflicted. However, these feelings were now conscious and integrated with feelings of sadness. After these conflicted feelings were summarized, the therapist inquired about the patient's headache. She smiled and said, "Isn't that funny—it's gone away". The fact that a headache, which had persisted for two weeks and proved intractable to medication, should lift within the hour that her repressed feelings of rage toward her father were faced directly, seems to provide compelling evidence for the psychodynamic factors implicated in symptom formation.

Summary

The process of restructuring in patients with regressive defenses, such as depression and somatic complaints, has been outlined and illustrated. Patients who rely on regressive defenses—including depression, panic disorder, and functional disorders—demonstrate a deep-seated inability to distinguish between feelings and the defenses against them. Consequently, a significant rise in feeling is accompanied by increases in regressive symptomatology. Therefore, any strategy designed to intensify affect would be clearly contra-indicated. Davanloo has developed a method for restructuring defenses in these cases. This circular process builds the ego in order to increase the patient's tolerance for the direct experience of feelings and the unconscious material associated with these feelings. Patients must be able to link their symptoms to the feelings and impulses being repressed before any further uncovering can occur.

Detailed clinical examples were given to illustrate this important innovation, making ISTDP possible with patients who had previously been considered unsuitable for most forms of short-term dynamic psychotherapy. It should be noted, however, that in cases such as The Woman with Headaches, treatment often takes 40 sessions.

5 DEEPENING ACCESS TO AFFECT

> It's a necessary condition of human
> health to be able to bear what has
> to be borne, to be able to think
> what has to be thought.
>
> *Semrad (Rako & Mazer, 1980)*[1]

Patients come to us because they are suffering and want to get well. In order to heal, they must experience the thoughts and feelings previously considered unbearable and unutterable. That which has been buried in the shadows must come to light. The process through which previously inaccessible feelings, memories, and ideas are de-repressed and made available for re-working will be the focus of the next few chapters.

In this chapter a process designed to facilitate the experience of grief-laden feelings will be elucidated.

The Centrality of Affect

Wachtel (1993) succinctly summarized the psychodynamic view of the cause and cure of neurotic suffering when he wrote:

> The patient's problems are understood as deriving most fundamentally from his having learned early in life to be afraid of his feelings, thoughts, and

DOI: 10.4324/9781003542131-5

> inclinations, and the effort to help him overcome his problems is focused very largely on helping him reappropriate those feelings and incorporate them into a fuller and richer sense of self and of life's possibilities.
>
> (Wachtel, 1993, p. 32)

While most in the psychodynamic community would agree with this statement, the methods for achieving this goal vary considerably from therapist to therapist.

Davanloo (1990) adopted an uncompromising stance on the central importance of affect in intensifying and accelerating the process of dynamic psychotherapy. Emotion is the lifeblood of existence and the fuel of all our endeavors. For those patients who repress their feelings, life becomes a sterile and mechanical exercise. In addition to the deadening of inner life that accompanies extensive repression of emotion, repression keeps patients blind to the source of their pain and prevents resolution of the underlying problem. Therefore, Davanloo (1990) advocated tenacious work on the defensive (repressive) barrier to achieve a breakthrough of feelings into consciousness. Once the feelings penetrate the repressive barrier, all the memories and traumas associated with them flow freely. This process provides the affectively charged material required to make meaningful interpretations about the repetitive dynamics operating in the patient's current life, in the interactions with the therapist, and in the past with significant others.

The Phenomenon of De-Repression

The outpouring of unconscious material from the past, following an emotionally charged reliving of recent events within a therapy session, has been referred to as "de-repression" (an alternative to the phrase "undoing of repression" used by Freud in 1917). This process, also referred to as "uncovering", seems to be facilitated by the patient's affectively charged involvement in the therapeutic process. "Since in most instances, anxiety is most strongly attached to a complex configuration of cues in which verbal, affective, cognitive, and motoric elements are prominent, verbalizing without the other cues being present is unlikely to have much therapeutic value" (Wachtel, 1977, p. 94). Davanloo's technique of applying pressure to the defenses, and challenging the patient to be affectively, cognitively, and motorically involved in the process seems to effectively achieve this end.

There is some agreement in the psychodynamic community (Alexander & French, 1946; Ferenczi & Rank, 1925; Gill, 1982; Strupp & Binder, 1984) that the most rapid and accurate route to the core conflicts underlying patients' symptoms and complaints is achieved through a focused examination of the patient's *current* affective experience. This is contrasted with an approach that begins with a long and detailed history, only understanding the patient's current difficulties within this historical framework. To acquire historical data early on in treatment, when anxiety and defenses are high, could lead to a highly distorted picture of past events. For this, and other reasons already outlined, clinicians like Davanloo (1990) have championed the view that it is essential to bring the patient's current experience, especially that with the therapist, into focus at the inception of treatment. Only those memories that surface as the current emotion is being experienced are deemed dynamically significant. This insight seems to get "discovered" and then forgotten repeatedly, as clinicians get caught up in a seemingly random search for memories about the past.

Ferenczi and Rank (1925) were the first clinical theorists to encourage an approach in which feelings and defenses currently in evidence are the focus of dynamic inquiry. Their work had little impact on mainstream psychoanalytic theory and practice at the time. Years later, Alexander and French (1946) expanded on this early work, re-emphasizing that a focus on contemporary experience, particularly in the transference, provides the most powerful tool for achieving rapid therapeutic change. More recently, Strupp and Binder (1984) have concluded that examination of the transference is a beacon linking the current dynamics to unresolved conflicts from the past. The treatment model being delineated here shares this view and endeavors to work in the present, only making links to the past as they emerge spontaneously from the contemporary experience of affect.

Research Support

In addition to the accumulating clinical evidence (Been & Sklar, 1985; Strupp & Binder, 1984) that the most rapid and effective route for obtaining access to the unconscious is through the direct experience of affect, empirical data on state-dependent learning also supports this hypothesis (Bower, 1981; Della Selva, 1991). State-dependent learning refers to the fact that subjects are most likely to retrieve a memory when in the same affective state as when the memory was encoded. Therefore, anything we can do to help patients experience their feelings as fully as possible should speed the process of memory retrieval. Once these memories become conscious, patients have a fresh opportunity to understand what has happened to them and how these recalled events have affected them throughout life.

Research on memory reconsolidation confirms this hypothesis. These findings suggest that, when long-forgotten memories are retrieved, they remain in a labile state for a short period of time, allowing them to be reconsidered and altered. This modified memory is then stored in a revised form. In this way, changes taking place in a focused and emotionally-charged therapy session can lead to permanent change (Ecker, Ticic, & Hulley, 2012).

Other empirical evidence supports the notion that emotional involvement in the therapeutic process enhances outcome. Some research has discovered a correlation between a rise in the complex transference feelings and an unlocking of the unconscious, with both symptom and cost reduction the result (Town, Abbass, & Bernier, 2013).

Integrating Cognitive and Affective Modes of Experience

As important as the free and unencumbered experience of affect is for the process of psychotherapy (as well as for life itself), this is not an end in and of itself. Rather, affective activation is an effective means for gaining rapid access to the unconscious conflicts responsible for the patient's difficulties. Once these conflicts come alive within the session, they can be dealt with directly. An examination of the transference pattern of behavior provides a pathway for achieving deep cognitive understanding of emotionally-felt experiences, a vital combination in facilitating rapid therapeutic change.

Those therapies based almost solely on the expression of affect (Janov, 1970) often ignore the vital role of defensive processes, irrational beliefs, and perceptual distortions of self and other that accompany these feeling. Other, more cognitively-based therapies, often give short shrift to the role of emotions in psychotherapy. That said, Aaron Beck (1976), the father of cognitive therapy, has acknowledged the vital role of affective involvement for successful outcome. Beck was a psychoanalyst who, like Davanloo, was frustrated by the lengthy course of analysis and variable outcomes. He set about to discover ways to enhance effectiveness and did so by identifying dysfunctional thoughts and beliefs that caused the patient grief. He added this type of intervention to his existing analytic understanding, while subsequent generations have focused more narrowly on "challenging distorted beliefs". As a result, the effectiveness of cognitive behavioral therapy (CBT) has decreased steadily over the past 40 years (Johnsen & Friborg, 2015; Wampold, et al, 2016).

According to Strupp and Binder (1984), who have conducted years of research on short-term dynamic psychotherapy (STDP), the key to therapeutic change is "conceived of as the affective experiencing and cognitive understanding of current maladaptive patterns of behavior that repeat childhood patterns of interpersonal conflict" (pp. 24–25). This is the essence of what Malan and Osimo (1992) have referred to as the T-C-P link. Their research, as well as that of others (Trujillo & McCullough, 1985), investigating the effectiveness of STDP, has generated data corroborating the hypothesis that successful outcome is highly correlated with the frequency of affectively meaningful T-C-P links.

There is a rather wide consensus in both the clinical and research literature that the most effective and efficient method for the facilitation of deep change is a two-pronged approach: (a) mobilize intense affect; and (b) examine the thoughts, memories, and beliefs associated with these feelings as they emerge through the affect-laden communications from patient to therapist (Ecker, et al. 2012). As affect is experienced and memories surface, the perceptual distortions of self and other that accompany them become available for reworking. Again, many forms of therapy seem to focus on one of these factors, to the relative neglect of the other. A large part of the power and grace inherent in the systems of short term dynamic psychotherapy (STDP) developed by clinicians like Malan (1976b; 1979), Malan and Osimo (1992) and Davanloo (1978; 1980; 1990) can be attributed to the ways in which the cognitive and affective spheres of experience are integrated and interwoven within each session.

Techniques for Activating and Deepening Affect

There is accumulating clinical and empirical evidence that creating an emotionally charged atmosphere in the treatment setting is a rapid and reliable route for facilitating therapeutic movement. Short-term dynamic therapists have developed a whole host of tools and techniques for achieving this goal. These include: (a) focusing on detail and specificity; (b) using imagery; (c) dealing with defenses to remove barriers that may block the activation and expression of affect; (d) acquainting the patient with the physical sensations accompanying affect; and (e) providing therapist empathy. Each of these techniques will be briefly described.

Although all these techniques are useful at times, specificity on the therapist's part is equally important for a successful outcome. In other words, examining feelings in general is of little therapeutic value. We must examine specific feelings toward specific people in specific examples to work in a therapeutic manner. For some patients, focus and specificity is sufficient to evoke strong feelings. For others, defenses prevent this kind of emotional activation and must be confronted. Finally, some patients are so out of touch with their feelings that they require an introduction to emotion; a process that is roughly parallel to the process of acquainting patients with their defenses. In these cases, a focus on feelings and sensations in the patients' body is the place to begin.

Focusing on Detail and Specificity

The Intense Short-Term Dynamic Psychotherapy (ISTDP) therapist conducts a tightly focused interview in which patients are expected to be quite specific about the people and events being discussed. The therapist is actively involved in a dialogue with the patient from the outset and asks clarifying questions when indicated. Any vagueness is challenged. If the patient speaks in generalities, the therapist asks for recent and specific examples of the issue being discussed. This procedure facilitates recall and tends to increase affective involvement in the process, both considered necessary ingredients for intensifying and accelerating the therapeutic process. Recent research (Bucci, 1985; Geiselman, Fisher, MacKinnon, & Holland, 1985) strongly confirms the notion that memory retrieval is enhanced by a tight focus on specific and concrete details.

Using Imagery

One technique for enhancing and intensifying affect is the active use of imagery. This technique is equally useful for facilitating the recall of emotional significant memories and for the expression of previously repressed feelings. Davanloo refers to this technique as "portraiting". The patient is asked to "paint a picture" of the memory or impulse being discussed. This frequently includes: (a) physical and temporal details; (b) the thoughts and feelings experienced by all the central characters in the memory or fantasy; and (c) the sequence of events. This technique provides an avenue for experiencing and re-living events in an emotionally meaningful way, without resorting to repression or acting on the feelings and impulses involved.

Encouraging patients to immerse themselves as fully as possible in their own experience provides an emotionally powerful tool for the reworking of traumatic situations from the past. In addition, a focus on the sights, sounds, smells, and sensations associated with a particular feeling seems to aid the integration of the experiencing and observing functions of the ego.

The case of the Woman on an Emotional Roller Coaster (see Chapter 4) provided a good example of this process. It was the breakthrough of complex transference feelings, achieved through a portrait of the patient's hostile impulses toward the therapist, that ushered in long repressed memories of these same mixed feelings toward her mother. The memory of an especially traumatic incident, accompanied by all the terrifying feelings and impulses involved, came rushing to the fore clearly and dramatically as the patient was asked to portray her angry impulse toward the therapist. This provided the patient with a new opportunity, as an adult, to deal directly with a situation that had been too overwhelming to deal with as a child. In addition, this revelation made clear what the central dynamic forces have been in her life. Then it became possible to work on the central conflict directly, at the source, eliminating the need to unconsciously recreate the situation with her husband, daughter, therapist, and friends. This method of rapid uncovering greatly reduces the likelihood of acting out and further repetition and speeds the process of working through.

Dealing with Defense Before Feeling

Rather than "fishing for feelings" in those patients who defend against the experience of affect, Davanloo (1990) advocated a focus on the defenses first. This preliminary work is designed to render the patient's defenses dystonic, to mobilize intense and complex mixed feelings toward the therapist, to facilitate the direct experience of these feelings, and, in so doing, promote the development of a full partnership in the therapeutic process.

Anger is often the first layer of feeling to surface. It is important to emphasize that, in practice, dealing with defenses against anger is rarely sufficient to expose the complex system of mixed feelings toward significant others. On occasion, the experience of previously repressed rage leads quite directly to the pain, grief, and longings for closeness that lie beneath it. More frequently, the therapist encounters defenses against the experience of guilt, grief, and longing as well. In fact, defenses against the painful feelings involved in mourning, and the bittersweet nature of tenderness and joy, can be quite tenacious and must be dealt with directly. Patients often want to revert to anger as a way of avoiding these other feelings. It is essential that the therapist follow the process and not get diverted by defensive anger at such times.

Again, the goal of this intensive treatment is to enable patients to fully experience all their mixed feelings toward others by increasing their capacity to bear them without resorting to splitting or other regressive defenses. The question is how this is accomplished.

Acquainting Patients with the Experience of Affect

For some patients, the aforementioned techniques prove insufficient to activate affect. If the patient's detachment is the result of defenses over a conflict, the techniques described tend to be successful at evoking strong feeling. What happens when there is a deficit of affective attunement and discrimination? When such patients say, "I don't know what I'm feeling", they may be making an accurate statement. As one patient said, "You keep asking me how I feel. How do I feel? I have no idea. I am not keeping anything from you, it's just that I have spent so much of my life ignoring and numbing myself to feeling that I don't know myself". In these cases, maintaining unrelenting pressure on defenses would be an error. Instead, the therapist should alert patients to subtle changes in their posture, tone of voice, and facial expression. In the case just described, the therapist noticed sadness in the patient's face as she talked about how little she feels. This was pointed out and was followed by an exploration of the bodily sensations that accompanied the dawning awareness of the emotion of grief. The patient noticed a slight heaviness in her chest. At the end of the session, the therapist suggested that she continue to notice her bodily sensations and use them as cues to what she was feeling. The patient found this very helpful. She began to "tune in" to her physical feelings and use them as information regarding the emotions involved.

Providing Therapist Empathy and Encouragement

Once the unconscious is accessible and communicating freely to the therapist, pressure and challenge to defenses are no longer required. In fact, such an approach would be contraindicated. Instead, maintenance of a focus on affect through gentle but firm encouragement, along with occasional interpretive links between past and present, will usually suffice to keep the work moving apace.

The techniques of pressure and challenge, so useful in the early stages of defense work when resistance in the transference is at its height, are not helpful once an alliance is in place and the unconscious is more freely available. At this stage, should defenses resurface, they can usually be brushed aside with relative ease, as the therapist has the unconscious therapeutic alliance to call on for assistance. For example, when resistance returned in the case of the Woman on an Emotional Roller Coaster, all that was needed to get her back on track was gentle encouragement ("You've been working really hard, let's not stop now") followed by a question about what else came to mind when the impulse to strangle the therapist came into consciousness.

The Unconscious Therapeutic Alliance

The breakthrough of feeling into consciousness seems to be the key in facilitating rapid de-repression. In addition to "unlocking the unconscious", this process solidifies what Davanloo (1987c) has referred to as "the unconscious therapeutic alliance". The unconscious therapeutic alliance (UTA) is just that—an alliance based on communication between the therapist and the patient's unconscious. The UTA is akin to an innate healing force that operates like an emotional immune system. Excessive reliance on defenses interferes with healing, while the process of relinquishing defenses and facing avoided feelings liberates the UTA and assists both patient and therapist on the path to healing. This alliance comes into operation once the resistance is in abeyance. According to Davanloo (1987c), these forces exist in inverse proportion to one another. When resistance is high, the unconscious therapeutic alliance is low and vice versa.

This type of alliance should be distinguished from a conscious therapeutic alliance (Greenson, 1967), which depends on patients' intellectual curiosity about themselves, as well as conscious positive feelings toward the therapist. Since negative transference feelings block the development of a conscious therapeutic alliance, traditional psychoanalysis is impossible in such cases. This is not necessarily so with ISTDP. If a patient enters treatment with negative transference feelings, they become the first order of business. All the patient's feelings toward the therapist are dealt with in a direct and straightforward manner from the inception of treatment. The ways in which the patient attempts to avoid the full experience of these feelings are addressed, until the resistance is broken through, and a genuine therapeutic alliance is created. Conducting a trial therapy is the only certain way to assess the patient's ability to establish both a conscious and unconscious alliance with the therapist. This alliance is the strongest weapon we have against the return of resistance and, hence, lends speed and clarity to the process.

Keeping the Therapeutic Goal in Mind

The goal of ISTDP, like that of all dynamically oriented treatments, is to gain access to the unconscious forces driving the patient's maladaptive behavior. Despite agreement on the goal, the therapeutic approach advocated here diverges significantly from a more traditional psychoanalytic approach. The therapist is active in questioning patients and encouraging them to have an honest look at the painful and anxiety-provoking feelings they typically avoid. In fact, any avoidance is noted and challenged. According to ISTDP, the spontaneous offering of memories, dreams, and associations are a signal to the therapist that the unconscious alliance is strong. Interpretations about the meaning of symptoms and behaviors can only meaningfully occur after the feelings involved have been directly experienced and the memories that surface on the heels of them come to light. This eliminates the need for the therapist to guess what the possible meaning of a defense or symptom might be, as the emotional truth is clearly revealed through the process of affective activation and de-repression. Patients frequently make their own interpretations at this point.

Grief Work

> I dreamed I was sad and sometimes cried. But through the tears and the melancholy, inspired by the music of the verse or the beauty of the evening, there always rose upwards, like the grasses of early spring, shoots of happy feeling . . .
>
> *William Trevor (1991, Two Lives, p. 84)*[2]

Thus far, the importance of achieving a high level of affective activation and involvement for the speed and effectiveness of dynamic psychotherapy has been reviewed.

In the following section, specific techniques for working with grief, and the defenses against it, will be examined and illustrated. As was demonstrated earlier, patients enter treatment in a state of ambivalence. They seek relief from suffering but dread facing the painful thoughts, feelings, and memories involved in the psychotherapeutic process. In ISTDP, the patient's defenses, which become a resistance in the treatment, are rapidly identified, clarified, and exhausted as the patient is encouraged to have an open and honest look at his or her emotional life. In many cases, the first emotion to surface is anger at the therapist for challenging and pressuring the patient to get actively involved and to face what has been vigorously avoided. In other cases, particularly those in which defenses against emotional closeness are prominent, grief over loss is the first emotion to surface. In most cases, the outpouring of grief is complex. There is grief for those who have been loved and lost, but there is also grief over the ensuing loss of freedom to re-attach. Patients become acutely sad over the lack of close relationships in their current life.

Many of the patients who seek psychotherapy, regardless of their initial presentation, complain of an inability to experience joy in their lives. As William Trevor (1991) suggested, in the quoted verse from the novella *Two Lives*, warded-off grief is often found beneath this lassitude. Unless the acutely painful feelings of grief and mourning are directly experienced, no joy or happiness is possible. As therapists, our job largely revolves around helping patients face pain and grief and to render the experience tolerable, reducing their need to resort to pathological defenses against these affects.

To design a therapeutic intervention that will aid the grieving process when it has been distorted or derailed, we must understand the natural course of mourning.

The Grief Process

Freud's Contribution

Freud was the first psychotherapist to discuss grief in clinical terms. In *Mourning and Melancholia* (Freud, 1917), he outlined four features characteristic of mourning the loss of a loved one: (a) a profoundly painful feeling of dejection; (b) an abrogation of interest in the outside world; (c) the loss of the capacity to love; and (d) inhibition of activity. The tasks involved in mourning include facing the harsh reality that the loved one is gone and then withdrawing "libidinal cathexis" from the deceased so that this emotional energy will be available for further attachments.

Freud has outlined the two areas of functioning—the cognitive and the affective—that must be addressed to complete the process of mourning. Exactly how to tackle these problems clinically was not addressed, however. What Freud did suggest was that the patient become conscious of every hope and memory "which bound the libido to the object" to achieve detachment from the deceased. Only then would the ego be free to attach again. It was assumed that a healthy individual should be able to complete the mourning process in a fairly rapid and complete fashion.

Subsequent theorists have suggested that these notions, based on drive theory and the hydraulic model, are out of keeping with the current evidence. For example, studies (Goin, Burgoyne, & Goin, 1979) of those who have successfully navigated the mourning process suggest that a strong attachment to the deceased is maintained over time. What distinguishes successful from pathological mourning is the nature of the attachment. In successful cases, attachment to the deceased is generally positive and provides a sense of unity and comfort. In contrast, in cases where the attachment to the deceased is hostile, highly ambivalent, or guilt-ridden, patients tend to do poorly. Still, the effects of loss are devastating in any case. There remains a tendency to "underestimate how intensely distressing and disabling loss is and for how long the distress, and often the disablement, commonly lasts" (Bowlby, 1980, p. 8). Bereavement can literally be fatal, with widowers being at particularly high risk (Jacobs & Ostfeld, 1977; Parkes, Benjamin, & Fitzgerald, 1969). In this sense, the feeling that one can't go on without the beloved has some basis in fact.

Lindemann's Work

Dr. Lindemann's pioneering work on grief, following the Coconut Grove fire in Boston, is widely heralded, yet his interest in adjustment to loss predated this event. In his work with patients suffering from ulcerative colitis, Lindemann (1945) discovered a clear link between the loss of a loved one and the onset of the disease. Of particular importance was the finding that patients suffering from ulcerative colitis were detached from their emotional reactions to the loss. In these cases, "Adequate mourning is replaced by an impaired mental state combined with a visceral disorder" (Lindemann, 1979, p. 45). In addition, "The course of the ulcerative colitis was strikingly benefited when this grief reaction was resolved by psychiatric technique" (Lindemann, 1979, p. 70). The patient's avoidance of the psychological suffering attendant to the grieving process manifested itself in gastro-intestinal symptoms. As patients were helped to face their grief directly, the need to avoid it through such somatic discharge was lessened considerably.

Because of his work on the link between loss and physical illness, Dr. Lindemann was primed for the study of acute grief reactions after the Coconut Grove disaster. Hundreds were killed in a nightclub fire, leaving many more to confront the sudden and traumatic loss of their loved ones. For the first time, a major study was undertaken to examine the process of grief as it occurred. The findings from this report (Lindemann, 1944) indicated:

1 Acute grief is a definite syndrome with specific somatic and psychological symptomatology.

2 This syndrome can occur immediately after a loss, or be delayed, exaggerated, or apparently absent.

3 In place of the typical syndrome, a distorted picture may appear, such as ulcerative colitis or an exaggerated identification with the deceased.

4 With the application of appropriate techniques, these distortions of the mourning process can be transformed into normal grief so that the reactions can be resolved.

The Acute Grief Syndrome

Lindemann (1944) outlined five features he considered characteristic of an acute grief syndrome:

1 Somatic distress, including tightness in the throat, deep sighing, a heavy feeling in the chest and abdomen, and an overall feeling of muscular weakness.

2 A preoccupation with the image of the deceased.

3 Guilt.

4 Anger and hostility.

5 Restlessness.

What he found most compelling about mourning was not only the number and variety of symptoms involved, but the way they tended to conflict with each other. For example, the desire for reunion coexists with anger at the deceased. Anguished cries for help occur alongside rejection of any attempts at comfort. Helping someone grieve requires a great deal of skill as well as sensitivity to all the complex and conflicting emotional states involved.

Kübler-Ross's Findings

Elizabeth Kübler-Ross (1969) was a pioneer in the study of death and dying. She focused most of her attention on the experience of those facing their own death, rather than the bereaved they leave behind. Still, her work with dying patients has relevance to our understanding of the grief process. She has outlined five stages of the process: (a) denial; (b) anger; (c) bargaining; (d) depression; and (e) acceptance. She found that those close to the dying patient go through very similar stages of adjustment. In addition to those stated, guilt is often prominent in the bereaved. For the dying, there is an end. For those who remain, grief is a long and difficult process, which frequently feels endless. According to Kübler-Ross, the greatest help for the bereaved is human contact—providing the support necessary to render the emotional turmoil bearable.

Her work with the families of dying patients supports the notion that it is the defenses against the experience and shared expression of the feelings around the impending loss that cause most of the difficulties in the end. "If they had been helped before the death of their partner to bridge the gulf between themselves and the dying one, half of the battle would have been won" (Kübler-Ross, 1969, p. 143).

Bowlby's Contribution

Bowlby (1980), who studied the effects of separation and loss, mostly in children, repeatedly focused on the "long duration of grief, on the difficulties of recovering from its effects, and on the adverse consequences for personality functioning that loss so often brings" (p. 8). He identified four phases in the mourning process: (1) numbing; (2) yearning and searching accompanied by periods of sobbing and angry outbursts; (3) despair and disorganization; and (4) reorganization.

Numbing

C. S. Lewis (1961) described many of these experiences in his personal account of the grief he suffered following the loss of his beloved wife. He started by describing the anxiety and restlessness characteristic of the early phases of grief: "No one ever told me that grief felt so like fear. I am not afraid, but the sensation is like being afraid. The same fluttering in the stomach, the same restlessness, the yawning. I keep on swallowing" (p. 1). He also describes the somatic distress so characteristic of grief. He then goes on to say, "At other times it feels like being mildly drunk, or concussed", which seems to describe that state of numbness so characteristic of the initial stage of grief.

Yearning and Searching

Bowlby contended that yearning is a powerful and highly painful affective state in its own right and can't be reduced to guilt or fear of retribution, as classical psychoanalytic theory might hypothesize. Others (Shand, 1920) have focused on the survival value of yearning and searching during the early phases of mourning. Since the irretrievable loss of an attachment figure during childhood is such a statistically rare event (a parent can only die once, and in most cases, the "lost" figure returns following separation), feelings and behaviors that get mobilized during unwanted separations are the first to appear when a loss is confronted. The yearning and searching, so highly adaptive in prompting reunion following separation, only wane slowly as the reality of the loss is accepted. In addition, these feelings and behaviors tend to elicit strong caretaking responses in others during a time when the mourner is most in need of support. Kübler-Ross has emphasized the crucial role of social supports for the survival and adaptation of the bereaved. Because our highly technological society tends to isolate the dying from the living, people today are often ill-prepared to deal with the reality of death.

Despair and Disorganization

As the phase of yearning and searching subsides and the full impact of loss begins to be felt, despair and a state of disorganization often set in. In this regard, Engel (1961) has pointed out that normal grief involves both acute suffering and impairment in the person's ability to function for days, weeks, or even months. Left alone, those who mourn are at high risk for death themselves. An active and responsive support system that supplies basic care is crucial for the survival of the bereaved.

The Process of Reorganization

What is required for the process of grief to proceed to resolution? Many feel it is essential for the bereaved to endure the emotional upheaval involved:

> Only if he can tolerate the pining, the more or less conscious searching, the seemingly endless examination of how and why the loss occurred, and anger at anyone who might have been responsible, not sparing even the dead person, can he come gradually to recognize and accept that the loss is in truth permanent and that his life must be shaped anew.
>
> (Bowlby, *Attachment and Loss*, 1970, p. 93)

Many in the field have emphasized that grieving tends to be a long and gruelling process; something we tend to underestimate.

Pathological Mourning

Lewis (1961) wrote, "Aren't these notes the senseless writhings of a man who won't accept the fact that there is nothing we can do with suffering except to suffer it? Who still thinks there is some device (if only he could find it) which will make pain not be pain" (p. 38). Most agree that the differences between normal and pathological grief are relative, based on the degree and intensity of reaction. No clear line between normal and pathological can be drawn. Bowlby (1980) has suggested that pathological mourning is an exaggeration or distortion of normal behavior due to defensive efforts that have interrupted or distorted the normal course of mourning. Because defensive processes almost always accompany grief at some point in the process, Bowlby (1970) suggested it is not the occasional employment of defenses that suggest a pathological course, but the "scope, intensity and tendency to persist" (Bowlby, 1970, p. 35) that is so deleterious.

Any mental process that minimizes or avoids the pain of grief can be considered a defense. All mourners resort to such strategies at times, but if these defensive attempts at excluding painful thoughts and feelings become rigid and fixed, the mourning process will be distorted, resulting in symptoms. The most important factors in differentiating normal from pathological grief are the flexibility within the defensive system and the individual's awareness of behaving in ways that temporarily avoid the pain of mourning. Flexibility and awareness are hallmarks of adaptability. Conversely, rigidity and a lack of awareness suggest pathology.

Frequently, the defenses adopted against the painful feelings of grief get encrusted and prevent future adaptation. Consequently, the patient seems to get stuck in one phase of mourning—say numbness (chronic detachment) or despair (chronic depression and hopelessness). Fixation at one phase of mourning prevents the patient from moving through the process required to achieve acceptance and resolution. When this occurs, the characteristic defenses against mourning take on a life of their own and come to resemble character pathology, as they effect all areas of the patient's functioning. This was the case with the Detached Observer (see Chapter 3), who became immobilized in the phase of numbness and detachment. The patient's chronic avoidance of grief prevented him from becoming emotionally attached to anyone.

Davis (1988) has called pathological mourning "the great deceiver", as it rarely appears in a clear and direct form and is often disguised as an affective disorder, anxiety and panic, or a psychosomatic disturbance. Others have suggested that post-traumatic stress disorder may be a form of pathological mourning (Horowitz, 1979).

Susceptibility to Pathological Mourning

Most in the field (Bowlby, 1980; Lindemann, 1944) agree that the following three factors greatly influence susceptibility to pathological mourning:

1 Premorbid personality adjustment.

2 The nature of the relationship to the deceased.

3 The manner of death.

In other words, someone with a fragile or depleted ego will be more likely to succumb to a pathological course of mourning than someone with a strong, flexible ego. Disordered mourning is also more likely to occur in cases where lives have been "deeply intertwined" (Bowlby, 1980), or when the death is traumatic and/or untimely (Parkes, 1970; 1975). Any combination of these factors greatly increases the likelihood of a pathological outcome (Parkes, 1975).

Davanloo's Studies on Pathological Mourning

While training as a psychiatric resident in Boston, Davanloo studied with Dr. Lindemann and was profoundly influenced by his work on grief and mourning. His own studies (Davanloo, 1988) have identified six factors that predispose individuals to a pathological course of mourning:

1 A highly ambivalent or hostile relationship with the deceased.

2 A sudden, unexpected, or untimely death.

3 A feeling of responsibility for the death.

4 Witnessing a death by accident.

5 Low ego-adaptive capacity.

6 Ego depletion due to caretaking prior to death.

Implications for Treatment

Lindemann (1944) suggested a tightly focused approach to grief work. The therapist guides patients to review their relationship with the deceased in detail, focusing on both positive and negative feelings and impulses. In so doing, patients are encouraged to face and accept, rather than avoid, the emotional pain of bereavement. In addition, patients need to become aware of the maladaptive defenses they have used to avoid the experience of grief. This is especially important in increasing patients' ego-adaptive capacity (i.e., to respond flexibly and realistically) and preparing them to endure future losses without resorting to pathological defenses. In the end, patients should be able to acknowledge all their mixed feelings for the deceased and have a new perspective from which to view their life and death.

Bowlby (1970) has found that "only to a non-judgmental companion who shows himself sympathetic and understanding are these latent responses likely to be expressed" (p. 239). Obviously, this need not be a therapist. Isadora Duncan lost both her children in a car crash. She had a friend who, rather than offering platitudes, encouraged her to talk about her children, review her memories, bring out pictures, and cry over the untimely loss (Moffat, 1986). In her autobiography, Duncan (1927, 1955) wrote, ". . . for the first time since their death, I felt I was not alone". Such experiences allow the intense grief and anger of mourning to be directly felt and shared and seem to prevent a lapse into despair.

Pathological mourning often presents itself in subtle and disguised forms. It can masquerade as anxiety, depression, psychosomatic illness, or character pathology. Because of the hidden nature of the problem, traditional analysis has had very little success in treating this disorder (Davis, 1988). Davanloo has suggested that the same defenses employed to ward off the pain involved in the grief process are also used in the therapeutic relationship to keep the therapist at an emotional distance. Davanloo's techniques of defense analysis and rapid identification of the transference pattern of behavior create psychic disequilibrium. This greatly increases the likelihood of transforming pathological mourning into acute grief (Davis, 1988).

In fact, much psychotherapy, even that not explicitly directed toward resolution of grief, is concerned with undoing the denied losses experienced throughout life. As the patient faces the impact of these losses, all the disavowed feelings of anger, despair, and longing can be directly experienced. A feeling of liberation from the past is frequently the result of this therapeutic work.

Stark (1994) believes that most of the resistance encountered in therapeutic work is the result of the patient's unwillingness to face grief and loss. In her opinion, "the defended patient, the resistant patient, is someone who has not yet grieved . . . " (p. 123). By activating the process of acute mourning in the therapeutic setting, patients are given the opportunity to deal with the reality of painful losses and the effects these have had on their lives. Through this process, patients abandon chronic detachment and regain the capacity to make emotional contact with others and to experience joy in living.

Clinical Examples

The Man in a Fog

In the following case, the patient arrived for treatment complaining that he was preoccupied and "in a fog". This 30-year-old married man reported a significant decrease in his ability to focus or concentrate at work. Consequently, his job performance was suffering. His gait and speech were slow, and his physical movements were stiff and restrictive. He immediately struck me as being among the "walking wounded". Inquiry quickly revealed that the onset of these symptoms coincided with the death of his dog. He had decided to carry the dog into the vet's office and hold him while the lethal injection was administered. As this experience was explored, the patient reported that his first child, a son, had been stillborn some three years earlier. This information was communicated in a detached and "matter-of-fact" tone. In fact, the "fog" had descended right after his son's death, yet he had not previously made that connection.

Since the original onset of symptoms followed the death of his firstborn child, it became clear that the primary therapeutic task would involve focusing the patient's attention on the painful events and feelings surrounding this tragic loss. The sudden, unexpected, and untimely nature of this death were predisposing factors to a pathological outcome. We would only find out later that there were others as well.

Many studies have confirmed that the death of a child is among the most devastating losses anyone can face (Bowlby, 1980; Friedman, Chodoff, Mason, & Hamberg, 1963). In the case of a stillborn, the baby is often whisked away quickly, depriving the parents of the opportunity to face the reality of their loss (Peppers & Knoff, 1980). In fact, that is what took place in this case. In addition to undermining his ability to come to terms with the reality of the death and his feelings about it, the quick removal of the baby was another contributing factor preventing the couple from sharing their grief. Studies suggest that marital and sexual difficulties frequently follow the loss of a child (Raphael, 1983).

In this case, the patient's use of defensive detachment, initially employed to avoid the experience of grief over his son, became a habitual way to avoid emotional closeness with anyone. If the pathological course of mourning was not translated into acute grief, this detachment could harden into character pathology. Reviewing the painful events surrounding the baby's death while in an emotionally detached state would be of little therapeutic value. The first step of treatment involved the identification and clarification of all the patient's defenses against closeness with the therapist. He was then guided to focus on the consequences of maintaining such a stance.

The defenses of detachment were directly linked to his presenting complaint of being in a fog and unable to function. Linking these defenses with his presenting complaint increased his motivation to approach the painful memories and feelings he had previously avoided.

As the patient's ego began to turn against its defenses, the therapist was able to capitalize on the strengthened therapeutic alliance and guide the patient, gently but firmly, toward the most painful aspects of the loss. Imagery and visualization proved powerful tools in this process. Once the avoidant defenses were punctured and the sadness and grief began to be felt, the therapist asked what picture came to the patient's mind. Now mind, body, and emotion were all activated and involved, contributing to a deep experience of grief.

Feelings of Sadness

THERAPIST: So now we see that you have never faced the feelings about your son.

PATIENT: I've had a hundred feelings but never faced them. The first feeling is sadness.

THERAPIST: You feel that now?

PATIENT: Yes, I feel a lot of sadness. Usually, I wouldn't think about myself. I'd think about my wife.

THERAPIST: You have sadness too. What's the image that comes to your mind?

PATIENT: One that comes back most is seeing the baby in the blanket when it was all over. He definitely looked like me.

THERAPIST: Could you describe his face?

PATIENT: It's hard to describe a face. A baby is a baby.

THERAPIST: But you said he looked like you. You knew it wasn't just any baby, but yours.

PATIENT: I remember his eyes. His lips were all red, very red, like lipstick, almost purple. The color was definitely not right. I can remember (arms shaped as if holding the baby) feeling him and he was warm—after the delivery, you know. Then I felt like, maybe he's sleeping and he's going to wake up (tearful). I know it's stupid and doesn't make sense to feel that, but inside you want to believe it. I think that's natural. I remember his eyes being closed and wishing he would wake up.

THERAPIST: His lips tell you something is not right. The pain and grief are so intense you want not to believe it.

PATIENT: Everyone said he looked like me. That made it more real—that this was my child. This happened to me.

THERAPIST: What's the feeling inside now?

PATIENT: I want to keep the baby. I don't want to let him go. I want to keep him forever, but I can't. I just feel that loss (cries). I think about the future—the things that will never be (more tears).

THERAPIST: The loss of all those hopes and dreams.

PATIENT: Feeling of wanting to hold on was so great—the hardest thing was to let go (makes grabbing motions with his hands and is crying).

This material is very sad, almost heartbreaking. A gentle but persistent focus on the patient's painful feelings of grief proved very effective. Painting the scene and returning to the delivery room were techniques used to heighten the patient's awareness of his previously avoided emotions. The specificity and detail, especially of the baby's face, were especially important in bringing the experience to life in the here and now. It was so moving, in fact, that the therapist's eyes filled with tears. At that point, the patient seemed to physically recoil, and he fell silent. He had previously mentioned an inability to cry at the time of his son's death, fearing that his grief would intensify that experienced by his wife. His hypersensitivity to the therapist's reaction suggested a link between the two (C and T) that was vital to expose and work through rapidly. The following excerpt will illustrate the shift in focus to the patient's experience of the therapist and her emotional reaction.

Feelings and Defense in the Transference

THERAPIST: It looks like you're having a reaction to my welling up with tears.

PATIENT: I wasn't thinking of anything. I'm just trying to get myself together.

THERAPIST: Why now? It seems to be a response to my emotion.

PATIENT: I guess if I were to share this with the average person, they'd tear up too.

THERAPIST: What comes to mind?

PATIENT: I guess I think I feel your sorrow, your reaction, and maybe it stops me from going on.

THERAPIST: Yes, I sensed that. You stop and pull back. It's as if my having a reaction frightens you.

PATIENT: It's like how my wife felt. I tried not to think about myself. I didn't want to lose it because then she would lose it.

THERAPIST: That fear, of the woman losing it, gets in the way of sharing the grief. You stay alone with it.

PATIENT: Yeah, I guess you're right—it's not necessarily desirable to keep it all inside (long pause). I feel cold. My whole body feels cold. I'm going back to the hospital (starts to cry).

This brief vignette revealed a very important dynamic in this man's life, illustrating how his defenses against his own true feelings created an emotional distance from others. While the affective shifts may not be readily apparent in the transcript, there was a noticeable change in this man's demeanor in response to the therapist's emotional reaction. He stopped crying, sat up in his chair, and said he was trying to "get himself together". Attention to this type of non-verbal communication is extremely important to notice and highlight. Allan Abbass (personal communication, 2020), a master ISTDP clinician, suggests that we must learn to "listen with their eyes", as well as their ears, to be highly effective. The unconscious often speaks through the body, so noticing even subtle physical changes enhances the work.

By examining the transference pattern of behavior, the patient gained insight into the parallel between his reaction with the therapist and that with his wife. As he evaluated the cost of this strategy (emotional detachment and interpersonal distance), his position shifted once again from avoidance and repression to connection and activation. He spontaneously returned to the scene in the hospital, signaling that he was ready to resume the work.

Resuming the Portrait

THERAPIST: We ended with the feeling that you didn't want to let go. You go cold, like the baby. Did you let him go or did they take him?

PATIENT: The doctor took him, and I handed him over.

THERAPIST: But what you wanted to do?

PATIENT: Hold on.

THERAPIST: Can you put it in words?

PATIENT: I was so shocked I didn't have words.

THERAPIST: But now?

PATIENT: "You can't have him, he's mine". I hold him tighter (clutches his chest) and say, "Stay away, he's mine, you can't have him". I just want to hold onto him (more tears). I felt so helpless—I wanted to change the situation.

THERAPIST: What's it like to hold on? How does it feel to say no?

PATIENT: Maybe the more I hold on, the harder it will be to let go. The emotions get stronger and stronger. I wouldn't let anyone near him. Maybe I'd think crazy things like the baby is OK and it was all a mistake. I just couldn't believe it.

This communication suggested that the patient had learned to be afraid of intense emotion and equated these feelings with "going crazy". We discovered the source of these fears when a link to the past was made.

THERAPIST: Their coming in so quickly interfered with the process—for it to become a reality to you.

PATIENT: But my poor wife—to have to physically go through that—giving birth. I guess I was really concentrating on her (very tearful). I was devastated. She was even more. I wish I could spare her that pain.

Dispelling Pathological Beliefs

To aid the process of working through, we must deal with the pathological beliefs that accompany the affect-laden experiences our patients have had. Stern (1985) has hypothesized the operation of an innate drive operating in all humans to form and test beliefs about their interpersonal world. Research findings suggest that infants regulate their behavior according to these beliefs about reality. It is the babies' interpersonal reality, their interaction with primary attachment figures, that supplies this vital information. Because infants are totally dependent, they must adapt to parental demands and expectations, or their very survival will be threatened. As Wachtel (1993) has put it, a child will "trim his sails to meet the prevailing winds".

These ideas have been confirmed by Emde (1989) and Weiss (1993), both of whom have gathered data supporting the hypothesis that we are powerfully motivated to unconsciously assess external reality in terms of safety and danger before commencing with action. In other words, people take action to master their environment and optimize the chance for a successful outcome, and not simply to express an impulse, defense, or compromise between the two. Yet these things affect a person's ability to reach that goal of mastery. Defenses can impair the accurate assessment of reality and predispose people to failure and frustration.

This research has direct relevance for understanding the therapeutic process. It is not enough to reactivate the painful emotions involved in the memories that surface during the treatment process. The pathological beliefs associated with them must be elicited and corrected as well (Ecker, Ticic, & Hulley, 2012; Weiss, 1993). Weiss has developed a rationale for therapeutic intervention based on Freud's (1920) theoretical shift from an emphasis on centrality of the pleasure principle to that of the reality principle. This shift was accompanied by the suggestion of the operation of a motive toward mastery—not just of our inner drives and instincts, but of the external world. In *An Outline of Psychoanalysis*, Freud (1949) wrote that man, "after taking its bearings in the present and assessing earlier experiences, endeavors by means of experimental action to calculate the consequences of the courses of action proposed" (p. 199).

Our patients frequently suffer from distorted and pathological beliefs acquired in early life and need to be assisted, through fresh experiences, to change these beliefs. This is most likely to occur within the therapeutic relationship (Strupp & Binder, 1984; Wachtel, 1993). In fact, "Most people who have undergone psychoanalysis feel that they have learned and gained from the contact with their analyst, from the kind of person he or she is and the way the analyst functions" (Pine, 1985).

These theoretical revisions, and the research data that support them, have not been adequately translated into standard practice. ISTDP attempts to do so. The type of intervention being suggested here is multifaceted. The initial focus on defenses liberates affective expression, leading to the rapid de-repression of memories, ideas, and beliefs acquired early in life. This process facilitates the uncovering of unconscious conflict, increasing the unconscious therapeutic alliance and decreasing reliance on maladaptive defenses. Further, this work increases the patient's tolerance for the experience of strong mixed feelings toward significant others. As the process unfolds, working models of self and other become more realistic, complex, and multidimensional. Past and present, although clearly linked, also become distinct.

Three Sessions Later

The patient entered this session reporting that feelings of grief were welling up spontaneously throughout the week. Of interest, he also reported that other feelings, including happiness and joy, were beginning to emerge. He was noticeably lighter and brighter in appearance. I asked if he was able to share all these feelings with his wife, and he said he was keeping the sad feelings to himself. We began to explore, in greater detail, where he got the idea that to share feelings is to burden someone.

Examination of Distorted Beliefs About Self and Others

PATIENT: Feelings have been coming up all week. It feels good to release it.

THERAPIST: And were you able to share it at all?

PATIENT: No, I'd only let it come up when I was alone.

THERAPIST: What we've learned about this so far is that you tend to be very protective of others. You've gotten the idea that your emotions are a burden to others. You're afraid to burden them so you keep the feelings closed up inside.

PATIENT: It's hard to get away from that. Part of me wants to open up, but I'm still afraid and hold back.

THERAPIST: Where did you get this belief? It must have come through experience.

PATIENT: I'm sure. What comes to mind is my grandfather. He passed on, and I thought I shouldn't let my upset show because my mother was so devastated. I didn't want to add to her sense of loss.

THERAPIST: So you were just a boy?

PATIENT: That was just a few years ago.

THERAPIST: But wasn't there an earlier loss?

PATIENT: Oh, that was my grandmother, but I don't remember much about that.

THERAPIST: Wasn't your mother also very upset then?

PATIENT: Oh, definitely. She had a nervous breakdown.

THERAPIST: What happened?

PATIENT: I was about seven. My grandmother was sick, and we expected her to die. I remember feeling really sad, but not crying, because my mother was so upset. My father never showed any feeling—especially in those situations. He'd try to be light and say, "It's all for the best".

THERAPIST: But your mother was very upset? What's the picture?

PATIENT: I can see her sitting in the chair with a tissue—bawling and sobbing. She let everything out—crying really hard. It was too much to control.

THERAPIST: How do you feel going back to that?

C-P Link

PATIENT: Sad that she had to go through that—to experience all that pain. I wish I could help her. I felt helpless, like I did with the baby.

THERAPIST: So there it is all over again. You have your own loss—your grandmother and your son—but you are so preoccupied with the sadness of the woman and feel such a pressure to do something about it, that you don't experience your own grief.

PATIENT: Maybe it gets me away from my own grief. I was confused. My mother was so upset and then my father, not at all. I thought that was the male role. All the men in the family were like that.

THERAPIST: Then your mother couldn't bear it. What kind of breakdown did she have?

PATIENT: She was hospitalized and had shock therapy. They took her out to Long Island, and we would visit. I was hoping she'd come home soon.

THERAPIST: So right after losing your grandmother, you lose your mother to depression and hospitalization.

PATIENT: I can feel my body tense. I feel a reaction in my body but I'm not sure what it is. I feel like I want to do something physically—like reaching out.

THERAPIST: That separation is gut-wrenching. Again, you don't want to let go (as with the baby). What's the feeling?

PATIENT: I didn't want her to go. I see myself as a little boy by the screen door (very tearful). I'm sad and confused, feeling so helpless.

In this case, the patient's mother, wife, and therapist were initially linked. They were all viewed as women who might break down in the face of grief and abandon him. As the work progressed, and the patient dealt with his feelings toward his mother directly, he was able to see how he had been misperceiving other women over the years. At this point in the treatment, we were able to establish that this earlier ungrieved loss was another factor rendering him vulnerable to pathological mourning of both his son and his dog.

Following this work, the patient was able to distinguish between his mother, his wife, and the therapist. In particular, he determined that both the therapist and his wife were capable of experiencing grief without decompensating. Changes in the patient's characteristic mode of attachment followed. He was finally able to share his grief with his wife and tolerate her grief without undue anxiety or the need to withdraw. It is important to note that this change did not take place spontaneously once he experienced all his own feelings about the loss of his son. This change only transpired when attention was paid to the transference pattern of behavior. Having an experience with the therapist in which she was moved, but present and engaged, seemed to provide a corrective emotional experience once that was juxtaposed to his expectations from the past. It is just this kind of juxtaposition that has been found to alter emotional patterns on a permanent basis (Ecker, et al., 2012).

Effects of Loss on Self-Image

Bowlby (1970) and others (Stern, 1985) who have studied the effects of early relational patterns on the formation of a self-image, have paid particular attention to the effects that separation and loss have on the child's ongoing sense of self. Mann (1973) has placed special emphasis on the relationship between the patient's current and chronically endured pain regarding separations, losses, and disappointment in relationships and a persistent negative self-image. He has stated, "I came to understand that the repetitive series of separations and losses that every human being endures forms the outline of the self-image that each person constructs" (Mann, 1991, p. 18).

Engel (1961) has stated the opinion that the loss of a loved one is, in and of itself, traumatic. Multiple losses result in cumulative trauma and grossly affect the individual's sense of self and the world. "The affective result of trauma blurs a person's perception of time, which in turn increases negative affect, which increases the sense of hopelessness" (Mann, 1991, p. 28). Even those in the mental health field often grossly underestimate the devastating effect of loss on our patients and how long and difficult the path to resolution really is.

In this case, the material suggested that the patient learned to be afraid of strong affect in himself and others as a result of several early losses. In his mind, intense feelings lead to breakdown, hospitalization, and loss. The patient remarked that his mother was never the same after the shock treatments, so there was a sense of loss even after physical reunion with his mother.

The patient was given a new opportunity to understand the impact of these early experiences on himself and to appreciate how they affected his reaction to subsequent losses. This created a fresh opportunity to evaluate, as an adult, whether strategies developed as a child were currently required. Again, the experience of affect was a necessary but insufficient step to achieve permanent change in his adaptation to loss. We also had to expose and then critically assess the accuracy of the distorted and pathological beliefs that accompanied these experiences for character change to occur.

It became apparent that this man's tendency to keep his feelings to himself and to assume a caretaking role for others, especially the women in his life, was a strategy adopted at an early age in order to prevent further loss. Although this strategy was maladaptive in adult life, it was adaptive as a child in relation to a mother who was quite fragile and unable bear grief. In contrast, he discovered that sharing grief with his wife and therapist increased his feelings of closeness with them.

A Man with Sexual Difficulties

While evidence of pathological mourning was readily obtained in the case of the Man in a Fog, in many cases it is more difficult to ascertain. In the following case, a middle-aged man was referred for psychotherapy by his Urologist, who could find no organic basis for the patient's erectile dysfunction. Inquiry revealed an 18-month history of anxiety and depression in addition to the presenting problem of erectile failure. When asked what was happening in his life at the time these difficulties began, he reported that his mother, a chronic psychiatric patient, had died. However, the patient attached no significance to this "coincidence", saying, "not that that could have anything to do with it". There is no therapeutic value in trying to convince a patient, on some rational level, that symptoms have symbolic meaning. The emotional significance of his mother's death was the very thing he was defending himself against. Thus, we initially focused on the patient's emotional detachment.

The first several sessions of treatment were spent acquainting the patient with his defenses against emotional closeness. When his detachment was noted, he reported being afraid of letting himself feel; mentioning that he had a lot of anger inside and was worried about losing control. By linking the patient's presenting complaint (lack of sexual desire and an inability to maintain erections) to the defense of emotional detachment, the defense became increasingly dystonic. The session being recounted here began with an exploration of this issue.

Anger toward His Boss

PATIENT: I have two feelings when it comes to anger—I either tense up and keep it inside or I erupt.

THERAPIST: So what you're saying is that when you feel angry, the aggressive impulses that come with it are so strong, you're afraid, if you don't squelch it, you'll act on it. To keep yourself in check, you don't let yourself feel the anger.

PATIENT: With the exception of the last month, since coming here. I've been able just to talk to certain individuals and say "I'm angry"—be firm and to the point and it works out well. But these people are reasonable to begin with.

THERAPIST: But when someone is unreasonable, like your boss, you become enraged. There's no dealing with this guy—words don't work.

PATIENT: That's true. And it's worse right now. Others feel this way about him too and are losing their cool.

THERAPIST: So you're not the only one. The anger is stronger than ever.

PATIENT: Yeah.

C-P Link

THERAPIST: So, if this came out, in your imagination?

PATIENT: If I ever let go, I would hit him and beat him, continue to beat him with my hands in his face, and continue to beat him until he says he understands and would change.

THERAPIST: How likely is that?

PATIENT: Not at all. But that's what I picture—just hitting him until he stops acting the way he acts.

THERAPIST: So what point would that be?

PATIENT: Probably kill him because it never worked with my mother so why should it work with him (puts his head in his hands and rubs his eyes).

THERAPIST: That's who comes to your mind?

PATIENT: Yeah. I wish I had killed her 20 years ago—maybe I wouldn't have the problems I have today.

A link between the boss and his mother emerged spontaneously following the breakthrough of the murderous impulses. This is a clear example of a strong unconscious alliance providing a bridge from a current conflict to an unresolved emotional conflict from the past. No interpretation is required, as the patient makes their own connections.

Facing the Rage toward His Mother

THERAPIST: So, as you get in touch with the impulse to beat this man, you see your mother and realize you had a murderous rage toward her. He's another unreasonable person you just can't get through to in any civilized way. You feel so enraged you want to kill him. Where would this take place with your mother?

PATIENT: In the apartment next door.

THERAPIST: Where?

PATIENT: In the dining room where she would sit smoking. That's where I'd try to talk to her, but I couldn't get through. I imagine talking to her quietly and trying to resolve our problems, but she would just talk, talk, talk, but make no sense, jumping from subject to subject. In fact, it's just like this guy—he's just like her.

THERAPIST: So as you think about this, you're trying to talk to her, but you can't get through, and the feeling of anger rises. If those feelings came out toward her?

PATIENT: Yeah, I feel it (voice up, hands mobilized). I'd start hitting her and choking her and punch her and, if I was smart, I'd kill her.

THERAPIST: How?

PATIENT: I'd just beat her until she stopped talking. You couldn't stop her talking. I'd punch her and choke her until she couldn't say anymore, until she was dead, so she would just shut up.

THERAPIST: How do you see her?

PATIENT: Laying on the floor dead.

THERAPIST: What does she look like?

PATIENT: A poor soul, at rest now.

Facing the Guilt and Grief

THERAPIST: Physically?

PATIENT: Her face would be swollen, she'd be bleeding, and like a jerk, I'd feel sorry about doing it.

THERAPIST: So there are feelings of remorse?

PATIENT: Sure. I don't know why I should . . .

THERAPIST: But you do.

PATIENT: Yeah, I do (tears up).

THERAPIST: There's a deep feeling of sadness that comes over you.

PATIENT: Yeah, because she had a shitty life—she did (starts to cry). And then to have it end like that would make it worse.

THERAPIST: So there are tender feelings underneath all this.

PATIENT: Yes, but I resent those feelings.

While acknowledging feelings of grief and guilt, the patient preferred to stay angry with his mother rather than face all the complex mixed feelings toward her. The therapist followed the feelings as they emerged, while simply sweeping away his conscious resistance ("I resent those feelings"). Experiencing grief and tenderness toward her inevitably activated guilt about his murderous impulses. In patients like this, who are clearly punishing themselves, getting to the guilt that drives their need to suffer is essential therapeutic work (Carveth, 2006).

THERAPIST: But they are there. As angry as you have been with her, you also feel for her and have compassion for her suffering. So, what would you do with her body?

PATIENT: I don't know, it would depend. I could picture myself sitting down and thinking it through. Would I admit it or hide it? I would probably cover it up.

THERAPIST: So you would bury her yourself.

PATIENT: If I could get away with it (laughs).

THERAPIST: What's funny?

PATIENT: I see myself burying her behind the house in the woods. I see myself covering her up with dirt. I'm only laughing because, through the years, she would make comments about how she didn't want me to go to any fuss when she died, and I'd say, "Don't worry Mom, I'll just dig a hole in the back and throw you in".

THERAPIST: So there's some truth in that.

PATIENT: I guess so (laughs again).

THERAPIST: You're saying that for 20 years, at least, you've been enraged with her. She was such a pain in your neck, you just wanted to kill her, dig a ditch, and throw her in it. When the anger is spent, then sadness comes. You don't like it, you want to resist that feeling, but it's there. So, to face throwing this lifeless body of your mother into a ditch . . .

PATIENT: At this point my main concern would be to cover up what I did.

This last response provided a clear indication that evasion of guilt had been interrupting the grief process and was a significant factor in creating his presenting complaints. This mechanism also contributed to his need to withdraw from others. His desire to hide the secret that, with her death, he had gotten his wish to be rid of his mother, required emotional withdrawal from others, including his wife. Sexual closeness became impossible.

THERAPIST: But what happens to these sad feelings?

PATIENT: I think it would bother me a lot. If I covered it up, I wouldn't get a guilty conscience and confess later, but I'd suffer internally with my own guilt.

THERAPIST: So what would that be like, to suffer internally?

PATIENT: Phew (big sigh). I don't know, it would bother me for the rest of my life. I'd think about it all the time and my stomach would bother me—you know the way my stomach gets—and I would never have any peace.

THERAPIST: So, let me ask you, isn't this exactly what you've been experiencing inside? Ever since she died, you've been filled with anxiety and guilt and there's been no peace for you. You've isolated yourself, and no one knows what you're suffering inside.

PATIENT: That's true.

The source of this man's suffering became quite evident following the breakthrough of murderous rage, guilt, and grief. The breakdown of defenses, and breakthrough of feelings, provided an opening into the unconscious, shedding light on the origin of his difficulties. On an unconscious level, he had considered himself a murderer and was punishing himself ever since he got his wish (his mother's death). Once he became consciously aware of the link between his repressed rage, guilt, and grief and his symptomatic suffering, he was able to reassess his relationship with his mother and whether the punishment fit the crime. In fact, he had been an extraordinarily dedicated son to his seriously disturbed mother. All in all, he left the session feeling good about the way he had treated his mother and very sad about the suffering she had to endure because of her illness (she was alternately diagnosed as having paranoid schizophrenia and manic-depressive illness).

Other memories surfaced, helping us to understand the origin of his conflicts. He recalled times when his mother would open their apartment window and scream that he was going to kill her. She was seriously mentally ill, with paranoid and manic episodes, requiring repeated hospitalizations. He had internalized her voice and was afraid to admit his murderous feelings, lest he prove her right. Following this work, he was able to distinguish between feelings and actions. Furthermore, he was able to understand that these wishes were a reaction to the real neglect and abuse he had suffered at his parent's hands. The eventual compassion he was able to have for his mother, he was also able to feel for himself. The harshness in him softened. Others at home and at the office commented on how approachable he had become.

A pervasive sense of guilt and the assumption of a caretaking function for his mother throughout life were two of the factors that had predisposed this man to a pathological course of mourning. By activating acute grief, he was able to acknowledge and integrate his disparate feelings toward his mother. This led to changes that were fundamental and far-reaching. His whole demeanor and characteristic way of dealing with his own feelings and interacting with others changed significantly. Closeness with his wife was restored and the couple resumed what had been a rich and satisfying sexual relationship.

The Woman with Panic Attacks

The following case is another in which pathological mourning was initially disguised. This middle-aged mother of two entered treatment because of anxiety and panic that had plagued her since moving from her hometown to a new city. Not only were they in a new city, but her husband had changed his profession and was working long and erratic hours. The patient became highly anxious and panicky when her husband was gone for long periods. She was also increasingly angry with him for leaving her alone with no clear idea of when he would return. The patient wondered whether these separations were especially difficult for her because her mother had been in and out of hospitals most of her life. She died when the patient was 12. All this was reported in a highly detached manner. The patient said she had no memory of her mother's death.

The therapeutic work began in the transference, highlighting the defense of detachment and the self-defeating effects of this strategy for our work. Over time, the patient became an active collaborator in the process and was especially motivated to face all the mixed feelings toward her husband, which she viewed as the source of her anxiety. In this, the sixth psychotherapy session, the patient reported an incident in which her husband arrived home considerably later than expected. Although he agreed to call when detained, he failed to do so. She reported feeling furious with him, but as soon as he came in the kitchen door, she was filled with anxiety and retreated behind a newspaper. Our focus was on the experience of anger toward her husband.

Anger toward Her Husband

THERAPIST: You hid behind the newspaper, but how do you feel toward him?

PATIENT: I am furious.

THERAPIST: How do you experience this anger toward him?

PATIENT: I start seeing myself pushing him but then it goes away. I start to get real upset and then I stop (getting tearful). I don't see the point of this.

THERAPIST: You don't seem to let yourself really feel the anger. You have a thousand ways to avoid it. There is nothing more terrifying to you than experiencing your own rage.

PATIENT: (nods in agreement). Yeah, I'd like to get rid of my own rage (smiles).

THERAPIST: But you're so terrified, that as soon as it starts to rise, you bury it and then the tears come.

PATIENT: Then I'm up all the time, can't sleep, and I try to figure everything out, and then say I'm going to leave. I can't stand it. I just can't stand it.

THERAPIST: So do you want to bury it or look at it?

PATIENT: Let's look at it!

THERAPIST: So if this anger came out toward him, what would this look like?

PATIENT: I see me pushing him (motions with her arms) on his chest.

THERAPIST: And you're in the kitchen?

PATIENT: Now I think about a knife. I push him until he falls down, and I think about (brother). The kitchen made me think of the knife.

THERAPIST: Who has the knife?

PATIENT: If I could, I would probably take the knife and stab him (voice up, hand making a stabbing motion)!

THERAPIST: Where?

PATIENT: In the heart . . . because I don't want things the way they are.

THERAPIST: This is very frightening to face and I'm sure it runs deep—thoughts of your brother came.

PATIENT: But I don't want to talk about that. I told my husband I don't want to talk about my family and the past. I just want to know why these things happen to me now.

THERAPIST: But I'm sure there's a link. It's as you face your anger toward your husband that your brother comes to mind.

PATIENT: Well as a kid, he wanted to kill me—he slashed my wrists with a knife.

THERAPIST: That must have been a terrifying experience, no doubt, but it looks like that also evoked a reactive rage in you toward him which is equally frightening. How much are you going to take until you strike back? It's the same pattern with your husband. You put up with his being late, breaking promises, leaving you alone with the children, and your anger toward him builds and builds.

PATIENT: Yeah, it's true, but it's scary because if I'm going to react, I'm not going to mess around. I'm saying I wouldn't want him just hurt.

THERAPIST: So what happens?

PATIENT: He's dead. If he's dead, he's dead.

THERAPIST: How does this happen?

Sudden De-Repression of Post Trauma

PATIENT: I push him, then stab him. How he's lying on the floor. He's flat on his back.

THERAPIST: How does he look?

PATIENT: Quiet. Dead. White. No, orange. I don't want to see orange (becomes agitated and highly distressed, shaking her head and covering her eyes). I want to talk about something else (breathing rapidly, eyes darting around). I don't want to see. I want to go home now.

THERAPIST: Tell me what's happening inside right now. You seem to panic.

De-Repression of Mother's Death

PATIENT: I see my mother in the coffin—lying on her back, dead. Her skin is orange, her fingers are black. She doesn't talk to me. Well, I just want her to talk to me (uttered in a childlike voice). But dead people can't talk (starts to cry), and I don't want my husband to be dead because I want him to talk to me.

Lowering Anxiety

The patient's anxiety had become too high to proceed, so lowering her anxiety became the first order of business. She was speaking in a childlike voice and almost seemed to be in a dissociated state. Working to reduce anxiety so that she could face her feelings without resorting to regressive feelings was indicated.

THERAPIST: Let's look at what happens inside.

PATIENT: I'm scared.

THERAPIST: You seem to panic.

PATIENT: I'm just scared right now, and I don't want to be around anybody.

THERAPIST: What happens physically? You hyperventilate.

PATIENT: I can't breathe.

THERAPIST: What else.

PATIENT: I get shaky. I don't want to be bad, I wanna' be good (crying). I wanna' stay married. I don't want to go away.

THERAPIST: You think your mother went away because you were bad?

PATIENT: She went away because she wouldn't go to the doctor. By the time she went it was too late—it had gone through her body.

This powerful and rather unexpected de-repression of feelings and memories regarding her mother's death surfaced spontaneously as the patient faced the anger she was feeling toward her husband. He, like her mother, had left her alone repeatedly, with no idea of when he would return. On what turned out to be the last visit to her mother in the hospital, she found her in a coma, unresponsive. The patient reported feeling so furious that her mother wouldn't wake up and talk to her that she stomped out of the room saying, "If you won't talk to me, I'm never coming back to see you again". The next thing she knew, her mother was dead. The feelings of guilt were too much for her to bear as a child. She repressed the entire series of events surrounding her mother's death and funeral, as well as all her true feelings about them. It was only on the heels of this current emotional experience with her husband that these long-buried memories returned, allowing her to assess the situation anew. From an adult's point of view, she was able to understand that her anger did not cause her mother's death. In fact, the mother's death was largely due to her fear of doctors and refusal to seek treatment. The patient was able to feel compassion for herself as a little girl who had to face her mother's death alone. Having no one to talk to about her guilt and grief contributed significantly to the development of her anxiety and depression, as well as a passive, compliant character structure.

Following the grief over the death of her mother, she was able to face all the grief and anger she experienced while her mother was alive, but chronically sick and unavailable. Death is not the only kind of loss that needs to be mourned.

Grief work can be nearly as difficult for the therapist as it is for the patient. We must be able to bear the sorrow of our own losses and disappointments if we are to help our patients deepen their own experience of pain and grief. If we defend against these painful feelings, we'll keep a distance from the grieving patient. Conversely, the attuned therapist's compassionate attitude in the face of grief can often, in and of itself, deepen the patient's experience of painful longing. We often overlook the fact that repressed pain and sorrow are frequently triggered by the experience of positive, loving feelings. When patients find the compassionate understanding they have always longed for but never received (Schnarch, 1991), the contrast between past and present responses intensifies these feelings.

Saying Goodbye

The tenaciousness with which we want to hold onto loved ones can prevent us from coming to terms with loss and moving on to new relationships. Helping our patients say good-bye to loved ones once they have experienced all their mixed feelings toward the deceased can be a very freeing experience. Following this work in therapy, patients sometimes find their own highly personal and meaningful ways to say good-bye and pay tribute to their loved ones.

In the case of the Detached Observer (see Chapter 3), the patient had a dream about a young boy riding down a river on his mother's coffin. This dream clearly depicted his enduring attachment to his mother and inability to say good-bye to her. A young woman, with arms outstretched, was waiting at the shore. He wanted to jump off the coffin and swim to her, but he felt he couldn't leave his mother. He was holding on, not just to spare himself the pain of loss, but to spare his mother her fear of being alone. This dream graphically depicted the price he was paying for holding onto his mother (i.e., he was unable to attach to available women and remained alone).

The Detached Observer

THERAPIST: It looks like you've never said good-bye to your mother. You're like the boy on the coffin, drifting. It's a barren scene, but you're still holding on.

PATIENT: It's a hard thing for me to see. To say good-bye to someone you never knew is what makes it harder.

THERAPIST: It means facing all the regrets. It looked like you had a reaction to something I said. Was it the image of the little boy on the coffin? (Patient nods and starts to cry.)

This is a common phenomenon observed in clinical practice. It's not those who have had a good relationship with a parent that can't seem to let go, but those who didn't have enough of the good. At one point in the session, he said it very precisely: "There just wasn't enough good to hold onto. How do you say goodbye to someone you never really knew?". As he got in touch with the grief and the resistance to saying good-bye to her, I asked him to imagine talking to her about his struggle.

THERAPIST: Can you imagine telling your mother about all that's been lost and how you've been holding on for dear life to a corpse?
PATIENT: (crying). I can't imagine telling her.
THERAPIST: What happens?
PATIENT: I can see her, like, in heaven. Not how she was here but I can see her up there, fully aware of everything I've been going through and how sad it makes her. That she wishes she could help . . . but she can't (sobbing).

This is another illustration of how, once the unconscious is open and fluid, minor defenses can simply be brushed aside. When first asked to imagine talking with his mother, the patient says he couldn't do it. The therapist simply continued with another question ("What happens?"), and the patient responded with a spontaneous image of his mother in heaven.

THERAPIST: What's that like for you, to get an image of your mother as calm, knowing what's happened, and feeling for you?
PATIENT: Well, it's a connection, seeing me and feeling for me.
THERAPIST: She can't actually do anything, but what is it you think she wishes for you?
PATIENT: Oh shit (head in his hands) . . . to be happy and get what I want.
THERAPIST: What happened just now?
PATIENT: That feeling that she would want me to be happy. That's something I never felt from her—that it mattered how I felt.
THERAPIST: But why the "Oh shit"?
PATIENT: For her to want me to be happy even though she wasn't. That's sad.

This material speaks to the patient's identification with the deceased. For this man to embrace life, there needed to be a significant alteration in the quality of the maternal introject, from depriving and frustrating to warm, nurturing, and gratifying. Even though he did not have interactions of this kind with his mother to build upon, the interaction with the therapist provided an experience he could use to imagine what it would have been like had his mother been healthy and emotionally available. In a sense, imagining her wanting him to be happy gave him permission to move on and develop satisfying relationships. He had been remaining connected and loyal to his mother by staying alone or choosing women who were like her—cold and aloof. Following this work, he found himself attracted to women who were outgoing and affectionate.

Survivor's Guilt

Those who have assumed a caretaking role for the deceased seem to have special difficulty in saying good-bye. There is a kind of survivor's guilt (Weiss, 1993) that prevents them from embracing anyone who might in some way replace the deceased. In the case of The Detached Observer, his guilt was overcome by imagining that his mother would want him to have happiness. In this scenario, he didn't have to choose between loyalty to his dead mother or the arms of a warm, available woman. When the parent has actually been possessive and jealous and has demanded exclusive loyalty, this transition is much more difficult (just such a case will be presented in Chapter 6).

Summary

These rather diverse cases demonstrate both the magnitude and variety of psychological sequelae stemming from unresolved grief—from symptoms such as panic attacks and sexual dysfunction, to ingrained character patterns of isolation and detachment. In addition, techniques designed to transform pathological mourning into acute grief were demonstrated. For this reason, Davis (1988) referred to pathological grief as "the great deceiver".

Throughout this chapter, it has been repeatedly emphasized that helping patients get in touch with the experience of guilt and grief is a necessary but frequently insufficient condition for permanent change in defensive patterns and character style to take place. To achieve those ends, the pathological beliefs that have accompanied the feelings and memories associated with loss must also be examined and re-worked; allowing a fuller, more complex and contemporary view of self and other to evolve.

Notes

1. Ranko, S., & Mazer, H. (1980, 1983). *Semrad: The heart of a therapist.* Northvale, NJ: Aronson.
2. From *Two Lives* by William Trevor.

6 WORKING WITH POSITIVE AND EROTIC FEELINGS

Deep oh deep is grief,
but deeper still is joy.
Gibran, 1923,
The Prophet

One of the central goals of any psychodynamic psychotherapy is to increase patients' awareness of and tolerance for a mix of strong and conflicting feelings toward significant others. In Intensive Short-Term Dynamic Psychotherapy (ISTDP), the therapeutic process typically proceeds in a kind of spiral from the outer layer of defenses against emotional closeness, to anger, underlying pain and grief, and, finally, longings for closeness. The goal of treatment is to enable patients to acknowledge, contain, and integrate the full range of human emotion. All the layers of feeling must be accessed, experienced, and woven together in such a way that patients can see themselves and others clearly. Such emotional integration is a prerequisite for what is sometimes referred to as "whole object" relationships, in which both gratification and frustration are expected and tolerated. Basic needs for attachment and closeness are met without compromising the need for autonomy. Ultimately, an inner sense of personal freedom and a renewed or expanded capacity for joy should be evident.

DOI: 10.4324/9781003542131-6

Anxiety and Defenses against Positive Feelings

The process of de-repression reveals the factors that have been responsible for the avoidance of strong internal feelings and close emotional involvement with others. Anger and grief are not the only emotions that are capable of evoking anxiety and, hence, fuel avoidance. In many cases, there is considerable anxiety, guilt, shame, and inhibition around the experience and expression of warm, tender, loving, and sexual feelings. What is responsible for this? There is a good deal of debate about this matter. On the one hand are the drive theorists who view difficulties with closeness and the experience of positive feelings largely as an epiphenomenon (the result of defenses against reactive sadism and unresolved grief). This view posits that, to contain the forbidden feelings of anger and the painful feelings of grief, the patient maintains an emotional distance from others—for it is close contact that evokes these frightening affects. Because warm, tender, loving feelings lie beneath these other emotions, they get lost in the process. Davanloo (1990) seems to fall into this camp.

There is no indication in Davanloo's writings, clinical case reports, or presentations that he believed positive feelings can be directly associated with anxiety. With the oedipal situation, for example, Davanloo (personal communication, 1990–1991) developed the view that anxiety and inhibition regarding sexual feelings, impulses, and fantasies are secondary and indirect. It is not the sexual feelings themselves that are forbidden, he has argued, but the murderous feelings toward the rivalrous parent accompanying the sexual longings that are taboo. Therefore, working through the anxiety and guilt associated with the sadistic impulses should be all that is required to free the patient's sexual inhibitions.

Other theorists (Fairbairn, 1954; Winnicott, 1965), who have expanded and revised classical psychoanalytic theory to include theories of attachment and object relations, have suggested that affects are not *intrinsically* good or bad, safe or dangerous, but are *deemed* so as the result of direct experience with primary caretakers in early life. Those emotions that were freely expressed and responded to are more likely to recur than those that met with punishment and censure. In some families, rather harsh and violent behavior is sanctioned, whereas warmth and tenderness are forbidden. Children raised in such an environment would be expected to express anger and hostility with relative ease but to become anxious, defensive, and avoidant when positive feelings are aroused. Similarly, sexual feelings and behaviors can be accepted or prohibited, with direct consequences for the child's sense of comfort or anxiety in the presence of such feelings. If this is true, then dealing only with anger and aggression would not necessarily strip sexual feelings and impulses of their attendant anxiety, nor render their expression more likely.

Although a fusion of sexual and aggressive feelings is often discovered in patients who have serious difficulties with intimacy and closeness, my clinical experience suggests that dealing with anxiety and defenses against aggressive feelings is often insufficient for achieving ease and comfort with one's sexuality. To accomplish this, all the prohibitions against sensual contact must be explored. An integration of sexual and loving feelings does not necessarily emerge spontaneously, as these are actively kept apart in some cases. Direct therapeutic intervention aimed at achieving an integration of the two is usually required in those who have long kept them split. The case of the Man with Primary Impotence (in this chapter) will illustrate this type of work.

Sexual Feelings in the Therapeutic Relationship

Although longings for closeness and tenderness will most likely emerge following the experience of reactive rage and grief, their full expression may still be defended against if the danger associated with them is not exposed and critically evaluated. Again, the interaction with the therapist, which is a living example of the patient's characteristic mode of attachment, will provide the most direct information regarding those feelings, impulses, and fantasies that have become fraught with anxiety and dread.

The Early Emergence of Sexualized Feelings

Sexualized feelings can emerge very early in treatment. When this occurs, it either indicates fairly severe pathology or the fact that sexual feelings are being used as a tactical defense. On several occasions, male patients have raised the issue of their sexual attraction to me in the opening phases of defense work when pressure toward closeness is beginning to be exerted. The patient might say, "Well, I can't discuss that with you because you're an attractive young woman". Tactical defenses such as these must be immediately targeted with a statement such as, "What does my appearance have to do with this? You are here because of your difficulties, and to help you, I have to understand the problem. Now you tell me you can't go into it. How can I be of help to you?" In most cases, this approach is sufficient to turn the patient's ego against this defense. Inquiry can continue, and the sexualized content typically disappears.

Occasionally, however, the patient's focus on sexual impulses is strong and indicates a primary area of difficulty. In one such case, a young man came to treatment because of serious difficulties in relationships with women, most of which had a sado-masochistic quality. He reported feeling very anxious and upset to find that I was young and attractive. He had hoped I would be "old, heavy, and unattractive" so that he would not have to struggle so directly with his conflicts over sexual impulses. Inquiry revealed that his concerns were warranted. As an adolescent, he had sexually molested his sisters and was caught "breaking and entering" into the home of a young woman he planned to molest. More recently, he had been expelled from college for writing a threatening note (in blood) to a classmate who had insulted him. This historical information, along with the anxiety and disorganization apparent in the session when we addressed his attraction to me, all indicated serious deficits in ego functioning and were contra-indications for this type of treatment. He was referred to a male psychiatrist who specialized in the treatment of sex offenders.

Positive Feelings During the Midphase of Treatment

Positive feelings toward the therapist, marked by a heightened desire for closeness, sometimes have an erotic and sexualized flavor. These feelings typically emerge during the mid-phase of treatment, as reactive anger and grief get worked through. The therapist is often a target for these feelings, just as he or she had been for anger and grief earlier in the process.

It should be emphasized that warm, tender feelings are sporadically present from the early stages of treatment. It is not unusual for patients to comment on the relief and gratitude they feel toward the therapist at the end of the evaluation process. Facing thoughts and feelings that had long been avoided results in a feeling of mastery and a sense of safety within the therapeutic relationship.

As treatment progresses, and reactive anger and grief get worked through, positive feelings and longings for closeness emerge more clearly. If these feelings and impulses are not frightening to the patient, they will get expressed freely. In such cases reports of greatly improved interpersonal relationships will follow. Little, if any, work is required in the transference in these cases. However, when anxiety and defense accompany positive and erotic feelings, the therapist will likely become a target for the working through of these conflicts.

In this form of treatment, positive and sexual feelings are dealt with in the same direct and matter-of-fact manner as feelings of anger and grief. The patient is encouraged to face them directly, experience them fully, and "portrait" the impulses these feelings mobilize. In addition, getting such longings out in the open prevents the development of resistance, dependence on the therapist, and the development of a transference neurosis.

Clinical Examples

The Detached Observer: Part 2

The clinical material to follow is suggestive of an Oedipal conflict. As already detailed in previous chapters, the Detached Observer required a period of intensive pressure and challenge to facilitate a shift from a highly resistant stance to one of affectively charged involvement in the treatment process. During the mid-phase of treatment, following intense experiences of rage and grief regarding the loss of closeness with his mother, as well as her eventual death, positive and erotic feelings toward the therapist emerged. These were eventually linked with similar feelings toward his mother. Rivalrous feelings toward the therapist's husband, as well as toward his own father, were also revealed. As the triangular relationship conflicts were addressed, the pre-existing dyadic problems with both his mother and father emerged. Then the ways in which the pre-Oedipal situation affected the patient's adaptation to these intense and conflictual Oedipal feelings became clear.

The Emergence of Longing and Desire

The case of the Detached Observer, presented in Chapters 3 and 5, proceeded in a fairly straightforward manner from pressure and challenge to the patient's defenses against emotional closeness to a breakthrough of reactive sadism. This was followed by deep grief over longings for closeness with his mother that were never met.

Many sessions were spent on grieving both the ultimate loss of his mother by death and, even more so, the loss of what would have been possible had she been emotionally available when alive (see Della Selva, 1993, for a detailed account of this phase of the work). This patient tended to be attracted to women who were cool and aloof, as his mother had been toward him. As treatment progressed, he became more interested in women who were warm, friendly, and responsive. He wanted to date but found that, as soon as his desire for physical contact started to rise, he would get anxious and withdraw.

A similar pattern was discernible in the therapy sessions. As soon as we would begin to explore his sexual feelings and impulses toward women, he would become anxious and avoidant with the therapist. His defenses against sexual feelings were becoming a resistance in the transference, suggesting the presence of these forbidden longings for the therapist. When asked, the patient acknowledged that he had been having warm, loving feelings toward the therapist. As with other feelings, the therapeutic focus began with the actual experience of these feelings and desires.

Defense Before Feeling

PATIENT: It's just a longing to spend more time.

THERAPIST: You want to be with me, not to be separated. What is that yearning like inside?

PATIENT: I have these feelings, but what good will this do? I'm not going to have all the things I want from you, so why is this a good thing?

THERAPIST: Let's look at the effects if we don't examine these feelings. How is this any different from your angry feelings, for example? Now, obviously, we were not going to enact them—you were not actually going to sever my head and smash it against a brick wall, but the feelings were there and, if we didn't get to them and face them, they would become another brick in the wall. So, there's a big difference between experiencing a feeling and acting on it.

PATIENT: I draw a parallel to my mother. I couldn't touch her either.

THERAPIST: There's a desire to touch me.

PATIENT: Yeah.

THERAPIST: How?

PATIENT: To hold you on my lap. Your arms are around my neck and your head is on my shoulder.

Patients will attempt to rationalize their avoidance of loving, sexual feelings. In this case, the fact that these longings would not be gratified was initially used as an excuse to avoid the whole topic. The therapist dealt with this defense by pointing out that these feelings are no different from any other. By focusing on his past success in dealing with previously dreaded feelings (sadistic rage, in this case), while noting the disadvantages of avoidance, the resistance was successfully diminished and the work continued apace.

The images that accompany loving feelings and impulses are just as important as those that accompany anger and grief. These spontaneous images frequently contain direct links to the past, as will be revealed in the next vignette. Such images contain a wealth of unconscious meaning and are by no means arbitrary.

Next Session—Dangers Associated with Sexual Longings

PATIENT: The last time we were talking about sexual feelings, and I left feeling very agitated. Then at night, I had strong thoughts of someone

> breaking in—coming right through the glass doors with machine guns to get me. I also had thoughts of me having my own gun and blowing them away—it would be a fight.

Aside from the content being reported, which is of great significance, the ways in which this man related to the therapist was also of note. As is characteristic of patients in ISTDP, he took the initiative in sessions and got right down to work. The patient was fully involved, not only within sessions, but in between meetings, coming prepared with important material to work through. Because of his high level of involvement, the patient was encouraged to make his own interpretations about what is emerging.

THERAPIST: What do you make of it?

PATIENT: I related it to our session—talking about sex. It's like it's dangerous. It's life or death—kill or be killed. There's no scaring away. Even if I have the edge, if they turn around, I'll shoot them in the back so there's no coming back.

THERAPIST: So who are these men who are after you?

PATIENT: There are two. It's my father and, I guess, your husband.

Transference First

As a general rule, feelings, impulses, and fantasies regarding the therapist should be the first order of business. Often, therapists collude in the avoidance of the transference (the most anxiety-providing area for therapist as well as patient) by moving too rapidly to genetic figures (Gill, 1982). Failure to attend sufficiently to the transference has several consequences. First of all, feelings that are evoked but not expressed are, by definition, being defended against and will contribute to increased resistance over time. Conversely, by dealing directly with feelings in the transference, the possibility of transference neurosis and increased resistance is eliminated. This approach reduces resistance and, in so doing, speeds up access to the unconscious conflicts from the past that are being enacted in the transference. Therapists can become intensely uncomfortable about the patient's positive feelings toward them and must guard against discouraging their direct expression.

Herein lies another important distinction between ISTDP and traditional models of dynamic psychotherapy. Whereas the transference is avoided in the early stages of traditional analytic work and eventually becomes the focus for working through, the initial work in ISTDP is largely transference based. As the transference feelings are experienced and directly linked with genetic figures, transference distortions steadily decrease. The real relationship and the therapeutic alliance assume increasing precedence over time.

In this case, feelings and fantasies about the therapist were dealt with before shifting focus to the material regarding past figures. The patient imagined killing the therapist's husband, which would, he surmised, evoke despair and rage in her.

De-Repression of the Primal Scene

THERAPIST: How does the scene develop? What do you see happening as you shoot these men, who you say represent my husband and your father?

PATIENT: You wouldn't want anything to do with me. I would feel like I messed everything up. I'd end up alone again.

THERAPIST: So you end up alone again—the loser. That's happened before, huh?

PATIENT: With my mother. I had almost given up, but I wanted her.

THERAPIST: Because you remember a real closeness between your parents and how your mother would respond to your father.

PATIENT: Yeah, I remember watching them kiss passionately when I was five or six and wanting that. I also remember, in our last house, I was about 11, and I walked in on them. She was in his arms—they were naked and smiling. I said, "Oops", and walked out. My father was sitting on the edge of the bed, and my mother was sitting on his lap, with her arms around his neck. They were smiling.

The longing to hold the therapist on his lap is directly linked to the memory of the primal scene. His desire to take his father's place will be imagined in fantasy. This will also make his beginning remarks about guns and a fight to the death very meaningful.

THERAPIST: So your mother's body was very exposed then.

PATIENT: I saw she had beautiful breasts. She looked really sexy with smooth skin, and smiling.

THERAPIST: So she was clearly enjoying herself—smiling, with no tics or signs of anxiety.

PATIENT: My father was too, which I rarely saw.

THERAPIST: So there was something very special there, and you wanted some. What is the impulse?

PATIENT: I wanted her, there's no doubt about that.

THERAPIST: How would you get her?

PATIENT: I would look at him and say, "OK, you've had enough". I'd grab my mother and say, "She's mine now". He'd say, "Hey, that's my wife. You don't know how to treat her, what she needs".

THERAPIST: So he would put you down. How do you feel toward him?

PATIENT: It's bullshit—he didn't help her, didn't treat her right.

THERAPIST: You feel you could do better.

PATIENT: I would beat him out the door. I'd punch and disable him. Knock him unconscious. Kick him, then drag him out, and leave *him* out in the hall and close the door. Then I'd grab her and make love to her. I want to touch her all over. I want to be the one who makes her feel great.

The patient went on to detail a scene of mutually satisfying love-making. In his fantasy, his mother gives herself over to him and did not resist the satisfaction of his wishes. His father was the barrier and needed to be removed.

Further De-Repression

PATIENT: This is what I wanted—how I see it. The actual contact with my mother is great. The problem is that my father is lurking in the hallway.

THERAPIST: So you are still haunted, like the other night at home—listening for every sound, looking over your shoulder.

PATIENT: I can't let him keep lurking. I'd shoot him. There's a 22 caliber in his closet.

THERAPIST: You knew about this gun?

PATIENT: Yeah, I shot it.

THERAPIST: When?

PATIENT: Not until I was 11 or 12.

THERAPIST: So, the same age.

PATIENT: I had just killed something for the first time. My eyesight started going at that time (myopia). I wanted to shoot but didn't want to kill anything. I was out with a friend, who was trying to get a bird. I said, "Let me have a shot", but I never thought I'd hit it.

THERAPIST: So you knew about this gun, how to shoot, and that you could kill.

PATIENT: I used to take it out and play with it—just take it out of the case and look at it. I was interested in it.

THERAPIST: And now we can see why. It's all coming together—the rage toward your father for keeping your mother all to himself, your wish to get rid of him so you can have her to yourself, and your fear of these powerful feelings and impulses.

PATIENT: The way I see it is that, after I'm done with my mother, I realize he'll be back and then I go get him. He'd be lying on the carpet, naked. I'd shoot him in the chest a couple of times. His arms are splayed, his mouth open.

THERAPIST: How do you feel when you look at him?

PATIENT: A mix. Powerful but sad. I didn't want this. I felt I had to. He wouldn't let me near her. I wanted him to let her love me. I didn't want to kill

> him to get it. And I wanted her to give me some of the love and attention she gave him. It's the only time I ever saw her relaxed and happy.

This material, along with a wealth of developmental data gathered throughout the course of this man's treatment, suggested that his mother was very detached from him and that his father actively encouraged this distance. In fact, when, as a young boy, he attempted contact with his mother, she would become anxious and symptomatic. The patient's father would literally pull him away from his mother and say, "See what you're doing? Go to your room, leave her alone".

As such, this is a case in which detachment was actively encouraged, while affectionate contact was punished. It is no wonder that reaching out and directly expressing his desires for affectionate contact would be experienced as dangerous and avoided at all costs. His initial detachment from the therapist was a replication of this pattern. Although ultimately self-defeating, this pattern of interaction ensured safety. For him, being unobtrusive—appearing to need little contact—was the only way of gaining any proximity to his mother. For the patient to achieve deep insight, an understanding of how that pattern of attachment was developed, what it was designed to preserve, and how it currently backfires all had to become conscious. In addition, having an experience with the therapist that directly contradicted this experience was deeply affecting. The therapist's active and persistent attempts to know him in an intimate way, while simultaneously pointing out the pain and self-defeat in detachment, constituted a very specific corrective emotional experience and was experienced as profoundly healing.

There was every indication that this young man had been deprived of the loving, affectionate care of his mother and was taught to be tough, manly, and independent very early in his life. In addition, his mother was very ill and frequently left the home for days and weeks at a time, deactivating the normal attachment behavior between mother and child. He maintained whatever proximity he could to his mother by requesting nothing of her.

When, at the age of 11, he found his parents in bed together, what seemed to surprise him most of all was that they were relaxed and smiling. He repeatedly talked about her smile as he recounted this memory. I believe this is what he craved most. In his fantasy, he talked about having uninterrupted access to her, which *she* found pleasurable. He wanted to touch her and "make her feel great". He wanted to be the one to bring a smile to her face. He had never found a way to do this. From this experience, he concluded that sexual contact was something, perhaps the only thing, that would evoke a warm response from her.

In order to gain access to his mother, he would have to get rid of his father. It is striking that he de-repressed the memory of the gun in his parents' bedroom and how he had shot and killed a bird for the first time right after discovering them naked together. In fact, when he found the bird, it had been shot in the chest. In the fantasy of killing his father, he shoots him in the chest. Clearly, the bird unconsciously represented his father. Following this incident, his eyesight deteriorated rapidly and significantly. This is as close to the Oedipal myth as possible. After our work on the guilt he felt about these wishes, he had surgery to correct his extreme near-sightedness. He no longer needed to stay blind to his own desires or deprive himself of their satisfaction.

In the subsequent session, the patient spontaneously reported the fantasy of himself as a baby and child, lying on a blanket in a field next to his mother. What he felt most strongly was a desire to be suckled at the breast—to be able to touch, smell, and taste his mother. This longing was experienced as far deeper and more primary than the genital sexual longing he initially became aware of and, in many ways, was more difficult and less socially acceptable for a grown man to acknowledge. These two levels of desire need not be mutually exclusive. Most marriage and sex therapists (Schnarch, 1991; Zilbergeld, 1992) agree that an integration of these longings and desires deepens adult attachments and is a sign of health. In sexual ecstasy, boundaries are blurred, and blissful regression is experienced. Adults must be secure in themselves and their relationship to be able to achieve this.

A Taboo on Tenderness?

In our society, power, toughness, and a lack of sentimentality are viewed as hallmarks of maturity. To be tender, gentle, and sentimental is considered "babyish". There seems to be an especially strong prohibition against these feelings in men. Since sexual prowess is equated with power and toughness, men frequently sexualize their longings for closeness.

Ian Suttie (1937, 1988) suggested that there is a taboo on tenderness far more stringent than that against sexual feelings and impulses. Suttie is considered by many to be one of the most pivotal figures in the movement away from mechanistic drive theory to an object-related attachment theory. He hypothesized an impulse toward tenderness and affection that was social rather than biological in nature, and has been derived from self-preservation instincts rather than genital appetite. The aim of this impulse was considered truly interpersonal and required, for its satisfaction, "the awakening of an adequate response of appreciation and tenderness in the other person" (White, 1937).

This was graphically depicted in the Detached Observer's fantasy. He imagined awakening a response in his mother that he had not been able to evoke during his life. Suttie hypothesized that being pushed away by one's mother at an early age (which he referred to as "psychic weaning") would be particularly distressing because it constitutes the deprivation of contact which had been enjoyed "from time immemorial" (1937, 1988, p. 87). This was contrasted with the pain of being deprived of sexual gratification, something that might be desired but had never been experienced.

Suttie felt that, whenever this primary need for succor was frustrated or thwarted, anxiety and "neurotic maladjustment" would result. One of the distortions Suttie observed was that of sexualization of a desire for affectionate contact. The other, also evident in this case, was that of detachment. It is important for us, as clinicians, to help our patients sort out their longings and expand their repertoire of expressive behaviors, so that sexual activity becomes but one of many ways for expressing loving feelings.

The Man with Primary Impotence

Where there is a history of sexual dysfunction, working with sexual feelings and impulses, particularly as they emerge in the transference, is of critical importance. The man described here reported a history of primary impotence. His first experience in attempting intercourse, at age 16, resulted in the loss of his erection and inability to penetrate his girlfriend. This became a consistent problem that had plagued him for many years. The success achieved in this case is especially notable, since primary impotence has been a sexual dysfunction associated with severe psychopathology and carries with it a poor prognosis (Singer-Kaplan, 1974).

It became apparent from the beginning of treatment that the source of this man's difficulty had to do with a fusion of sexual and aggressive impulses. During the initial evaluation, his pervasive defenses against any meaningful closeness with the therapist were targeted. This resulted in an outpouring of grief over how superficial his relationships had been. Later in the session, following a ten-minute break, the resistance against meaningful contact with the therapist returned. This time, pressure on the defenses resulted in the experience of anger toward the therapist. The patient reported an impulse to "knock you over in the chair, flip you over and fuck you up the rear". The spontaneous expression of an impulse toward rape indicates a fusion between sexual and aggressive feelings. Before we can attempt to remediate such a problem, we need to understand how the fusion develops.

The material that emerged in this case provides a possible answer. Following the breakthrough of the sadistic impulse toward the therapist, the patient began to weep and recalled how his mother had insisted on wiping his bottom, even when he was seven and eight years old, by laying him across her lap in the bathroom.

Although there was something stimulating and gratifying about this contact, he also became aware of a fury toward his mother for using him for her own gratification. The patient's father worked nights, and because his mother was afraid of being alone, she had the patient sleep with her. One night, when he was about five years old, he witnessed marital rape. He woke up to hear his mother screaming and imploring him to go get a hammer and clobber his father.

The genesis of the fusion between sexual and aggressive feelings couldn't be clearer. He had learned, in an intense and direct manner, to associate sex with violent aggression. In his experience, both at home and in his tough city neighborhood, the notion that men take women aggressively was repeatedly reinforced. Being tender and loving was equated with being "soft" or "a sissy"—something to be avoided at all costs. He split loving and sexual feelings and kept them actively apart. He was unable to orgasm inside any attractive, age-appropriate partner and could only ejaculate inside women who were "old and ugly". At the start of treatment, he was both baffled and embarrassed by this pattern. Only once these feelings were faced in the transference and linked to unresolved conflicts from the past did the need to develop a kind of "Madonna and Whore" split become apparent.

Memories of these early experiences were highly traumatic and had been largely excluded from his conscious memory. The fantasy of raping the therapist served as a disguised memory of sorts. As the fantasy of raping the therapist faded and the memories of trauma from the past came into focus, the feelings associated with these early incidents could be approached directly.

If his sexual difficulties were the result of intense and terrifying feelings associated with past trauma, the reliving and reworking of these feelings in a direct manner should result in a relief of symptoms.

Therapeutic Strategies for Dealing with the Fusion of Sexual and Aggressive Impulses

When there is a significant fusion of sexual and aggressive impulses, the first task is to disentangle the two by draining the reactive sadism. This frees up the sexual feelings and impulses, which then need to be integrated with loving feelings. This session, from the mid-phase of treatment, will illustrate the beginning integration of sexual and loving feelings. This work also served to enhance the patient's sense of separateness from his mother and helped him to consolidate a sense of self based on his own needs and desires rather than those internalized from his mother.

The Emergence of Sexual Longing in the Transference

THERAPIST: That's a big smile.

PATIENT: I'm a little nervous about seeing you, but it's nice to see you. It's both. I'm nervous but it's nice to see you—a friendly face.

THERAPIST: So you have some warm feelings toward me.

PATIENT: Yes (uttered in an exaggerated tone with laughter).

THERAPIST: You get nervous about the positive feelings.

PATIENT: (now in a genuine and thoughtful tone). Yes. Yes I do. I'm very nervous. Maybe it has to do with you being a woman.

THERAPIST: What's anxiety-provoking about having positive feelings toward a woman?

PATIENT: With a woman, well, a potential lover.

THERAPIST: When did you become aware of these feelings toward me?

PATIENT: When I came in and saw you. I looked at you and, in fact, I looked at your legs. I said to myself, "Nice legs".

Integrating Sexual and Loving Feelings

THERAPIST: So there's a sexual flavor to these warm feelings.

PATIENT: Yes, and it's very difficult to talk about. With women it's difficult to let them into what I'm feeling. Not to digress, but isn't this separate from feelings of friendship and warmth? Isn't the sexual a separate kind of thing? I've always separated them.

THERAPIST: So this is really important, isn't it, and maybe it explains some of the heightened anxiety. You try to keep sexual and loving feelings separate but you have both feelings here toward me.

PATIENT: Yes, in fact, I've been thinking about you and fantasizing about you in a sexual and romantic way.

THERAPIST: And how about today? You notice my legs. What's the impulse? Is there a fantasy?

PATIENT: It wasn't an image but a feeling. It's forbidden territory. From the neck up is OK, but below is forbidden.

THERAPIST: So, if you can't split the loving and sexual feelings, you'll split me in two. This is a very strong tendency in you.

PATIENT: They've never gone together. I could never masturbate to the thought of a girlfriend. It was something forbidden, taboo, violating. I would imagine a friend's mother or a teacher.

THERAPIST: But now they exist together. You have both warm, loving feelings toward me and sexual feelings.

PATIENT: I look at your body and your face, but I almost separate them. Your face looks beautiful to me, you look beautiful to me. But when I go down past the neck I go, "WOW, that is sexual!"

THERAPIST: How do you experience these feelings?

PATIENT: It's a feeling of longing and desire, to take you, your arms, your shoulders, to hold you and fondle you. It's luscious—it's wonderful. I'm allowing myself to feel this.

THERAPIST: You say it feels luscious. So now it feels good—not so scary or forbidden.

The anxiety attendant to his sexual feelings was being stripped away, as he allowed himself to enjoy these feelings and desires—all of which composed a new experience.

T-P Link

THERAPIST: And what is it like to let me know about them?

PATIENT: Usually, I fear rejection—that you will resist me and say no. Very specifically, I picture rubbing you along your shoulders and your arms. It feels great to me but feels dissociated from you. As soon as I see your face, I think of rejection (suddenly sits up in his chair). It's like I'm fucking my mother! Oh shit, you know what I mean?

THERAPIST: How did that come to your mind?

PATIENT: That's the most taboo. Suddenly, I got an image of my mother in a blue dress with white polka dots. I loved that dress; it had a sheen to it. I remember sexual feelings, and it comes back to me, the feel of her belly—seeing her in her girdle.

The patient's initial comment, "It's like fucking my mother", certainly surprised me. I was suspicious that he was being provocative or sarcastic, as he could sometimes be. However, the immediate and specific memory of his mother in a particular dress, followed by a spontaneous link with his current fetish-like preference for women to wear silky slips and nightdresses, indicated a genuine unlocking of unconscious feelings and memories.

THERAPIST: Just like now, you love the feel of silky fabric over a woman's body.

PATIENT: Yes, and how the feel of her belly gives me excitement.

THERAPIST: So it starts here with letting yourself feel the sexual arousal toward me and then your mother comes to mind, along with memories of those feelings from the past.

PATIENT: I can see her in the bedroom and remember holding her, the warmth and softness of her belly—the hips and buttocks too, which I go crazy over now.

THERAPIST: So what do you want to do?

PATIENT: Rub her behind with my hands. I get aroused. Feeling the soft, fleshy contour of her hips and I move into the vaginal area, and I want to fondle and finger her. That feels like a building excitement and a hunger. It's funny, in the fantasy, I look up at her, so I'm small.

THERAPIST: And what do you see?

PATIENT: I see her face, like a Mona Lisa smile—a knowing, understanding smile. She's not angry. She says to me, "Now you know you're supposed to . . . " Oh, I mean . . . (Freudian slip).

THERAPIST: What's that like—if she's not angry and rejecting but wants you?

PATIENT: Very uncomfortable.

It is very important to follow the out-pouring of material and not to make assumptions about the direction it will take. Although the patient, and probably the therapist, expected the mother to be viewed as a sexually rejecting figure, the slip of the tongue in the previous vignette, along with other supporting material, indicated that the patient felt his mother had sexual desires for him. It was these desires that frightened him.

THERAPIST: Later you did feel she had sexual feelings toward you, and you remember those lascivious looks. What about in the fantasy, is she lubricated?

PATIENT: She's lubricated, yeah, ready. Wow, that's wild. Right now I don't feel upset about it. I don't even feel bad about it. I can imagine it feeling wonderful and I don't feel so much the prohibition and horror. There was a lot of sexual feeling there. She used to wipe my ass, and my cock was on her lap. I picture fondling her vagina. She's wet. I'm getting hotter and hotter exponentially. I'm erect and I enter her and we're having intercourse, and it feels great. Then I look at her face. It's my mother's face, and it's old and pale. I don't like it. It doesn't feel good. Her body and her face don't go together. I look at her face and it's, "Oh, yuck!"—a definite turnoff.

Again, the spontaneous flow of associations provided the context for understanding his earlier experience in the transference. The focus on the split between the therapist's face and her body "below the neck" reflected an existing split between feelings and perceptions associated with his younger and older mother. This got played out in his current life. He reported being unable to function sexually with attractive partners and could only have intercourse with women who he considered "old and ugly". He remained highly attached to his mother and has been unable to free himself to love and sexually enjoy a desired partner.

Erotic Attachment to Mother as a Defense against Grief

THERAPIST: What's the feeling now?

PATIENT: Real sadness. I feel real, real sad (starts to cry). I'm holding back, pushing it down, and I want to go back to when I'm fucking her.

THERAPIST: So you go back to her young body and the sexual feeling now to avoid looking at her. She's old and the feeling is sadness. To face her deterioration and death is painful, and you're tempted to go back to the warm, comforting body you remember when you were a boy.

PATIENT: The pain and anguish of watching her deteriorate—seeing her die a piece at a time. Watching someone you love to deteriorate is a terrible, terrible thing. This goes deep (crying). I've been having this feeling about young bodies. There's a resentment. I like to look at these young bodies but there's something scary about it—something taboo.

THERAPIST: You've just allowed yourself to face the feelings and fantasies toward your mother, which you sensed she also had toward you. What was really taboo was you having those feelings toward a young, age-appropriate woman. Like in your masturbatory fantasies as a boy—you couldn't let yourself imagine wanting your girlfriend sexually and you would substitute a mother figure. You've been true to her, holding onto her, and it's been very hard to let go. As you see her as she is and say good-bye, it seems to feel like a betrayal.

The preceding material suggested that his mother's eroticized attachment to him, and preference for him over his father, contributed greatly to an unresolved Oedipal conflict. Being the "Oedipal victor" cemented his unhealthy bond with his mother while interfering with his relationship with his father. Furthermore, his mother's jealousy of age-appropriate girls, and insistence that he sleep in her bed (displacing the father), undermined his ability to separate from her.

PATIENT: Yeah, I wonder about that.

THERAPIST: Facing the loss is very hard—you want to find a substitute (patient had recently started an affair with a woman in her mid-40s who, like his mother, had an old face).

PATIENT: It feels like my mother is inside of me. I've been worried about getting too old. I remind myself that I'm only in my 30s. It feels like my mother. She's dying and beyond help.

THERAPIST: So even if you have to die with her, you stay true. Both of you had difficulty saying good-bye. It seems you can't bear to leave her behind and go on with your life with a young woman. Would she want this?

PATIENT: She's always been so fucking selfish. She never had my best interest in mind. She only thought of herself and when I tried to do things for myself, like take music lessons, she'd curse me. I feel like I'm possessed.

THERAPIST: Do you want her inside of you or do you want her out?
PATIENT: OUT!

Ousting the Parental Introject

THERAPIST: How do you imagine that?
PATIENT: I picture allowing myself what I want. Being with a beautiful woman who is not neurotic. (In the past, he had displayed an uncanny ability to find women who were just as intrusive, controlling, and abusive as his mother had been.) I want to talk to her directly on the outside. "Get out of me. I'm not your baby boy! I'm not your baby boy!" (He starts to cry.) "There's nothing I can do for you. I don't want to die before I have lived. I won't let this happen".

This last vignette seems a powerful example of the role of pathogenic beliefs in the maintenance of psychopathology:

> Pathogenic beliefs warn the person who holds them that the pursuit of desirable goals, for example, to be independent, happy, or relaxed, or to have a good marriage or satisfying career, will endanger the person or others. To avoid these dangers, the person may renounce valued goals, and may develop inhibitions and symptoms.
>
> (Weiss, *How Psychotherapy Works*, 1993, p. v)

The origin of this patient's sexual conflicts was complex. He had unconscious guilt about wanting to displace his father and possess his mother sexually. He remained tied to his mother while simultaneously punished himself by choosing old, ugly women and depriving himself of the young, attractive women he actually wanted. In addition, there was evidence that had introjected his mother. She directly blamed him for her own deterioration and damned him to a life of misery and suffering as punishment. "You should live the life I lived!", was a declaration he heard repeatedly and a command he had lived out quite faithfully. She also told him she would die without him.

Through the therapeutic process, the patient came to realize that he had been keeping his mother alive inside of him. He said, "It's like she's in here and I just want her out. I want her out! I am not your baby boy! I am not your baby boy!" This ousting of the hostile introject, and declaration of freedom and independence, led to a transformation in his sense of himself as an autonomous being, capable of choice.

Whereas, in the case of the Detached Observer, the patient was able to reconcile his needs and desires with what he imagined his mother would want for him, in this case, the patient's mother cursed him and declared her wish that he live a life of misery and suffering. There was no way to undo this painful reality. It had to be faced and dealt with in some way other than the slavish compliance that had dominated his past.

In addition to experiencing and integrating his complex mixed feelings toward his mother, psychotherapy was necessary to expose and then disconfirm the pathological beliefs adopted through the relationship with his mother. The de-repression of his mixed feelings toward his mother would not have been sufficient to eradicate the pathological beliefs associated with them. His understanding of the rules governing interpersonal relations had to be examined and repudiated. By the end of the session just described, he was able to declare, with feeling and conviction, that he would no longer allow himself to be controlled by the fears and beliefs he had adopted at an early age. In facing that which he could not control (his mother's happiness), he was able to focus on that which he could effect—his own. A new sense of freedom ensued.

Those patients whose parents have consciously or unconsciously wished them ill must find their own will to live. This can only happen when they face and work through the painful reality of their parents' destructiveness. As Marie Cardinal (1983) put it, "Until you learn to name your ghosts and to baptize your hopes, you have not yet born; you are still the creation of others".

Bettelheim (1983) has suggested that achieving a separation from the internalized aggressor requires "an appropriate life-affirming counterforce", like psychotherapy. Up until the time this man entered treatment, his conscious and unconscious goals were in direct opposition to one another. Consciously, he wanted to be free, happy, and healthy. Specifically, he wanted to be able to love and be sexually expressive with the woman of his choice. Unconsciously, this was forbidden. He continued to comply with his mother's wish that he live a life of misery as she had, and, in so doing, stay loyal to her. As the unconscious feelings and memories came into view, a new alliance could be formed between his conscious and unconscious wishes, such that fulfilment of his needs and desires would be possible. Following this work, the patient formed a stable, loving, and actively sexual relationship with a woman who was both available and responsive, for the first time in his life.

Increased Freedom of Choice

This vital work highlights the crucial element of choice in the selection of current attachment figures. The issue is not simply one of having the ability to establish closeness and intimacy versus isolation and detachment, but one of expanding the arena of conscious choice over these matters. Emotional closeness is not necessarily good and healthy in and of itself, any more than keeping an emotional distance from others is necessarily pathological. It is frequently just as important to solidify patients' ability (and right) to keep a distance from those who would be damaging to them, as it is to enhance their tolerance for genuine intimacy with those who are responsive.

Many patients suffer because they are unable to protect themselves from the intrusiveness of others. The patient described here had an exceptionally intrusive and controlling mother, from whom he was unable to protect himself. As an adult, he tended to re-create this interpersonal drama by choosing women who were intrusive, controlling, and frequently violated his privacy in grossly inappropriate ways. For example, one woman he was dating broke into his home after a quarrel. Since she cleaned his apartment, fed the cats, and left flowers, she denied the incident involved any hostility or violation of his rights. It became just as important for him to learn how to establish boundaries with such women as it was to be able to pursue and become intimate with the kind of warm, responsive women he desired.

The goal is for patients to learn to be his or her own gatekeeper—allowing in only those individuals who are loving, while keeping a conscious distance from those who are damaging. In the novel *Like Water for Chocolate* (Esquivel, 1989), the necessity for this deep understanding of oneself as a prerequisite for achieving healthy, mutually gratifying relationships is beautifully depicted:

> My grandmother had a very interesting theory; she said that each of us is born with a box of matches inside us, but we can't strike them all by ourselves . . . Each person has to discover what will set off those explosions in order to live, since the combustion that occurs when one of them is ignited is what nourishes the soul.

She went on to say that it was equally important:

> To keep your distance from people who have frigid breath. . . . If we stay a good distance away from those people, it's easier to protect ourselves from being extinguished.
>
> (Esquivel, *Like Water for Chocolate*, 1989, pp. 115–116)

Gender Differences in Response to Trauma

It has been noted (Herman, 1992; van der Kolk, 1987) that men who have been abused and traumatized as children tend to identify with the aggressor and become victimizers as adults. Women, on the other hand, tend to consolidate an identity around their victimization and repeat a pattern of being victimized in their intimate relationships. In both cases, there is a deep fusion of sexual and aggressive feelings. What differs is the outward manifestation and behavioral sequelae of this fusion.

Most in the field have attributed these differences to socio-cultural influences that shape gender-related behavior. For either gender, the tendency to act out and repeat traumatic interactions is often viewed as a way of defending against remembering and experiencing a whole range of painful and disruptive feelings associated with traumatic memories. As the defensive element of the behavior is stripped away, the expressive element achieves dominance.

In the case just reported, the patient re-enacted early trauma in which sex and violence were acted out by victimizing women he considered weaker than himself. He would use them and discard them without regard for their feelings. In the following case, a woman learned to associate love with pain and subjugation.

The Masochistic Artist

This 40-year-old professional woman of considerable beauty, intelligence, and accomplishment came for treatment because of a marital separation that had precipitated an intrapsychic crisis. She was questioning both why she was having such a difficult time extricating herself from a clearly unsatisfactory marriage and what had motivated her choice in the first place. She entered treatment shortly after leaving her husband of 12 years and resuming an affair with an old lover. She was tormented by anxiety and guilt regarding this affair, which reinforced the painful sense she had of herself as weak and immoral. That she was separated and had endured many years of deprivation and mistreatment by her husband did not seem to factor into her understanding of her own behavior. Each time she would begin to entertain the notion of choice regarding her marriage, she would be overcome with anxiety and guilt, insisting she must try ever harder to reconcile with her husband.

During her marriage, the patient had become very successful in her career while her husband floundered. As soon as she had become established, he quit his teaching post and never regained any semblance of financial or professional stability. He became increasingly demanding of her in every way—to stay slim and ever more successful in her career while remaining beholden to him. No matter how much she accomplished, he was never satisfied. In fact, all her accomplishments were diminished and devalued by him. This pattern of control through demands and criticism paralleled the relationship she had had with her mother, who was described as "crazy as a tic". From the outset of treatment, it was this mother–daughter dynamic that was most prominent, not only in her relationship with her husband, but also in relationship to the therapist. This particular T-C-P link was the focus of early interpretive work.

In contrast, the patient's lover seemed to resemble her father. She described both as "Boy Scouts"—sweet, kind, responsible, and unassuming. The patient was initially reluctant to examine the relationship with her father and tended to regard it as unimportant. In the session to be recounted here, she reported having seen the movie *Cape Fear.* Her reactions and associations to the film were directly connected to her father, who she was beginning to realize was very possessive of her. I decided to use this opening to explore her sexual life and relationships with men by asking about her masturbatory fantasies.

Exploration of Masturbatory Fantasies

THERAPIST: We haven't looked at your sexual development. When did you start masturbating and what are your masturbatory fantasies?

PATIENT: Well my fantasies started around the age of six. Really my sexual fantasies always have been pretty masochistic—rape fantasies—things that are self-degrading.

THERAPIST: Let's look at one of the rape fantasies.

PATIENT: Well they can go all sorts of ways, like let's say a motorcycle gang or a burglar, but the heaviest one is about a family. I've been having that one more frequently lately.

THERAPIST: How does it go?

PATIENT: I'm in the country, looking for a piece of furniture, for example. There's a person who looks a little strange and he owns an antique shop. He wants me to look at something in the barn, but it actually turns out to be a torture chamber. He proceeds to rape and torture me. Then we go up to the house and the family is all there. His wife is into this too. There are older children and younger children. I keep thinking, what is this all about?

THERAPIST: What's your idea?

PATIENT: Well, it's obviously about a father figure and a family. It seems indicative of a lot of things. If I examine it, I won't be able to use it as a fantasy. You see, I'm not blind to the dynamic in which I am always the victim. But it goes back so far. My worst fear is that I've been so damaged from an early age that I won't be able to change it. I feel kind of fatalistic about it.

This sexual fantasy reflected her own family constellation. There was a mother and father, and two sets of children—older children from her father's previous marriage, and she and her sister from her parents' marriage. Sexual fantasies seem to offer a kind of window into the world of internalized object relations, defined here as an organization of mental representation of self and others that has been established early in life through the interaction between the child and significant others. In a thinly disguised way, sexual fantasies often reveal how the patient views intimate relationships, as well as revealing the source of these assumptions in the early family dynamics (Schnarch, 1991). As the patient would go on to say, the fantasies were "symbolically fraught", and not understood as actual memories.

The patient arrived for the next session in a state of acute distress. She felt compelled to return to her husband, as if she were trapped and had no choice but to reunite with this depriving and emotionally abusive man. She then reported a dream that she felt was highly significant. Dreams are often offered during the phase of treatment when de-repression is at its height. The dreams are typically quite revealing, with little distortion evident.

Dream Work

PATIENT: I had this dream about my father. There was a man who was my lover. We made love and it was nice. Afterward, I sat and watched him—like Picasso's "Sleep Watchers". Then it was like a sci-fi film where the guy turns into a werewolf, except he turned into my father as a young man. He woke up and raped me—sodomized me. It was a dream within a dream. In the dream within the dream, I was trying to wake up and I thought "Oh, that's it, that's it". What this is, I don't know.

THERAPIST: When the man was a contemporary, the lovemaking was nice. Then he turned into your father, and he raped you. How did that go?

PATIENT: I remember it was sodomy—penetration of the rectum. The clearest memory is what he looked like. It was so vivid. You know you forget what your parents looked like when they were young.

THERAPIST: What was your feeling in the dream?

PATIENT: Victimized.

THERAPIST: Any arousal?

PATIENT: No. I was frightened, and I wanted to wake up. But it was more than that. It was a clue or a hint. It made sense. I felt like "I got it" that was the main feeling.

Defenses against Cognitive Clarity

In a sense, this patient doesn't let herself know what she knows about her father and his sexualized attachment to her. Although the patient had no memories of being sexually abused by him, a wealth of memories surfaced that suggested he was overly concerned about her interest in boys and tended to project his own sexual feelings and desires onto her in a highly attacking and critical manner. As early as age six (the age when her fantasies began), her father insisted that she had a prurient interest in boys and their bodies while at a basketball game. When she was ten, she and her sister ran into some strange men on an island in a lake on their property. They made a hasty return to shore and reported the incident to their father. The patient's sister became hysterical, while she remained the calm one who got them safely to shore. Her father failed to attend to his daughter in distress or to the men on the island. Instead, he focused on the patient and her lack of emotional upset, suggesting she must have been interested in the men and liked their attention. Numerous other memories of his anger and jealousy regarding boyfriends were reported. The dream, then, seemed like a clear depiction of the way she experienced the relationship with her father. He became angry when she was involved with age-appropriate boyfriends (satisfying lovemaking with a peer in the first part of the dream), and behaved in an attacking and possessive fashion toward her (graphically depicted as a rape).

It is essential that we, as therapists, not jump to conclusions and take too literal or concrete an approach to dreams and fantasies. Again, there was no evidence that this woman's father raped or physically molested her. Nevertheless, his reactions to her were experienced as harsh and punitive. In fact, this more subtle means of undermining her confidence as a young woman increased her confusion about its source. The patient internalized the message that she was perverse and viewed herself in accordance with her father's projection. In so doing, she remained blind to her father's role and internalized these projections as her own.

Patient Makes Her Own Interpretation

PATIENT: I've been thinking about this—there's something in these fantasies. My father was a prince because my mother was such a witch. He would come home and rescue me and my sister. He knew that. If my attention was diverted to someone else, then he would notice and tease me about it or diminish it, because then he couldn't be the only one to rescue me.

THERAPIST: Perhaps the dream was an expression of how you felt—that he was jealous and possessive. His taking you is graphically depicted in this dream. Unlike the fantasies, in the dream you are terrified; this is against your will, and there is no arousal. Let's look at how you feel toward your father for treating you like this.

PATIENT: The feeling is blocked. I think the awareness—the "Oh, that's it", is beneath that.

Here, the patient confirms that it is essential to get in touch with emotions first, before moving on to interpretations. She seemed to be saying that her inability to feel was a way to remain unaware. It was all a part of a numbed and foggy state she had maintained about her relationship with her father. Access to her feelings was the key to understanding.

Alice Miller (1986) has suggested that there is a special prohibition against awareness of parental deficiencies, particularly in cases in which the parents are narcissistically vulnerable themselves. In this case, the patient's mother was very disturbed and was a frightening figure for the patient. She clung to the idea that her father was a prince and would save her from her mother. It would have been too overwhelming for her to recognize the deficiencies in both, so she denied her perceptions of her father's difficulties and readily accepted his projections.

Encouraging such patients to focus on their internal experience and to articulate these feelings is an invaluable aid in clarifying perceptions of self and other. Miller (1986) has stated that change occurs much more rapidly than previously considered possible when patients can articulate the childhood traumas they've experienced. These patients, whom I've referred to as self-sacrificing (Della Selva, 1991), focus on the feelings of others at the expense of their own experience. They do this so automatically; they literally don't know what they are feeling. Helping them to access and attend to their own feelings proves a reliable guide to their internal truth. At the same time, it is this very thing that has been forbidden and feels dangerous. The danger involved becomes clear in the next vignette.

Assessing the Dangers Associated with Feeling

PATIENT: I feel I have to give in—if I don't submit, I'll lose him.

THERAPIST: Let's see how that would happen.

PATIENT: I feel I can't struggle against it—that I have to hold something down inside me that wants to struggle against him but oh (cries out in pain and reports that she's been having back spasms).

THERAPIST: What do you make of these back spasms coming now?

PATIENT: I feel like my body is punishing me, but that's a very upsetting thought—to think I need to be punished, if that's what it is. Or, maybe, that I'm just so used to it.

THERAPIST: This is all coming together now—you submit to this pain and hold down the anger inside you—the part that wants to fight against him. What would happen if that came out?

PATIENT: I feel like I'd want to kill him, really. I'd strangle him.

The Roots of Masochism

The question this patient raised was vital, and one that has been a point of contention in the field. Is masochism the result of the patient's need to suffer, or a re-enactment of traumatic interactions that have become an ingrained pattern of attachment? The ways in which we understand the origins of masochism will directly and profoundly affect our attitude toward our patients and the therapeutic endeavor.

Davanloo (1988) has articulated the belief that masochistic patients have a need to suffer as punishment for their own violent and sadistic impulses. According to his view, these patients suffer from superego pathology. Consequently, treatment is directed toward the patients' sadism, guilt, and need for punishment through masochistic suffering. The possible danger in this approach is that patients feel blamed for their own suffering and are re-traumatized by the treatment. Should this occur, their sense of themselves as bad and deserving of punishment could be reinforced instead of being dispelled.

Although the notion of pleasure in suffering has a long history in psychoanalytic theory, this assumption has recently come under intense scrutiny (Shainess, 1986). There is increasing evidence that those who behave in a masochistic fashion are treating themselves the way they were treated as children. Their behavior constitutes an enactment of early, unconscious attachment patterns. In this way, patients' symptoms serve as a disguised means of communication.

When patients' defenses against feeling and remembering are eroded, the situations they faced as children become increasingly clear. As they are encouraged to face the rage toward parents and experience the grief over all that has been lost, symptoms that had previously served as disguised communications are rendered obsolete.

Since this woman tended to take on others' feelings and perceptions as her own, and stayed blind to her own internal truth, a focus on the experience of her true feelings was an essential step in the consolidation of an authentic sense of self. The patient was encouraged to experience the growing rage against her father. She declared a wish to annihilate him and peel off his skin, layer by layer.

THERAPIST: So you're no longer the submissive little girl. You are angry and you want to fight back. What is his reaction?

PATIENT: He doesn't have a chance.

THERAPIST: What does his face look like?

PATIENT: I don't want to see his face.

THERAPIST: Why not?

PATIENT: I don't want to see fear. I don't want to care about that. I don't care. I don't care.

Although the patient can be understood as holding onto anger as a way to avoid grief over the loss of her father, the anger was important in and of itself. This woman had not been able to access and utilize her anger to protect herself in the past. This had rendered her quite vulnerable to being used and abused, particularly by men. Her determination to hold onto the anger rather than sympathize with her father was a safeguard against losing herself in the experience of another. Although the ultimate goal was for her to be able to experience her own feelings while maintaining some empathic contact with others, focusing exclusively on her own experience at this point in treatment seemed necessary to tip the balance. I decided not to push her to experience the grief at that moment and, as the material in the following session reveals, it was not necessary.

Re-Playing Versus Re-Living

PATIENT: Before I felt like I was re-playing a situation from the past—literally re-playing it out of compulsion because there was something wrong with me. I couldn't really make my marriage work because something was wrong with me, and I really am an adulteress, and I really can't be trusted. And also, the sense that when I go to someone who is loving, it's the wrong person—it's all a mistake. More recently, though, I feel like I'm actually re-living a trauma. Not just reconstructing a situation, but actually re-living a trauma.

THERAPIST: And allowing yourself to experience all the feelings in reaction to it.

This statement, along with the material that will be revealed in a subsequent session, lent considerable support to the hypothesis that the source of this woman's masochism was a compulsive re-living of the early relationship with her parents. What she had been unable to remember and directly experience in relation to the past was replayed in her current intimate relationships. Once that repetitive dynamic became clear, and she began to experience the feelings of rage and grief she had repressed, her whole demeanor changed. There were immediate and dramatic decreases in symptomatology, and even more impressive, dramatic changes in her sense of herself, others, and the world. These changes will be illustrated in Chapter 7.

Summary

As feelings of reactive rage and grief over losses are experienced and integrated into conscious memory, positive feelings toward the therapist, frequently linked to genetic figures, become prominent. These positive feelings can, and often do, include a sexualized longing for physical contact. In my experience, the anxiety and defensiveness that often accompany these feelings should not be minimized, nor should they be considered a mere consequence of unresolved anger. Frequently, these feelings and impulses are quite anxiety-provoking in and of themselves. The dangers associated with their experience and expression have roots in the past and need to be exposed and re-evaluated for therapeutic change to occur. As anxiety wanes, tolerance for positive feelings and longings for closeness increase. These changes enhance the quality of the patient's current relationships.

7 WORKING THROUGH TOWARD CHARACTER CHANGE

> Man's main task in life is to give birth to himself, to become what he potentially is. The most important product of his effort is his own personality.
>
> *Eric Fromm (1947), Man for Himself*

For the therapeutic process to achieve rapid and enduring change in a patient's character, the intrapsychic system must be in a state of disequilibrium. Frequently, an external crisis in the patient's life begins this process. When no such crisis has occurred, or the patient's ego is constricted by the rigid use of character defenses, Davanloo (1990) advocated creating an intrapsychic crisis using the techniques of pressure and challenge. Once achieved, continual pressure to remain highly emotionally and cognitively involved in the therapeutic process keeps characteristic patterns of adaptation from settling back in. This, in turn, facilitates the working through of core conflicts and solidifies character change.

DOI: 10.4324/9781003542131-7

What is "Working Through"?

Freud (1914) considered the process of working through to be the feature of psychoanalytic treatment that distinguished it from other, more suggestive forms of therapy. Despite the lip service often given to the crucial nature of working through for the ultimate success of therapy, less has been written about this process than any other aspect of psychodynamic treatment (Weinberger, 1995). In addition, the lengthy nature of most psychodynamic treatment has made any systematic research into the process of working through untenable. So, we'll begin with what has already been written about this vital process and proceed from there.

Early in his work, Freud discovered that catharsis was a necessary but insufficient ingredient for the achievement of stable and enduring change. The process that occurs *after* an insight is obtained and leads to stable changes in feelings, attitudes, and behavior has been called "working through". During this process, insights are translated into observable changes in the patient's ego functioning. These changes include improved modulation of anxiety and affect, alteration in the patient's defensive structure, and modification of internalized images of self and other. Because all defensive processes originate in the ego, the functioning of the ego is altered when defenses are dismantled through the process of working through. Greenson (1967) wrote that working through operates "only on the ego", and for treatment to be considered successful, "the ego has to give up its pathological defensive function".

Working through is the "meat" of dynamic psychotherapy and constitutes the mid-phase of treatment. It is the longest and least predictable phase of therapy and varies most widely from patient to patient and therapist to therapist. In part, such variability may be due to the lack of guidelines for conducting this crucial aspect of the work. This is especially troubling because this phase of psychotherapy seems to have the greatest impact on outcome. Wachtel (1977; 1993) has suggested that most failures in psychotherapy are attributed to a lack of working through and rarely, for example, to a lack of insight. He reminds us that, in psychotherapy, as in life, it is follow-through that makes the difference.

The Process of Working Through

Nearly all definitions of working through involve the notion of repetition. According to Greenson (1967), during the process of working through "a variety of circular processes are set into motion in which insight, memory, and behavior change influence each other". As this process occurs, it needs to be repeatedly reviewed to deepen insight and further the process of change. In Intensive Short-Term Dynamic Psychotherapy (ISTDP), this type of circular process is set into rapid motion and maintained within an affectively charged atmosphere, speeding up the process of working through.

We can only gauge the success of working through in a post-hoc fashion, by observing changes that occur subsequent to our interventions. The depth and stability of these changes are put to the test when the patient faces a conflictual situation and displays the following changes:

1 A reduction in anxiety.

2 Decreased reliance on defensive processes.

3 An increase in emotional activation and freedom of affective expression.

4 Cognitive understanding of the relationship between feelings, anxiety, and defenses.

5 A newfound sense of mastery that overrides feelings of helplessness.

6 Increased adaptive capacity suggesting psychological growth. Each of these elements will be briefly reviewed.

Reduction Changes in Anxiety

Although all dynamic psychotherapists understand the importance of the triangle of conflict (the relationship between impulse/feeling, anxiety, and defense), different schools of thought seem to place particular emphasis on one factor over the others when intervening in neurotic styles of behavior. The drive theorists view the strength of the impulses as the determining factor in neurotic maladjustment, and tailor their interventions to tame the impulses by increasing the role of secondary processes. In other words, "Where id was, let ego be". The ego psychological approach suggests that it is not the feelings or impulses themselves that cause the trouble, but the habitual use of pathological defenses against their full and direct experience. Consequently, their therapeutic strategy involves efforts aimed at an alteration of defense and resistance.

Yet another set of theorists (Dewald, 1972; Wachtel, 1977; 1993) have suggested that the *excessive anxiety* associated with feelings and impulses is the driving force behind neurotic behavior. This factor has been "relatively neglected" by psychodynamic theorists (Weinberger, 1995). Davanloo is an exception. The therapy he has developed, like many learning-theory based approaches to therapy, emphasizes the importance of *exposure* to anxiety-provoking stimuli. In ISTDP, patients are encouraged to face their problems very directly. As the anxiety originally associated with forbidden feelings and impulses is reduced or eliminated, the pathological defenses that were designed to avoid that anxiety will no longer be required. Then, the adult ego will be free to adduce new and more adaptive strategies for the expression and satisfaction of feelings and desires. Working through can be conceptualized as a series of extinction trials in which affects become detoxified (Wachtel, 1977). The result is increased freedom of expression.

A reduction in anxiety is undoubtedly a goal of psychotherapy, but how can therapists help their patients achieve this goal? Dewald (1972) suggested that the gradual elimination of anxiety, guilt, and shame, so essential in the remediation of psychopathology, is the result of the "repeated exposure to rational perception and conscious integration" provided during the phase of working through. Davanloo would agree. Anxiety increases as the forbidden feelings and impulses are approached. Once the feeling breaks through the repressive barrier and is directly experienced without the feared consequences occurring, anxiety is reduced. This is particularly powerful when it occurs within the therapeutic relationship (Teyber, 1992). Patients tend to become increasingly bold following such an experience, expressing themselves more freely. This typically results in positive interactions with others, further reducing the anxiety that was previously associated with affect.

Take the Woman with Panic Attacks (see Chapter 5) as an example. The experience of anger was highly anxiety-arousing for this patient, and she avoided it at significant cost. As the root of her dread was deeply unconscious, so an exploration of conscious reasons why she felt that her anger was dangerous would have yielded little of therapeutic value. Davanloo suggested that we expose the conflict by approaching it directly. As the patient talked about anger toward her husband, the therapist applied pressure on the defenses to facilitate the actual experience of her rage. It was the direct and current experience of anger toward her husband for being away from home for long periods of time that provoked the impulses to kill him. As she faced the impulse to stab him, the image of her dead mother appeared. Then, the memories of the trauma associated with her mother's death came into consciousness, providing an opportunity for the patient to relive (emotional) and then re-evaluate (cognitive) the situation from the perspective of an adult. As a child, she experienced an overwhelming sense of guilt about her mother's death. She was so filled with anxiety and dread, lest anyone find out about the death wish she harbored toward her mother, that she sealed off the entire experience from her consciousness. These feelings and memories only broke through into consciousness following the experience of murderous rage toward her husband.

As an adult, she understood that her angry wishes did not cause her mother's death and no longer needed to be feared and avoided. Instead of judging herself so harshly for the anger she felt toward her mother, she was able to feel some compassion for herself. Consequently, she was no longer anxious and panic-stricken about feeling anger toward her husband. Instead of avoiding the anger by creating distance from him, she was able to use her anger constructively by requesting that her needs be taken seriously. The de-coupling of anxiety and guilt from her anger, which came about as a result of the working through process, was a key factor in her recovery.

As this brief example illustrates, repeating in the present that which was experienced as traumatic in the past can create the opportunity to re-evaluate the danger of feelings, impulses, and wishes which were experienced as forbidden in the past.

Evidence of Decreased Reliance on Defenses

Malan and Osimo (1992) have suggested that symptom removal alone is insufficient to accomplish character change. Indeed, for the process of working through to be considered complete, every symptom and pathological defense must be replaced with something adaptive. Clinicians spend most of their time and effort detecting defects in the regulation of affect and cognitive processing of their patients, rarely considering in any depth what non-defensive ego functioning actually looks like.

Norma Haan (1977) filled in this gap by detailing the differences between coping (healthy adaptation), defending (neurotic solutions), and fragmenting (psychotic decompensation). Coping is defined by flexibility and conscious choice. Coping behavior is purposeful and adaptive. In contrast, defensive behavior is rigid, habitual, and propelled by unconscious forces. Defensive behavior is driven by the past and distorts the present, while coping behavior is aimed at the future and oriented to present reality. Patients with fragile egos and few internal resources can fragment when overwhelmed with anxiety. Becoming flooded with anxiety prevents adaptation and often leads to repeated traumatic experiences.

These definitions can help us to be specific about the kinds of changes we are looking for in our patients. The goal of working through is to help patients become more conscious and purposeful in their behavior, employing flexible and adaptive choices. The *process* of living often changes more noticeably for patients than their specific behaviors. For example, patients who feel anxiously driven to prove themselves, like the Masochistic Artist (see Chapter 6), may spend many hours at work. Following a successful treatment, they may be as busy and productive as before, but they report a sense of freedom and delight in their work, rather than feeling driven by a need to perform, please, and produce.

When changes begin to occur, and the patient deals directly with a feeling or conflict that had been avoided by defensive means in the past, the contrast between the two should be highlighted. This gives the patient another opportunity to critically assess the differing experiences and outcomes, which further solidifies the new changes.

Increased Freedom of Emotional Expression Along with Cognitive Understanding: The Role of Integration in the Process of Working Through

Affective activation provides an effective means for gaining rapid access to core conflicts. As these conflicts come to life within the therapy session, they can be dealt with directly. This process provides a pathway for achieving a thorough intellectual understanding of emotionally felt experience—a vital ingredient for working through aimed at rapid therapeutic change.

According to Strupp and Binder (1984), who have conducted years of research on the process of change in short-term dynamic psychotherapy, the key to therapeutic success is "conceived of as the affective experiencing and cognitive understanding of current maladaptive patterns of behavior that repeat childhood patterns of interpersonal conflict" (pp. 24–25).

Initially, as defenses are abandoned, patients experience considerable depth of feeling. Davanloo insisted that interpretive work, conceptualized as a cognitive reanalysis of the process, must *follow* these emotionally charged experiences within the therapeutic setting. At this juncture, the therapist can meaningfully focus on the repetitive patterns apparent in the patient's life and can begin to understand what one patient called "the elegant economy" of symptomatic behavior. What had seemed senseless now has meaning. With fresh insight into the meaning and function of patterns that have affected both past and current functioning, new options can be considered. Furthermore, having a different experience in the here and now solidifies change. As Freida Fromm-Reichman (1950) has reminded us, "The patient is in need of an experience, not an explanation". Understanding the patient's current patterns in light of past experience is rarely sufficient to facilitate change. Having a new and different experience in the here and now, facilitated by facing, rather than avoiding, one's true feelings, consolidates the process of therapeutic change.

There seems to be a fairly wide consensus in both the clinical and research literature that the most effective and efficient method for accelerating the process of working through is a two-pronged approach: (a) mobilize intense affect; and (b) examine the thoughts, memories, and beliefs associated with these feelings as they emerge in the affect-laden communications from patient to therapist. By including both affect and cognition in the process of analysis, the experiencing and observing functions of the ego are interwoven, facilitating integration of these two spheres.

Mastery and Competence

Achieving a sense of mastery and competence can be achieved by overcoming a sense of helplessness. All the elements involved in working through, discussed so far, increase feelings of competence and mastery. Greenson (1967) suggested that patients often deal with feelings of helplessness engendered by early trauma by actively repeating the unresolved conflict from the past over and over again in their current lives. In so doing, "The ego, which was passive in the original traumatic situation, actively reproduces the event at the time it chooses, in circumstances favorable to it, and thus slowly learns to cope with it" (Greenson, 1967, p. 178). This repetition frequently takes place within the therapeutic relationship. Patients test their therapists by doing their typical dance and waiting for a response. In order to achieve therapeutic results, therapists need to respond differently from significant figures in the past, so that the same old story has a new ending. According to Malan (1979), "What went wrong must go right, again and again". In fact, this is the essence of the Control Mastery theory developed by Weiss (1993). He suggested that therapists will only know if they have passed the test by the patient's response. He found that patients become more open and expressive when therapists pass the test, while deflating in response to a failure.

Regardless of the particular goals to be achieved in any given therapy, character change has not been complete until and unless a fundamental shift from passive to active involvement in one's own life has occurred. Research confirms the notion that enhancing a patient's sense of mastery is crucial to positive outcome (Weinberger, 1995). How is this achieved? In ISTDP, patients are encouraged to assume an active role in their own treatment from the outset. The therapist expresses an inherent confidence in patients' ability to face difficulties and cope at their highest level of their ability. In addition to this somewhat general factor, more specific elements are also required to facilitate patients' growing sense of mastery. As patients become conscious of the particular thoughts and feelings they had previously defended against, they are free to deal with them in a conscious and intentional manner, typically leading to more effective behavior. This effectiveness leads to a sense of mastery.

Research (Bandura, 1986; 1989; Hollan, Evans, & DeRubeis, 1990; Whisman, 1993) strongly suggests that a patient's attribution regarding the cause of change significantly affects long-term outcome. Those patients who attribute their therapeutic success at termination to their own efforts were able to sustain their gains, whereas those who attributed success to external factors, such as their therapist, tended to regress following termination (Bandura, 1986; 1989). These attributions relate to whether patients experienced a sense of mastery in dealing with their own problems or whether they felt "cured" by the therapist. Davanloo's techniques place a great deal of emphasis on patient responsibility. Patients often report that, while treatment was difficult, they feel proud of themselves for working hard and facing their problems. This seems to bode well for future success.

As patients gain experience with an active mode of dealing with situations and feelings they had passively avoided in the past, a new or renewed sense of enthusiasm for life emerges. New tasks are approached with vigor, while old conflicts tend to be re-visited from this active, competent position. One patient, who had always felt completely helpless and overwhelmed in the presence of her mother, began to feel her own strength as she allowed herself to experience anger over the harsh treatment she had received at her mother's hand. She spontaneously said, "I'm 36 now, not a little two-year-old. I could literally kill my mother with my own two hands". She then smiled and said she had started working out at a gym and was enjoying her newfound upper body strength. This feeling of mastery expanded her view of herself to include a power to affect her surroundings and interactions. She was taking stands at work and getting noticed by her boss. Such pervasive alteration in her functioning denoted genuine character change.

Authors from James Mann (1973) to Alice Miller (1986) contend that it is essential to acknowledge the very real helplessness our patients experienced as children. However, this must be contrasted with their current ability to affect the world. It is this crucial distinction in our patients' view of themselves—from a helpless child to an active adult—that must change for psychotherapy to be successful. It was just this sort of change that occurred, during the therapeutic process, in the case of the Man with Primary Impotence (see Chapter 6). When treatment began, he defined his problem as a pervasive sense of helplessness. He reported feeling small and weak, as if he had no solid center of being. He contrasted this with his perception of his colleagues, who he viewed as competent adults. After the session detailed in Chapter 6, he was able to declare that he was no longer his mother's baby, but a man willing and able to make his own choices in life. Follow-up studies suggest that this kind of change endures and expands over time; affecting future behavior (Abbass, 2015; Abbass & Katzman, 2013; Abbass et al, 2017; Shedler, 2010; 2012).

From Regression to Growth

Change occurs as the *result* of a process of integration and application of the knowledge obtained in therapy. When concrete and stable change in behavior occurs, we conclude that the conflict that had previously prevented adaptive functioning has been "worked through". In more operational terms, we can say that conflicts are worked through when there is evidence in each corner of the triangle:

1 A reduction in anxiety.

2 An increased tolerance for the experience of affect.

3 Decreased reliance on defenses.

4 Increased capacity for intellectual and creative functioning, and an increased ability to form and maintain intimate relationships.

As this definition suggests, working through has been accomplished when growth resumes. Menninger (1958) suggested that the process of working through facilitates the transformation from regression to growth. When this occurs, "The infantile aims and goals lose much of their compulsive force; the patient is then free to choose or to develop new techniques, aims and goals that are more adaptive and gratifying" (p. 75). He went on to say that such a transformation requires "strenuous effort" and involves the rarely mentioned dimension of change called the will. Davanloo frequently spoke about the central importance of the patient's conscious will to change and exhorted them to assume control of their own behavior in alignment with their own will (as opposed to complying with the will of others). He has emphasized that our patients feel helpless, not only in dealing with the external world, but in the face of their own internal feelings and reactions. Both must be mastered for success to be considered complete.

Implications for Treatment

Before we can begin to understand and treat neurotic maladjustment, we must be explicit about our assumptions regarding what constitutes healthy functioning. How do we understand human nature? Are our most basic feelings and impulses anti-social and in need of strict restraint? So say the drive theorists. An alternative view is that our feelings and desires are basically healthy and sound, but when associated with anxiety, guilt, and shame, their means of satisfaction become distorted and ineffective. The solution depends on the definition of the problem. In the first case, renunciation of wish fulfilment is the answer. In the second, finding appropriate avenues for the direct gratification of basic needs would be the goal.

Davanloo's treatment model (1980, 1990) was based upon the latter set of assumptions. His therapy was designed to boost the development of ego functions such that patients are able to operate at their highest level of ego-adaptive capacity. This includes the ability to relate to others in a clear and direct manner, to work productively, and to pursue their dreams and develop their potential.

When symptomatic, patients defend against painful and anxiety-provoking thoughts, feelings, and memories in a way that prevents adaptive functioning in current life. The goal of treatment, achieved by the process of working through, is for the ego to attain or regain its ascendance. Then, those feelings or situations that used to arouse anxiety and generate the deployment of pathological defenses are dealt with in a deliberate and adaptive manner. For this type of change in ego functioning to be maintained, each pathological defense must be replaced with an adaptive strategy for coping.

The power and strength of ISTDP is achieved by combining and integrating all the preceding strategies. Rather than focusing on one aspect of conflict, whether it be feelings, anxiety, or defense, to the relative neglect of the others, all of these vital ingredients are addressed as a totality. This involves linking the three corners of the triangle of conflict (feelings, anxiety, and defense). While in certain cases, one aspect of the triangle of conflict may be particularly troublesome and will require focused attention, it is the deep understanding of the inter-connectedness of feelings, anxiety, and defense that is considered necessary to resolve a conflict. To facilitate the process of working through, the triangle of conflict is then linked with the triangle of person (therapist, current figures, and past significant others). The goal is for patients to become cognitively and affectively aware of the repetitive patterns of interaction that have predominantly influenced their functioning. As patients viscerally experience the power of these dynamics in their lives, particularly in the transference, they become consciously aware of the central issue or conflict that has been perpetuating these repetitions. This awareness creates the possibility of conscious choice regarding the satisfaction of their goals in a way that will facilitate growth and satisfaction with life, rather than fuel regression and perpetuate misery.

To achieve this end, some patients need more work in one realm than another. So, even though ISTDP focuses a great deal on the experience of feelings and impulses, the emphasis on insight and understanding is equally strong. In fact, greater time and effort may be devoted to the cognitive re-analysis of the triangle of conflict than in achieving affect-laden breakthroughs, especially with more fragile patients. It has been Davanloo's ability to deal equally well with each of these elements and to rapidly determine which patients require what kind of emphasis, that has contributed to the rapid and dramatic changes in those he treats.

This process has been operationally defined by Malan for purposes of training and research. His studies (Malan, 1976; 1979; Malan & Osimo, 1992), along with others investigating the effectiveness of STDP (Trujillo & McCullough, 1985), have provided data consistent with the view that successful outcome in psychotherapy is highly correlated with the frequency of affectively meaningful T-C-P links. This particular interpretation has been designed to facilitate an integration of cognitive and affective levels of experience.

Technical Considerations in Working Through

Once again, the differences between traditional analytic treatment and ISTDP are in technique, not theory or goals. Greenson (1967) espoused the traditional view that working through must be, by definition, a long and arduous process. In his classic text, he described how one particular insight was worked through over a period of six months of almost daily sessions. He went so far as to state that any rapidity in the process of working through would, by definition, be superficial and transient. We have since learned this is not the case. In fact, this condensed form of treatment can lead to rapid, deep, and long-lasting change (Alexander & French, 1946; Malan & Osimo, 1992; Abbass, 2015; Abbass & Katzman, 2013; Coughlin, 2018, 2022; Coughlin & Malan, 2018).

Maintaining a highly focused approach is critical. Rather than maintain "evenly hovering attention", Davanloo has suggested that we return to Freud's initial therapeutic stance of "seizing the resistance by the throat". Paying special attention to the repetitive patterns in the patient's thoughts, feelings, defenses, and behavior in a selective fashion will accelerate the process of working through. Rather than finding patient's conflicts to be highly complex and "overdetermined", Davanloo has found that they tend to be quite elementary in nature (Bauer & Kobos, 1987). What may appear to be a complicated picture of symptoms and defenses can often be viewed as derivatives of basic conflicts around love and loss, anger and betrayal. The process of working them through is accelerated by such clarity.

ISTDP employs the following active intervention strategies to facilitate the process of working through:

1 A high level of therapist activity.

2 A focus on the patient's current life (the C corner of the triangle of person, so often ignored in treatment).

3 Attention to change within and between sessions.

4 Encouraging the patient to assume an active, rather than passive, role in his or her own treatment and own life.

In ISTDP, the therapist makes it quite clear that real change in behavior is the goal. We are not involved in an intellectual exercise or mere expansion of self-understanding. Patients come to our offices because they are suffering and want to change. The therapist positions him- or herself on the side of change, creating an alliance with the healthy part of the patient's ego. As soon as an insight is achieved or a declaration is made, the therapist applies some pressure on the patient to behave in accordance with these intentions. Questions such as "Then what are you going to do about the smiling, the diversion, and the avoidance of this feeling?" or "Let's see if you can take this opportunity to do it differently and let me know, directly, how you feel this growing anger toward me?", make it clear that change is expected to follow insight. This active encouragement to put insights into action within the therapy session provides a new experience—one of mastery—within a safe environment.

Although some may consider these interventions new and radical, they have a long history. Freud encouraged his patients to approach what they fear, not just in the analytic sessions, but in their daily lives. Freida Fromm-Reichman (1950) believed it was essential to "train" patients to test out any insight gained in therapy sessions by "investigating it in its relatedness to their practical living and to the conduct of their relationship with others" (p. 144).

The therapist not only encourages change but models persistence and follow-through by drawing the patient's attention to each change as it occurs and then processing how it feels to do things differently. This step is often neglected and may be partially responsible for the added repetitions often required to foster change. Focusing on a single instance of change in some detail and comparing it with past experiences enhances the contrast between the two. This provides another opportunity to assess the relationship between behavior and outcome—both how past defensive maneuvers have contributed to the perpetuation of suffering, and how the present experience of direct affective expression leads to feelings of strength and competence. Such an analysis yields further impetus to change.

The Central Importance of T-C Links

In traditional psychoanalysis, getting to the past seemed to be the goal. The transference pattern of behavior was used to achieve the end of reconstructing the past. All too often, the patient's current life outside the analysis gets neglected. Ferenczi and Rank were the first to caution against this relative neglect and suggested that a focus on T-C links; only going to the past as necessary to facilitate an understanding of the present conflicts. All three corners of the triangle of the person must be attended to for working through to be complete, but the transference and the past recede in importance over time, while changes in the present become the most significant aspect of the work.

Practical Application of New Learning

During graduate school, I had an opportunity to train in the martial arts. Most of the training sessions were spent honing skills and techniques through repetition and drill. Within the group setting, sparring was structured and safe. The real question was, would the techniques learned in this environment be generalized to life on the street, where one might actually have to employ them? The teacher did not leave this to chance. At the end of each session, he would say, "Now it's practical application time". He would portrait scenarios in which students might need to use the techniques learned in class to protect themselves. This was of enormous value when I was jumped from behind one morning while walking to class. I could hear my teacher's voice in my head and quickly ran through my options. I was able to scare away the attacker. Without the bridge from technique to application provided by my teacher at the end of each class, I might not have been able to apply what I had learned. This is what we need to do in a systematic way during the working through phase of therapy.

Therefore, in the practice of ISTDP, the therapist encourages active attempts at change within the hour and communicates quite directly to patients that changes in their current life are expected as well. When a change occurs in relation to the therapist, the implications for the patient's current life and relationships are addressed directly. This link is neither left to chance nor assumed to occur spontaneously.

For example, a woman came into a therapy session reporting fury with her husband, which she dealt with by withdrawing from him. During the session, she was helped to look at how this pattern of avoidance was being repeated with the therapist. The patient was encouraged to do things differently in the session, expressing her anger and frustration with the therapist in a direct manner. Following this experience within the therapeutic relationship, it was essential to return to the precipitating incident in the patient's current life and ask how she would like to deal with the anger toward her husband, having had this new experience as a viable alternative to her characteristic withdrawal. The new options were imagined and played out in fantasy.

Portraiting

The technique of "portraiting" or visualization, discussed earlier as a useful tool in facilitating affective expression in the transference and about past figures, can function like a role play for current conflicts, providing a bridge between insight and action. This technique allows the patient to practice new behavior in the therapeutic setting and anticipate the outcome, before instituting it in the outside world.

This kind of work expands the experiencing and observing functions of the ego and enhances the patient's ability to integrate the two. It should be noted that both positive and negative reactions to the patient's changes should be anticipated. Although therapists tend to encourage openness and honesty, many of those the patient will encounter in "real life" will not. To avoid unnecessary disappointment, it is helpful to ask patients how they would feel if their new changes were not welcome. A focus on self-validation, rather than excessive reliance on other validation, is another way to inoculate patients against reactivity should others fail to respond as the patient might wish.

Follow-Up Inquiries

The therapist needs to keep track of the process and to follow-up on changes from one session to the next. It is essential to check on possible delayed reactions to changes observed in the therapeutic setting, as well as to inquire about additional changes in their current life. It's not unusual for a depressive to feel buoyed by the direct expression of anger in a session, only to feel anxious and guilt-ridden later on, reverting to defensive self-flagellation before the next meeting. The therapist must be alert to these possibilities and catch any regression as quickly as possible.

It is not necessary to wait for spontaneous offerings of change. If the patient does not mention what had been discussed previously, the therapist might ask, "I'm wondering what happened after our last session. You were wanting to be able to talk with your husband in a direct and forthright manner. How did that go?"

So, in a sense, working through is the process through which intention becomes reality. Freud (1937) also emphasized the importance of follow-up, suggesting that working through was only successful if the work enabled the patient to cope with future difficulties. This information can only be obtained by follow-up inquiries. Clinicians like Davanloo and Malan do this continuously, both while treatment is in progress and following termination (Coughlin & Malan, 2018; Malan, 1976; 1978).

Clinical Examples

The Masochistic Artist: Part 2

In the case of the Masochistic Artist (see Chapter 6), a marital crisis created significant psychic disequilibrium within the patient and prompted her to seek treatment. The therapeutic work created further unconscious upheaval, as previously repressed feelings and memories began to surface. The patient began to face what she had always avoided knowing and feeling. Instead of dreading the reliving of the trauma, she reported a feeling of freedom and relief.

The Dawning of Hope

PATIENT: Things are coming to a crisis and I'm relieved. I was very upset after seeing you the last time. Then I drove around and went shopping for a couch, because I think a couch is going to make my life better (laughs with delight). I can invite people over. Slowly I began to feel better, then really better, then I actually started to feel happy! It's like a miracle. You know, the worst part of my feeling is that I'm completely alone and that I always will be and there's nothing I can do about it—and I always have been. The only thing I could do was find ways to avoid it. Only now I can admit I've always felt this way. In the past, I've denied it saying, "No, I'm really upbeat and a happy person". But it's really not true. I've always had this deep-rooted fear of being alone. I don't mean actually being alone, but feeling alone. And, for the first time, I feel optimistic about not feeling that way—for the first time in my life.

There is a dramatic change in this woman's sense of time—from existential time in which pain seemed ever present, to real time, in which feelings come and go in response to current events. This is something James Mann (1973) discussed in his writings. His time-limited psychotherapy focuses almost exclusively on the meaning of time and how this is affected by the inevitable losses that occur in our lives. The goal of his brief and focused treatment is to replace the patient's pervasive sense of helplessness and diffuse pessimism with realistic optimism.

In this case, the patient reported feeling realistic hope for the first time in her life, signifying major revisions in her view of herself and the world. This was not achieved through an intellectual or philosophical discussions but by facing, experiencing, and living through all the painful feelings she had previously avoided. Paradoxically, it was only when she was able to acknowledge that she had always felt alone, depressed, and powerless to do anything about it, that the possibility of change became a reality for her. She found freedom in speaking the truth about her own inner experience.

PATIENT: Now when I feel sad, I don't deny it. Like the other day, I just gave into it, and I put on candles and classical music, had a glass of wine, and took a bath.

The Development of Self-Care

For lasting change to occur in a patient's character, it is not sufficient for her to remember traumas from the past. In this case, the resulting sense of herself as damaged and, therefore, deserving of the poor treatment she received, needed to be dramatically altered to achieve lasting change.

In addition to the direct assaults many of our patients were subjected to as children, they were rarely protected from the abuse and consequently suffer from a deficit in self-care and self-protection. The development of this vital function must be facilitated therapeutically.

In this case, the emergence of self-care appeared after the patient expressed deep appreciation for her suffering as a child. In the following vignette, she eloquently describes the real benefit of facing the truth, however painful. She developed the ability to take care of herself and soothe the pain rather than trying to avoid it. Resisting the pain led to a festering of the wound, while after facing and experiencing her painful feelings, they could pass through and be replaced by contentment.

What is being referred to as "self-care" can be conceptualized as a new and adaptive way to reduce anxiety that involves a change in the patient's view of herself. This patient was able to confront and then master her internal upheaval, as well as deal with external events that may threaten her well-being.

PATIENT: I woke up this morning and thought, you know, this is a miracle, really, this whole process. It gives me this freedom for the first time in my life—that I don't have to repress this. I could actually move beyond it or accept pain because on the other side is something else. It's a feeling of self. I was going to say self-sufficiency but that's not it. It's like I'm inside with myself now. I'm not alone anymore. I'm in here with me. It's a funny thing.

Changes in Symptoms and Sexual Fantasies

The profound changes apparent in the patient's sense of herself and the world are translated into concrete and observable changes in behavior.

PATIENT: I see changes immediately. For example, I can't use the old fantasies anymore. This is really interesting, because these are fantasies that go back 35 years. I couldn't construct this whole scenario—it was too obvious, too painful to me. Actually, then I focused on making love with my lover and imagined coming to orgasm as he came to orgasm.

THERAPIST: So it was a fantasy of mutual pleasure. No one was getting hurt, being forced, or humiliated.

PATIENT: It was sweet. I thought the whole switch was really dramatic.

Now the patient could imagine giving and receiving physical pleasure without pain needing to be involved. There was no longer anxiety, guilt, or fear of punishment following pleasure with a man of her choice. Freud (1930) wrote, "We are so made, that we can only derive intense enjoyment from a contrast, and only very little from a state of things". The contrast between the avoidance of pain in the past and the ability to allow it in the present gave rise to pleasurable feelings as well.

De-Repression of Feelings and Memories of "Rape" by Mother

PATIENT: My mother was always poking and prodding at me. She and my father would hold me down and pick the lint out of my navel. And my mother had this thing about enemas.

THERAPIST: What do you remember about the enemas?

PATIENT: It was in my mother's bathroom. What I remember is she'd put a towel over her lap and lay me over her and insert this and then there's this sensation of water coming in and the feeling that something bad might happen, like getting too filled up. It was scary—is it going to get too full? And this is kind of interesting, because it's sexual in a way. I'd be lying there, and she'd be patting me and soothing me, waiting for a number of minutes.

THERAPIST: What kinds of feelings do you notice when you go back to that now?

PATIENT: It's a feeling I still have, of being forced to submit.

THERAPIST: And the feeling inside?

PATIENT: A feeling of being trapped by love—trapped by this thing that's supposed to be good for you (crying). And no one to go to who would protect me.

THERAPIST: So inside there's a terrible feeling of helplessness. But, what about the feeling toward her?

PATIENT: I can see how my feeling is blocked because I feel I'm not allowed to be angry because she's doing it for my own good. I know I felt that way then. I felt outraged really and violated, but I couldn't feel that way then.

THERAPIST: Well, you couldn't express it then—you kept it down inside. But if you let that rise within you now, how would it want to come out?

PATIENT: We'd be in the bathroom, and I wouldn't let her do it. I would kick her in the stomach, push her away, and scream as loud as I could and punch her and run away. Because that is, like, a fight for something—it's self-defense. This is where it hits now—in defending myself that way—you see, I would get candy for being good, so sometimes I must have been bad, whatever that means, and so maybe I even did this. I was accused of being mentally ill by both my parents for having tantrums as a child. So, to be really good and to submit was to be healthy.

THERAPIST: So your feelings were considered wild, dangerous, and crazy. Is that the way you see it now?

PATIENT: No.
THERAPIST: What is your feeling toward her now?
PATIENT: Rage.
THERAPIST: How do you experience it?
PATIENT: I go blank.

During an earlier segment of this woman's treatment, when we began to approach the rage she felt toward her father, the patient claimed she went blank. Her anger was so anxiety-provoking that she wouldn't let it register. Work was required to remove this block and liberate the buried feelings toward him. During this session, as we began to face the rage toward her mother, she reported going blank once again. When patients have trouble articulating their feelings, questions regarding sensations in their body often reveal that they are, in fact, feeling a great deal. This certainly proved to be the case here.

THERAPIST: What happens in your body?
PATIENT: I feel I have a hole around my heart. I feel this sense of diminishment and a kind of cavernous feeling (crying). It almost feels like a boomerang shape, almost pulling down from my heart. I don't feel empty now—I feel I want to hold onto that feeling because it does turn into anger.
THERAPIST: So now you won't let it be flushed out or pushed down?
PATIENT: Yeah, it's my body. It's my body! It means it's me. It can't be violated, can't be washed away.
THERAPIST: But it's going to be a fight. You couldn't just say "Mommy, I don't want you to do that". She didn't listen.
PATIENT: I feel that I'd have to kill her. I have to protect myself.
THERAPIST: How?
PATIENT: I'm bigger than her now. I see myself strangling her and hitting her head against the tile and hitting her again and again and again until she's limp and then dropping her there by the toilet. I feel really pissed off. I feel like she's a piece of shit. I don't understand how someone could do that to a child and not hear them being in pain and just to think it doesn't matter (sobbing). I think it's unforgivable, it's unforgivable. To do that out of cruelty or I don't know what—it was killing me, and I don't feel blank about it anymore. I feel I want to kill her in self-defense.
THERAPIST: It felt like she was trying to gut you—clean you out from the inside. There was no one to go to. Your father always sided with her. Your sister was glad it wasn't her on the hot seat, so it must have seemed like killing her would be the only way to spare yourself.
PATIENT: Exactly. Running away doesn't work. I want to get rid of her.
THERAPIST: Otherwise you stay in the struggle, like you have been.

PATIENT: It feels like I can have pleasure—physical pleasure. That my body doesn't feel pushed down, it feels opened up. It's empowering. It's like being inside your body in this way that's filling—occupying your body, your height, your mass—feeling your presence. That's the other side of it. It's odd. I see myself emerge from the bathroom, see myself in the mirror, and see I'm a woman. I get dressed up, put on perfume, and leave the house. I want to go out into the world now, as a woman. I don't feel like I'm going to get arrested. I'm free.

This fantasy illustrates the process of growth as it takes place in real time. It began with the deeply felt experience of rage. She moved from a helpless, victimized stance to that of a strong and capable woman. Not only was she able to express the anger she felt toward her mother, but in so doing, was able to separate from her and became a woman in her own right. She imagined leaving her mother's house and going out into the world. Love no longer needed to be torturous. She could seek pleasure for its own sake. Guilt and self-punishment had been replaced with a sense of self as whole, healthy and complete.

This case meets Malan's criteria for character change, as each pathological defense was replaced with something adaptive. Both internal changes, such as her view of self and her capacity for self-soothing, and externally observable behavioral changes underwent significant alteration. Follow-up confirmed the stability of these changes and will be reported in Chapter 8.

The Man with an Explosive Temper

This middle-aged father of three came to treatment for help in controlling his temper. During his opening statement, he reported a history of severe abuse by his own father and his resolution never to repeat this in his own family. While he never struck anyone, he was having verbal temper tantrums that frightened him and were causing an increasing strain on everyone. He was especially troubled because he did not know what triggered these outbursts. He described them as coming out of the blue and were beyond his control.

Evaluation of Impulse Control

Careful evaluation of impulse control is absolutely essential in cases such as these, where an explosive temper is a presenting complaint. Detailed inquiry during the trial therapy revealed that these occasional temper outbursts (verbal) were the result of the patient's more pervasive tendency to squelch his feelings. He was so terrified of anger that he habitually suppressed any experience of irritation. Over time, his anger and frustration grew and exceeded his capacity to contain it. Then, at some unpredictable moment, a small annoyance would send him over the edge, and he would have a verbal temper tantrum. This experience upset him greatly and further reinforced his sense that anger is big, bad, and dangerous and should be avoided at all cost. This set the stage for the next round of suppression and eventual discharge. As this pattern was elucidated, his problem was reframed. Initially, he identified anger as the problem. As the result of our work, he began to see that it was his *avoidance* of anger (as well as other painful feelings) on an ongoing basis that created his symptomatic disturbance.

The interpersonal consequences of his intrapsychic solution for dealing with affect were then enumerated. This man had a way of talking around any issue at hand and kept an emotional distance while appearing superficially engaged. He tended to get so derailed by the minutia of a story that he would lose the listener in the process. This became our focus, for if he continued to keep an emotional distance from the therapist, no progress would be possible.

Defenses against Emotional Closeness

THERAPIST: You've mentioned that several counselors you've consulted have fallen asleep during sessions. Not just one, but several. Are you aware that you have ways of losing people? You not only have various ways to distance yourself from others, but you discourage others from coming close and getting interested in you.

PATIENT: I know. I put them to sleep with my rambling.

THERAPIST: Do you want to do that here with me?

PATIENT: No. I want to open up. I don't want to spend my life this way, but I get very nervous.

THERAPIST: Your anxiety is our indication that a lot of feeling is stirred up.

PATIENT: Yes.

THERAPIST: There must be a certain feeling toward me.

PATIENT: I'm not sure. I'm anxious and a little testy.

THERAPIST: Testy means what?

PATIENT: A little frustrated. I want you to have the answers, but I know it's up to me. I've got a wall around me, and you can do anything you like but it won't make a difference.

THERAPIST: Yes, you could defeat me. Is that what you want to do?

PATIENT: No.

THERAPIST: So, could we look at the anger?

PATIENT: Well, it's only irritation.

THERAPIST: Now you want to water it down.

PATIENT: But it's only on the fringes—it's not a big anger.

THERAPIST: Isn't this a big part of the problem? You store up resentments and wait until you're in a rage and then there's the last straw and you explode.

PATIENT: You're right but it's difficult. The wall is high. It scares me, facing the emotion. I don't know what's down there.

THERAPIST: You're very anxious about the anger.

PATIENT: Yeah.

THERAPIST: How do you feel the anger inside?

PATIENT: (big sigh) I don't know. I don't feel it.

THERAPIST: What do you feel?

PATIENT: Frustrated. Like a mouse in a corner with a cat waiting.

THERAPIST: So you're playing a cat-and-mouse game here with me around the anger. Is that what you want to do?

PATIENT: No.

THERAPIST: Will you let yourself feel it?

PATIENT: Physically I do. It's tight inside and there's tingling then numbness. I get cold.

THERAPIST: The feeling of anger gets covered over—you go cold. There's something terrifying about letting yourself feel this anger toward me.

PATIENT: Whenever I've shown emotions, people have shunned me. There's always been a negative reaction. I get hurt. When I've turned to someone for comfort, I get chastised and berated.

THERAPIST: Any indication that will happen here?

PATIENT: I don't know. I know you're here to help, but it's happened so many times.

THERAPIST: So you've decided to give up? No one has a chance with you, huh? Then how are we going to find out?

PATIENT: We're not.

THERAPIST: So there's no potential here. You've decided it's a lost cause.

PATIENT: No, not a lost cause, just a difficult cause.

THERAPIST: What are you waiting for? Do you imagine it will be any easier two years from now? All you do is hold onto your suffering. In fact, you've been saying it's getting worse, and your wife is ready to walk out.

PATIENT: I know. But I'm embarrassed by the emotion. I go out of my way to avoid it.

THERAPIST: The cover-up spares you some feared hurt and humiliation.

PATIENT: Yeah, but it's short lived.

This last comment is of great significance, revealing an internal shift from an identification with the defense of detachment to a turning against it, as its cost is keenly experienced. This evoked grief and provided the first unlocking of his unconscious.

Breakthrough of Affect

THERAPIST: It looks like there's a lot of feeling right now.

PATIENT: Yeah, but it's not anger. (Patient puts his head in his hands and sobs. There are waves of sobs for three or four minutes during which time the therapist waited quietly.)

THERAPIST: It sounds like this pain comes from a very deep place. Could we look at this together?

PATIENT: I wish I knew where that came from.

This is where the process of working through, in which affect and understanding are integrated, begins. The patient had an emotional experience that he did not understand. This was a large part of his difficulty. He experienced intense feelings as if they had come out of the blue. Catharsis without understanding is of no lasting value, so the therapist guided the patient through the experience with the goal of deepening his cognitive understanding of what the emotion is all about.

Cognitive Re-Analysis

THERAPIST: It's vital that we understand it. What is the painful feeling like?

PATIENT: In my chest. I feel very sad as I listen to you and think about how I'm pushing my family away.

THERAPIST: You've been keeping all these feelings inside so no one really knows you.

PATIENT: I have such a hard time telling someone how I feel. I'm always afraid of their reaction.

THERAPIST: How about here with me? How did you see my reaction?

PATIENT: With you, I don't know.

THERAPIST: What's it been like to open up to me? You've been brutally treated in the past and it's understandable that you're afraid, but you've kept everyone out, not just the bad guys. So, what's it like to open up?

PATIENT: I feel a little better. The sadness comes because I see myself doing it over and over again. In the past week, I think of how often I've kept feelings in and backed off from others.

This spontaneous link between the experience in the transference and his current relationships signaled a deepening awareness of the meaning and impact of his defensive withdrawal. Now, an exploration of the underlying feeling, leading to its origins in the past, could take place.

THERAPIST: What came to you when the feelings surfaced?

PATIENT: How I've been berated. My father used to . . . (starts to cry again). My father made me feel like a baby if I cried (crying and voice is small and squeaky, like that of a small, frightened child). If you got hurt, even physically, he'd yell at you. We weren't allowed to cry. And my mother never consoled us. It didn't matter how bad it was.

THERAPIST: So, to cry would be to invite more assaults.

Linking the Triangles

At this point the two triangles could be meaningfully linked. The patient was aware that he was anxious about strong mixed feelings and would avoid them in ways that kept him in a lonely, isolated position. As the previously avoided feelings were approached in the transference, the patient linked this experience to his interactions with others in his present life. Finally, critical memories from the past were exposed, rendering the link between the triangle of conflict and the triangle of person complete. This is the essence of working through in ISTDP. As these patterns were worked and re-worked in an emotionally charged atmosphere, that which had been avoided was directly experienced. This provided both a corrective emotional experience and a living alternative to previous modes of interaction. This provided a new vantage point from which he could decide how he wanted to live life going forward. Conscious choice became possible.

De-Repression

The patient entered the next session without hesitation. He revealed that the opening in the previous session had provided him with access to long-buried memories and feelings.

PATIENT: I wanted to talk to you about two things that happened during the week. I had two flashbacks. I was driving home one night after our last session and, out of nowhere, I had a flashback to the time my father killed our dog and beat me. I know I was very young because I was still in the crib. The first thing I saw was my father beating my mother with a belt. I could literally hear her scream. I had visions of him killing the dog, even though I didn't see it. He beat him to death behind the woodpile because he had bitten me. I know I got beaten too, but I don't remember it. My mother tried to intervene, but then she got beaten—that's what I remember. I recall looking through the spokes of the crib.

Facilitating Recall of Pivotal Life-Events

The nature of memory, particularly with reference to memories that surface during the course of psychotherapy, has become a source of heated debate (Loftus, 1993; Trierweiler & Donovan, 1994). There have been serious concerns about how to ascertain the truth regarding memories that surface after many years. Strong opinions have been formed on both sides. One camp suggests that memory narratives are "at best, fallible representations of life episodes" (Dickman & Sechrest, 1985; Trierweiler & Donovan, 1994). Others (Herman, 1992; van der Kolk, 1987) have emphasized the harmful effects of our failure to accept the validity of memories presented in psychotherapy. There is a need to develop guidelines for practicing clinicians that are based on empirical evidence, as well as clinical experience.

Evidence is accumulating that the fallibility of memory may have more to do with poor investigative technique than with distortions in memory per se (Bower, 1981; Geiselman et al., 1985; Loewald, 1976; McCloskey & Zaragoza, 1985). To correct this, it has been suggested that therapists approach the work of memory retrieval with a tight focus, asking patients for elaboration, with an emphasis on concrete physical details, sensory experiences, and emotional activation (Trierweiler & Donovan, 1994). In other words, patients should be encouraged to talk about what they remember in great detail, including what they saw, smelled, heard, and felt at the time. Davanloo (1990) did this intuitively by asking patients to immerse themselves in recalled experience while extracting details about such things as the date and time of the memory being evoked, clothing worn, facial expressions recalled, and the like. This type of work serves multiple functions, including that of uncovering and working through, by encouraging patients to paint the scene in great detail, and re-live the emotional experiences associated with the memory.

In the case presented here, working on the triangle of conflict in the transference created an opening into the unconscious. The patient reported having a flood of strong memories of pivotal traumatic experiences that his character defenses had been designed to avoid. As these memories were explored in the therapeutic setting, the feelings that accompanied them became our focus.

THERAPIST: What's the feeling that accompanies this memory?

PATIENT: Very sad and upset. Emotionally, I plunged. There was immense sadness seeing my mother getting beaten. I wanted to talk to my wife about it. I feel I can talk to her lately and realize that, as I start to share with her, I'm not getting the negative response I anticipate. She's warm and comforting. She hugged me.

Cyclical Psychodynamics

This passage suggests that the patient has been able to use the insight gained by his experience in the previous session to make real changes in his current life—the ultimate goal of treatment. Instead of repeating the past by withdrawing and depriving himself and others of the opportunity for emotional closeness, he opened up to his wife. Instead of receiving rejection or humiliation, he found comfort, further reinforcing the new changes in him. Defensive withdrawal had been replaced by active engagement, signifying substantial character change.

This type of reciprocal interaction between insight and behavior change is at the heart of a theory called cyclical psychodynamics, developed by Wachtel (1993). This theory places particular emphasis on the dynamic interplay between intrapsychic conflicts and internalized object relations on the one hand, and current interpersonal dynamics on the other. To facilitate working through and character change, it has been suggested that changes need to occur in both the internal representations of self and other and in concrete, observable behavior. Further, it has been suggested that changes in one area can affect the other in mutually reinforcing ways. Although traditional psychoanalytic theory seems to suggest that internal changes must occur first, with behavior change to follow, there is also evidence that this process can happen in the reverse.

Interpersonal experience can have a profound effect on internal images, fostering revisions of existing internalized models of self and other. In this case, the patient allowed the therapist into his inner emotional world. He was not berated, as he had been in the past. Rather, he found that the sharing of himself was profoundly healing. Something changed in his assumptions about himself and others that was rapidly translated into his interactions with his wife. He opened up to her and found she was warm and receptive. This further solidified the changes that began in the previous session. Many clinicians feel that this type of experience facilitates the replacement of outdated, negative parental introjects with compassionate alternatives.

In addition to the impact of this corrective emotional experience on this man's internal representations of self and other, the experience of complex transference feelings created an opening into the unconscious, as vital memories of early abuse surfaced in a dramatic way. Now the intense and conflictual feelings associated with the abuse could be worked on directly, at the source.

THERAPIST: What's the feeling now, when you go back to that incident?

PATIENT: Anger. Anger at my father for his brutality. It's also the only time I can remember my mother stepping in. and she got a terrible beating.

Memory of Homosexual Rope

This opening into the unconscious included the memory of a highly traumatic incident from his adolescence.

PATIENT: The second flashback was the rape. I was so naive and unprotected. Should I have seen signs that he was capable of this? Why did I get into the truck with someone I'd only met once? The thing that bothers me most is the passive submission. I thought of fighting back but didn't. When it was over and we walked out, I had the gun. He said to me, "I'm not nervous because I know it's not loaded" but I know I had a bullet in my pocket. I can remember rubbing the bullet in my hand but being numb and feeling sick. When I got home, I burst into the house crying, "This asshole raped me! He fucked me up the ass!" I remember my father saying, "Watch your mouth—your mother is here. What's the matter with you?" Later, in the police car, he said to the officer, "All this started when the Beatles came out". I thought, "What in the world is he talking about?" I was terrified.

THERAPIST: Even there, your father is totally oblivious and insensitive. What else came to you about this flash?

PATIENT: Remembering his grabbing me from behind and pushing me on the bed. He threatened me—take your clothes off or I'll beat you up. He sucked on me, but I didn't get hard because I was so scared. When I look at it now, I get angry at myself for submitting.

THERAPIST: You had learned to submit to violence and wanted to come out with your life. Now you feel angry. Even then, you thought of the bullet in your pocket. What did you want to do?

PATIENT: I would have killed him—no doubt in my mind. Rage so bad I wouldn't shoot him. I'd beat him to death with the gun. The bullet wouldn't be enough.

THERAPIST: How do you see it?

PATIENT: I had a golden opportunity to hurt him, but I didn't. I was on the bed. He was bent over with his back to me. With a good swift kick, I could have rammed his head into the door jam and either run out of there or beat the shit out of him. He was a big, muscular man. I remember seeing him in court and being afraid of his size. It was totally isolated and secluded there and no one knew where I was.

THERAPIST: What's the impulse now?

PATIENT: That I would turn quickly and hit him in the head with the gun. Beat his head into the ground. No doubt about it because it's an image I've had in dreams before.

THERAPIST: What happens?

PATIENT: He dies. I beat him to death with the gun butt.

THERAPIST: What do you see?

PATIENT: Head smashed to a bloody pulp. A mess.

THERAPIST: What do you feel?

PATIENT: Relief. He violated me, hurt me, and I've retaliated.

Link with His Father

THERAPIST: Your father violated you too. You must be angry with him too.

PATIENT: I'm angry for all the times he beat us. I could kill him. I turned on him once when he kicked my brother, and he put my head through the coffee table. And I got yelled at by my mother! I'd beat his face in. No doubt. I'd beat his face in and be crying in a rage at getting back at him.

THERAPIST: What happens in this image of unleashing the rage toward him?

PATIENT: I'd be crying tears of rage. I'd want to yell and scream. Father always yelled and screamed. His mouth would go. Verbally berating us. I did this when I'd get into fights.

THERAPIST: What do you want to say to him?

PATIENT: "You rotten son of a bitch. Don't ever touch me again. Don't touch my mother or any of us". It's a relief. The weight of the world off my shoulders. I would love to say to him, right now, "You mope and cry over what's happened to your kids (with the exception of the patient, they are unemployed, alcoholic, or in jail), and you're too stupid to know it's all your fault".

THERAPIST: You want him to suffer with that.

PATIENT: Payback is a bitch, but it serves him right. I just had a flash. There's so much anger over the fact that we loved him and wanted him to treat us as a father, not another bully. "Damn it, I wanted you to love me like a father should. You cheated us out of something we needed desperately". If he had been loving and compassionate, we would have learned that instead of learning to turn on those we love.

It is of critical importance that all the mixed feelings toward significant others be experienced as fully as possible. This patient felt murderous rage and agonizing grief in relation to his father, but also a deep longing for closeness—a yearning to love and be loved by his father—that he had also defended against in such a way that adversely affected the relationship with his own son. The next session will clearly reveal the impact the previous work has had on his current ability to form an intimate bond with his son.

P-C Link Regarding the Father–Son Relationship

There was a two-week break between the last session and the one reported here. The patient continued to work at a high level of ego-adaptive capacity. The roles assumed by patient and therapist had changed profoundly. The patient was doing most of the active work now, with the therapist observing and responding.

PATIENT: I want to tell you about Valentine's Day. I thought it was ridiculous that there were no cards for sons. I finally found the perfect card. I made a conscious effort to add something personal, and I spent a lot of time on this. I acknowledged that I've been hard on him but love him. I gave him the card and he started to cry. I asked, "What's the matter?" He was bawling—tears rolling down his face (patient begins to cry). He said, "Thank you so much", and sat on my lap (more crying). I just held him while he cried. We sat for 10 or 15 minutes. My emotions were so mixed. I felt so bad that I had caused him pain and uncertainty—that a card could unleash that. At the same time, I was elated—it was a door that I opened. From that point on, I noticed that, even if I feel angry, I stop and talk to him about it.

This man's harshness with his son had been replaced with compassion, love, and emotional connection. The entire family had benefited from his treatment.

The Repetition Compulsion

The notion of repetition is included in nearly every definition of working through available, with more traditional analysts assuming this will be a time-consuming endeavor. In large part, this is attributed to the strength and tenacity of the resistance. Although various types of resistance have been catalogued, the "repetition compulsion" is considered the most difficult to deal with therapeutically.

The tendency for patients to repeat and re-enact their internal conflicts externally in one situation after another has been referred to as the repetition compulsion. The repetition compulsion is "a theoretical construct consisting of two elements: (a) the unconscious instincts (sexual and aggressive) seeking expression, and (b) the ego's attempt to master old traumatic conditions or events associated with an infantile neurosis" (Strupp & Binder, 1984, p. 22).

According to drive theory, it is the first of these two elements, the strength of the impulses, that is the culprit in creating and maintaining psychopathology.

Kernberg (1975; 1976) is a contemporary advocate of this theory, suggesting that patients with borderline personality organization have exceptionally strong innate aggressive drives. Yet, it is the second element mentioned by Freud, regarding the ego's repeated attempts at mastery, that has received the most clinical and empirical support over the years. Initially, Freud considered the tendency for patients to repeat in the present what has occurred in the past as a resistance to remembering. Eventually, as his focus shifted from the primacy of impulses and the operation of the pleasure principle to a theory based on the ego's adaptation through the reality principle, the notion of repeating in an effort to achieve mastery gained prominence.

How can repeated exposure to traumatic events in dreams, fantasies, and behavior be explained? The nearly universal nature of this phenomenon suggests that it contains an adaptive function. Traumatic events are, by their nature, outside ordinary experience. Accordingly, repeating in the present traumatic events and reactions from the past may be driven by the individual's need to assimilate and integrate powerful yet discrepant information into one's ongoing theory of how the world works (Epstein, 1994; Janoff-Bulman, 1992). If, as hypothesized (Epstein, 1994; Stern, 1985), there is a fundamental motive to assimilate emotionally significant experiences into a coherent conceptual system of how the world works, material that can neither be ignored nor readily assimilated will keep re-appearing in an attempt at integration. Conceived of in this way, the repetition compulsion is adaptive because it creates opportunities for assimilation and adaptation to current reality, taking unusual and traumatic events into account.

A good deal of research data supports the view that we humans are hypothesis testers who need to assimilate new incoming information into our ongoing view of the world (Stern, 1985). It seems we will not rest until a problem is solved. As early as the 1920s, Zeigarnik (1927) found that there was consistently greater recall of unfinished than finished tasks. Lewin (1951) suggested that tension arises within the system when a task has not been completed. This tension creates energy that drives the organism toward completion. When the goal is accomplished, the tension is released, and the material is forgotten. He also found that the more emotionally involved the individual was in the problem and/or the more emotionally significant the outcome, the greater the tension created when the problem was unsolved or the task unfinished. Again, this tension creates the energy that drives the system toward mastery and completion of the task at hand.

Although resistance to change poses a problem in psychotherapy, Janoff-Bulman (1992) has suggested that resistance to change in our operating assumptions about self, others, and the world is adaptive most of the time and is, therefore, revised or abandoned with great reluctance. She refers to this "cognitive conservatism" as a trait characteristic of the species, designed to provide the kind of stability, coherence, and predictability that foster the feelings of security so necessary for daily survival. We seem to develop theories of unity and consistency to make sense of a complex and frequently chaotic world. We are then highly motivated to maintain consistency and to support our own hypotheses (Aronson, 1968). This need contradicts the desire to change that brings many to psychotherapy. Janoff-Bulman's point is that this resistance cannot simply be chalked up to psychopathology. In fact, she has asserted that, in most instances, it is healthy and adaptive to cling to our familiar guiding principles because they work most of the time. The question then becomes how to help patients overcome this resistance to change when necessary.

When Insight Does Not Lead to Change

In the two cases presented in this chapter, the work in the transference was effective in unleashing previously repressed memories and feelings regarding significant figures and events from the past. The implications of these revelations for the present rapidly became clear, and the patients made dramatic changes in their current lives, which further reinforced the internal changes that began in psychotherapy. Things do not always progress so smoothly. Sometimes insights, even emotionally experienced insights in the transference with links to the past, do not lead to changes in the patient's current functioning. How can this be explained?

Most dynamic psychotherapies subscribe to the notion that increasing patients' understanding (insight) of their repetitive patterns of interaction with others will help them more clearly define their difficulties and, in so doing, will facilitate problem solving. When this does not occur, even after a period of working through in which the pattern and its negative consequences are elucidated in many different situations, resistance is usually considered the factor responsible for the impasse. In particular, a transference resistance is suspected. Perhaps the gratification of the relationship with the therapist outweighs the patient's motivation to get well. Alternatively, getting well would mean facing separation and loss. If this is avoided, treatment could go on indefinitely.

In ISTDP, the transference relationship is monitored throughout treatment. Particularly at the inception of treatment, analysis of the transference pattern of behavior, with a strong emphasis on the negative consequences of defense and resistance, occupies a good deal of time and energy. As treatment progresses, the transference distortions are reduced and largely eliminated. A working alliance based on a collaborative relationship becomes ascendant and work on current and past relationships takes center stage.

For example, if a tendency toward dependency is noted early on in treatment, it could be anticipated as a potential barrier to rapid movement. This kind of anticipation can be pivotal in preventing an impasse or an aborted treatment. Davanloo (1986a; 1986b) has paid particular attention to self-defeating patients who seem motivated to destroy their chances for success and sabotage treatment in the process. This is most likely in cases where there is a history of failed relationships, including previous attempts at therapy. I treated a young man who complained of being unable to sustain a relationship with a woman. During the initial evaluation, it was revealed that three previous psychotherapies had been aborted after several months of treatment. As soon as things started to heat up emotionally, he would bolt. I asked him how this treatment would be any different. During that first session, when motivation was high, he declared his intention to address these feelings as they arose, rather than cutting and running, as he had done in the past. In fact, he did not break off treatment, but completed it successfully by facing, experiencing, and integrating all his complex feelings toward others. In cases like this, no substantive work can occur until the potential for self-sabotage in the treatment has been directly addressed.

Others (Crits-Christoph & Barber, 1991) have suggested that these explanations are insufficient to explain the numerous instances in which insight fails to lead to behavior change. It has been hypothesized that symptoms can assume "functional autonomy", becoming habitual and gradually independent of their original source (Wachtel, 1977). For example, a young boy may become passive and subservient with authority as a compromise between his anger at being controlled by authoritarian parents and his need to defend against it to avoid punishment and maintain the bond. Yet, over time, this pattern of passive-aggressive procrastination can become habitual and embedded in his character. Consequently, responses no longer occur just in response to anger, but become a habitual mode of functioning that is independent of circumstances or stimulus. These authors suggest that mere insight into the original source of this dynamic will be of little value in facilitating change.

Instead, a laser focus on the negative, self-defeating consequences of a reliance on character defenses provides us with a powerful alternative strategy. In particular, the ways in which these character traits will sabotage treatment if not abandoned are enumerated. Again, the focus is directed toward the vicious cycles infecting the individual's current functioning rather than toward the vicissitudes of the basic drives. Since patients often retreat to the past to justify their present behavior, such an approach would reenforce, rather than dismantle, defenses. Instead, the ISTDP therapist focuses on the ways that patients avoid responsibility for perpetuating their own suffering. The focus should remain on patients' behavior in the here and now, with some pressure to change, lest the therapeutic relationship end in another failure.

Summary

In ISTDP, the process of working through—in which both affective and intellectual modes of experience are integrated and lead to stable changes in behavior—begins with the initial evaluation and continues throughout treatment. According to Davanloo, affect must come first, but should be followed by a cognitive re-analysis of the process, in which both the triangle of conflict and the triangle of person are meaningfully linked. Research confirms the hypothesis that such interventions are significantly associated with enduring character change.

8 TERMINATION

May the spirit never die
Though a troubled heart feels pain
When this long winter is over
It will blossom once again

Loreena McKennitt[1] *(1989)*
"Breaking the Silence"

It seems fitting to approach the subject of termination by coming full circle, ending with the last verse of the song "Breaking the Silence", quoted at the start of Chapter 1. When psychotherapy comes to a successful end, the painful process undertaken by someone with a troubled heart leaves the person feeling renewed. At the same time, ending any significant relationship, including that with a therapist, evokes mixed feelings. The harsh truth is, we will lose everyone we ever loved, in one way or another, at one time or another. Living and loving on life's terms requires us to face this difficult truth and all the attendant feelings that accompany it. Some find it easier to be lonely than to take the risk of loving and losing. Yet, those are the only two choices we have on this planet. We can be open to love, attach deeply, and then feel our hearts break when loss occurs. Or we can harden our hearts and refuse to love. While the latter choice serves to avoid the searing pain of heartbreak, it renders one empty and alone. When we let our hearts break, and travel through the stages of grief, what remains are the happy memories and a positive identification with the deceased. When grief is avoided, an inner deadness can result. Isolation, cynicism, and negative memories often haunt the one who refuses to mourn.

DOI: 10.4324/9781003542131-8

Since the experience of loss is one none of us can avoid, and is so important for long-term health and resilience, facilitating the process of healthy mourning is a central task of the termination phase of therapy. A failure of the patient and/or therapist to deal with this painful reality head-on can undermine previous progress and set the stage for relapse.

The issue of termination involves two basic questions: when and how? There are both practical and existential elements to these questions. The longer and more protracted dynamic psychotherapy has become, the more often innovations tailored to reducing its length have appeared. In fact, in his paper entitled "Analysis Terminable and Interminable", Freud (1937) lamented that analysis was frequently a protracted affair and advised that we should attempt to shorten its duration. In this spirit, Freud, Ferenczi, Rank, and Alexander all experimented with setting a termination date to accelerate stalled treatments.

In Intensive Short-Term Dynamic Psychotherapy (ISTDP), the length of treatment, while relatively brief (1–40 sessions), is open-ended. Termination is tied directly to the achievement of therapeutic goals. Therefore, in contemplating the end of treatment, we must return to its beginning. We can only decide whether the patient is well by understanding the nature of the presenting illness. It all gets back to the goals of treatment. According to Freud (1937):

> First, the patient must no longer be suffering from his former symptoms and have overcome his various anxieties and inhibitions and, secondly, the analyst must have formed the opinion that so much repressed material has been brought into consciousness . . . that no repetition of the patient's specific pathological processes is to be feared.
>
> (Freud, 1937, p. 320)

Once these goals have been achieved to the satisfaction of patient and therapist, the issue of termination needs to be addressed.

Davanloo (1990), following Freud's lead, considered termination when therapeutic goals have been met. Ultimately, however, those goals can only be considered stable if the patient proves capable of weathering *future* storms without regression. Routine follow-up interviews with patients who have terminated treatment are required to make this assessment. Freud discussed a few incidental follow-up reports on patients previously treated, but did not make follow-up a standard practice. Malan and Davanlo routinely conducted follow-up visits at one-, five-, and ten-year intervals. This practice allows the therapist to identify failures, learn from mistakes, and track effectiveness over time.

Malan (1976b) reported encouraging findings which suggested that those patients who responded well to treatment not only maintained their gains over time but were better still at five-year follow-up. Such findings indicate that the brief, accelerated form of dynamic psychotherapy being described here does, in fact, remove obstacles to development and that the process of change continues well after treatment formally ends. So, most short-term dynamic psychotherapists, like their colleagues engaged in traditional long-term psychotherapy, consider termination when the stated goals have been reached.

How the actual process of ending treatment should proceed is a matter of debate, however. Whereas Firestein (1978) found no consensus about how to handle termination in the analytic community, there is greater agreement among the short-term dynamic psychotherapists. In general, practitioners of ISTDP continue the same technical approach of working the triangles right up until the last session. As termination approaches, interventions are geared toward facilitating feelings regarding separation and loss and understanding how these are related to losses from the past. With a few exceptions, there seems to be agreement that patients must face all their mixed feelings about ending, though the magnitude and importance of this phase of treatment for the outcome of treatment is quite variable, depending on the case.

Both the when and the how of termination will be discussed in this chapter. Special problems associated with termination and techniques to facilitate a healthy process of separation will be outlined. Clinical vignettes will illustrate the process. In addition, long term follow-up (up to 20 years) will be included.

How Important is the Termination to Outcome?

Malan's Research

Malan (1979) has suggested that termination, per se, is of variable importance for outcome, depending on the patient and the presenting complaints. He warns that "termination should not be over-valued into a fundamental principle". He found that a "radical" approach, in which the transference pattern of behavior was interpreted early and repeatedly, resulted in uncomplicated terminations, as the psychic conflicts responsible for neurotic interactions had been worked through during the mid-phase of treatment. Once these conflicts were resolved, and noticeable changes had occurred in the patient's life, the topic of termination tended to arise naturally and be dealt with easily.

The following factors seem to be responsible for this:

1 The focus on defense and resistance early in treatment.

2 Intensive working through in which the triangles of conflict and the person are repeatedly linked to consolidate insights.

3 Examination of the transference pattern of behavior from the inception of treatment.

4 The highly collaborative effort between patient and therapist.

Consequently, patients frequently report feelings of satisfaction about a job well done. While they often experienced some sadness about saying goodbye to the therapist, who had been a valued ally in their journey, it was typically mild and associated with good feelings.

In contrast to the uncomplicated termination just described, Malan found that, with those patients for whom loss was a focal issue, the handling of termination was absolutely crucial to outcome. The final phase of treatment in these cases tended to be longer, requiring three to five highly focused sessions.

The concept of a corrective emotional experience is highly relevant during termination. Malan (1979) made it clear that we must help patients come to a new ending. This new ending is not an attempt to provide for patients what they were deprived of in the past, but rather to help them face past and current failures directly. The therapist helps patients to bear all the rage and disappointment following these failures (including the limits of psychotherapy). This is what is new and corrective—having someone who will bear all the feelings with them. According to Malan, this type of experience helps patients give up impossible longings for endless nurturance or restitution and facilitates their ability to enjoy the satisfactions available in their current life.

Sifneos's Findings

Sifneos (1979) was in general agreement with Malan regarding the process of termination. He has emphasized that the therapist must be alert to signs of progress and make a point of recognizing evidence of change. This is an important and often neglected issue. We, as therapists, can become so focused on defenses and symptoms that we fail to recognize and respond to the therapeutic changes evident in the patient. The therapist's lingering doubts about the possibility of rapid and enduring change can slow down the pace of growth as well.

His research suggests that symptom removal is not the factor most likely to change following short-term anxiety-provoking therapy. Rather, the patients' *concern* about their symptoms or attitude toward them is the factor that undergoes significant change. Most successfully treated patients leave therapy with increased self-esteem and a sense of understanding themselves better (Sifneos, 1979).

The therapist expects patients to feel ambivalent about termination and communicates this, normalizing such a response. Feelings of accomplishment are acknowledged, as well as the inevitable sadness that will accompany the end of therapy. Additionally, Sifneos (1972; 1979) helped patients anticipate the future, and how they would apply what they have learned to conflicts and difficulties they will inevitably confront in life.

According to Sifneos (1979), 50% of the patients treated with brief dynamic psychotherapy raised the issue of termination spontaneously, once progress on their presenting difficulties had been made. In the other 50% of the cases, it was the therapist who brought up the subject of termination when progress had clearly been made. In these cases, there was some initial reluctance, followed by agreement.

Mann's Findings

Termination has been a major focus in Mann's (1973) time-limited psychotherapy and is highlighted from the start of treatment. In his model, therapy is strictly limited to 12 sessions. The date for termination is set at the end of the first session, so the end is in view from the start. "Mann believes that throughout treatment, patients are aware of the inevitability of termination and organize their defense mechanisms to guard against the pain of the loss" (Bauer & Kobos, 1987, p. 276). At the same time, the awareness of the end, from the beginning of treatment, tends to evoke feelings and memories about past losses, which can be reworked during the therapy. The theory underlying this treatment model suggests that all the rage, guilt, and grief attendant to separations and losses from the past were not able to be experienced and expressed at the time of their occurrence. Any such avoidance must be eliminated if therapy is to be considered successful. The therapist actively encourages the full experience of all these mixed feelings about the impending loss. It is believed that this new ending will be a maturational experience for the patient (Mann, 1973; Nacht, 1965). Mann stressed that this work could be as difficult for the therapist as for the patient. He contended that: "The therapist must not hesitate to examine with the patient all the feelings and fantasies" that arise during this phase of therapy. In fact, he considered the therapist's resistance to dealing actively with the feelings around separation the primary cause of "analysis interminable". He also suggested that the work of termination is the most difficult to teach trainees. We, as teachers and supervisors, must consider whether we contribute to this difficulty by our failure to focus on this phase of treatment and all that it demands from both patient and therapist.

Davanloo's Findings

When considering preparedness for termination, Davanloo (1979) looked for "total resolution of the central neurotic structure of the patient's problems manifested by the total replacement of the maladaptive neurotic pattern with an adaptive pattern associated with cognitive and emotional insight into the dynamic structure of his difficulties" (p. 21). He has suggested that such radical goals, amounting to cure, can be achieved in 1 to 10 sessions for a highly functioning neurotic, and in 20 to 40 sessions for those patients with a character disorder. Patients who have significant ego fragility and low ego-adaptive capacity can require 100 sessions or more. Termination is less of a distinct phase in ISTDP, than an integral part of the work. The aim is to work consistently at the patients' highest level of ego-adaptive capacity and to reach therapeutic goals as effectively and efficiently as possible. Each insight is worked and re-worked in a focused manner before moving on to another area of conflict. As each area of difficulty is worked through, the core neurotic structure is disassembled. By the end of treatment, patients are functioning very well, with a great deal of insight into their own internal workings. Consequently, the chance of regression at termination is very limited. This has been substantiated in research that suggests low levels of relapse and increased growth at follow-up.

Because termination is tied to the goals of therapy, it is impossible to set a date at the start of treatment. Still, the idea that treatment will be brief and accelerated is communicated, in both word and deed, from the inception of treatment. When patients call to schedule their initial appointment, they are told they will undergo an extensive evaluation requiring several hours. This evaluation will determine the nature of their difficulties and whether this form of treatment is indicated. They are also told that, should they be selected for therapy, they will be seen on a weekly basis until their problems are resolved. This clearly communicates that the aim is to *resolve* their problems and to do so in an efficient manner. In this way, the end is present from the beginning.

In uncomplicated cases, where there is an absence of ego fragility or traumatic early losses, termination tends to be a brief and straightforward process lasting one or two sessions. Where there has been early or traumatic loss, the termination phase is particularly important and typically requires three to five sessions.

According to Davanloo's (1978) clinical research, termination is broached by 70% of the patients with an Oedipal focus and only by 20% of the patients with character disorders. In the latter case, patients tend to cling to the therapist despite clear progress. It is up to the therapist to call this to patients' attention, and to deal directly with the pain and anger being avoided by holding onto the relationship. Davanloo (1980; 1990) emphasized patient activity and responsibility throughout the process, preventing pathological dependence on the therapist and minimizing prolonged terminations.

Davanloo's approach to psychotherapy is radical in many ways, including his decidedly optimistic view of the power and strength of dynamic psychotherapy (Bauer & Kobos, 1987). He communicated an inherent belief (based on a careful assessment of ego functioning) in his patients' capacities and urged them to work at their highest level of ability. This optimistic stance extends to the process of termination, which he viewed as no more difficult than any other stage of therapy. In fact, because defense and resistance are persistently and thoroughly dealt with early in therapy, a strong therapeutic alliance takes over as therapy continues. In most cases, the therapist's role becomes easier as the process progresses and patients do more and more of the work on their own. Rather than assuming that termination will be experienced as a traumatic loss, Davanloo tracked the patient's reactions as another opportunity to "explore and deal with unresolved feelings concerning past and current relationships". Often there is a celebratory air to the ending of treatment as both patient and therapist revel in the gains that have been made.

The Effect of Therapist Expectations

Most of the material written on termination focuses on patient variables (Novick, 1982). In particular, the patient's previous experiences with loss are considered a primary factor in determining how he will respond to termination. It is also essential to consider therapist variables. The therapist's theoretical orientation and expectations about how termination (not to mention our own feelings about and defenses against loss) will be experienced are very likely to influence the process (as well as outcome). If we expect the termination to be traumatic, we may search for confirming evidence of such a reaction. Conversely, our confidence in the patient's ability to deal with this loss in an adaptive way will also have an impact.

Need for Specificity and Flexibility

When planning termination, it is essential to be case-specific. The therapist must be flexible when determining when and how to go about termination, rather than relying on a rigid set of fixed criteria. Occasionally, a patient will have an unexpected reaction to the termination once a date is set. Allowing for an extra session or two to work this through tends to solidify change in the patient.

The real question is how to determine what would be best for a given patient. Malan (1979) has suggested that the therapist be aware of how separations were handled by the patient's parents and to use this as a guideline, by making sure the ending goes differently this time. Doing so prevents the possibility of re-traumatizing the patient and provides for a corrective emotional experience.

In a couple of cases, patients quite consciously decided to continue in treatment despite clear and profound changes in all areas of their functioning. In one case, a young woman decided to allow herself the "luxury" of some extra sessions once the work had been completed because, as the first of eight children, she had always been forced to grow up and be independent prematurely. In response to my comment that we be "as efficient and effective as possible", she said, "Efficient and effective? Forget it. I've done that all my life. I'm paying for this, and I'm going to allow myself to have a little longer than is absolutely necessary. I've had it with always making do with the absolute minimum".

This statement, in and of itself, was evidence of profound change, as she had been subservient and self-sacrificing in the past, and would never have directly declared her needs to another in such a forthright manner. That she could stand up to me and declare her intent to allow herself some leeway was extremely important. She was able to have a new experience during the termination phase of treatment, rather than repeating the old, in which she would move along at another's insistence.

Recognizing this communication as a sign of growth, and accommodating to it, rather than pushing for termination, was necessary in order to avoid re-traumatizing the patient. This is an example of how crucial the handling of the termination can be. Failure to allow the patient to take some extra time could well have resulted in a therapeutic failure.

This brief example highlights the importance of understanding the patient's experience of separation and loss within the context of all that has materialized during the treatment. Specificity is never more important than when determining a means for terminating treatment that tends to solidify the changes made throughout the course of therapy. More detailed cases in which a deep understanding of the patient's central conflicts influences the work of termination will follow.

Clinical Examples

Uncomplicated Termination

Patients who enter treatment with a clearly demarcated focus and erect few barriers to meaningful communication with the therapist work rapidly, effectively, and consistently right up until the end of treatment. They meet their goals and tend to raise the issue of termination themselves. The end of treatment tends to be viewed as an achievement and the primary feeling toward the therapist is that of gratitude.

The Gentleman Scorned (see Chapter 2) finished treatment in only ten sessions. The work was focused on helping him gain access to his anger, particularly toward women, and expressing it in direct and appropriate ways. In the past, he had alternately internalized his rage and become depressed or acted out in a defiant manner. Even in the second case, he would end up feeling guilty and like a failure, with depression the final result. So, in addition to being able to freely and appropriately express his anger, the patient wanted to be able to do so and maintain a good feeling about himself. He felt significantly improved and as if he had achieved his stated goal in coming for therapy. By taking the initiative in broaching the topic of termination, he was displaying evidence of significant change from a position of passivity and smoldering resentment toward women, to one of assertiveness. Even though I had some reservations about the depth and stability of his changes at first, his interaction with me suggested the changes were robust. Termination was a fairly straightforward review of the process and only required one session. At follow-up a year later, the patient reported continued progress.

Mother's Little Angel

This middle-aged mother of three came to see me at the urging of her primary physician who was unable to convince her that, despite all medical evidence to the contrary, she was not dying of cancer. Inquiry revealed that the onset of her symptoms—which included anxiety, panic, depression, and a host of somatic complaints—began six months prior to consultation, following the wedding of her eldest son. She also reported that her daughter had recently become engaged, and her youngest son would be graduating from college in three months. As we explored her reactions to the loss of her role as mother, she told me that her mother had died of cancer just as she was preparing to leave home and become independent at the age of 18.

The patient displayed some intellectual insight into the meaning of her current difficulties by saying, "I feel I'm somehow re-living the traumatic experiences of loss from the past". The following developmental material was revealed. She was conceived in an attempt to assuage her parents' guilt and grief over the death of their youngest son, who died at the age of four when he wandered off and fell into a gully that was ablaze with leaves and debris. Her mother called her "my little angel", a role she also played for her father and two brothers, nine and eleven years her senior. She recalled a happy childhood in which she was doted on and was frequently the center of attention.

Until the age of nine or ten, her home was a safe and happy place. All this came to an abrupt halt when her oldest brother returned home from the armed services in a state of paranoid psychosis. The brother she had adored was now a terrifying figure who would fly into uncontrollable rages without provocation. Her father refused to have him hospitalized, leaving the rest of his family in an unprotected state. Her father would escape to work, leaving his psychotic son alone with his wife and younger daughter. In a fit of anger, her mother banned her husband from their bedroom. During this time, the patient's mother became anxious and physically ill. Again, the patient was recruited to compensate and replace the lost object—in this case, her mother's husband. She became her mother's mate and protector, even sleeping in her bed every night. Since her mother refused medical care, the patient watched helplessly as her mother was eaten away by breast cancer.

This patient had a solid early childhood and showed no signs of ego fragility. She had developed a compliant and subservient façade in response to parental demands, caring for others while repressing all feelings of anger toward them. In psychotherapy, she was able, for the first time, to directly experience her rage toward her mother for using her as a substitute husband, withdrawing from life, and committing a slow and excruciating suicide. The direct experience of anger toward her mother, while anxiety-provoking at first, was extremely liberating. Her fears of dying of cancer disappeared, and she was able to deal with her feelings regarding the separation from her own children in a new and healthy manner. This was achieved by developing an adult relationship with them, rather than repeating the past in which she would hold onto them by being sick and needy, as her mother had done. In addition, having access to her anger enabled her to be assertive with her husband and co-workers. She was no longer everyone's caretaker. Her newfound energy was focused on her own life, revitalizing her marriage, solidifying friendships, and taking on more responsibility at work. Her family, friends, and physicians all noticed and applauded the substantial changes in her, which further reinforced them.

After 12 psychotherapy sessions, she felt ready to end treatment. The termination was uncomplicated and marked by feelings of gratitude and pride. Can substantial change occur this rapidly or was this a mere flight into health? Let's evaluate her progress vis-à-vis her presenting complaints. All symptomatic disturbances had disappeared and were replaced by adaptive strivings. She was no longer depressed and reported that her sense of humor had returned, that she felt spontaneous and flexible in her dealings with others, and had a deeper sense of closeness with family and friends.

The Emergence of a "New Self"

In the last session, she said, "I don't just feel like my old self, I feel I'm better than ever. I'm proud of myself for facing all the pain from the past and I feel it's strengthened me so that I'm better prepared for difficulties in the future". All these results seemed to indicate real progress and did not constitute an avoidance of deeper work through a flight into health. The termination was uncomplicated. She expressed her gratitude toward the therapist but also felt proud of herself for taking advantage of what the therapist had to offer.

At the time of termination, there was every indication of a full recovery. This case exemplifies the type of change in ego functioning that Menninger (1958) described when referring to criteria for termination. He stressed that, rather than the patient becoming his "old self", he'll become "an enlarged, an improved, indeed a new self". By the end of treatment, Mother's Little Angel had accomplished the task of becoming whom she could potentially be and was a woman in her own right.

The Manic-Depressive's Daughter: Part 2

It has been said that the central goal of psychoanalytic treatment is to release the patient from reliance on pathogenic defenses so that she can "confront the realistic problems of his life as a mature human being" (Munroe, 1955, p. 323). Just this sort of transformation, from reliance on avoidant defenses, to dealing adaptively with the daily problems in life, is illustrated in the following case. Treatment consisted of 25 psychotherapy sessions.

Review of Current Changes

PATIENT: My life seems to be getting in order. There's an improved quality of life. Even this week. My husband was gone on business, and it was last minute, but the children coped.

THERAPIST: And so did you.

PATIENT: Yeah. I felt like I did a great job. I was tired but it was a physical tired, not emotional, like being drained or frazzled or depleted. It was different. It felt different.

THERAPIST: You even feel good about the way you handled it and are more confident as a mother.

PATIENT: Yes, much more confident. It's really amazing how . . . maybe I've been preparing, and last week was like a final exam with him gone all week. It was ok so I feel pretty good about that.

As was noted in Chapter 7, symptomatic and characterological difficulties must be replaced with adaptive alternatives for a patient to be considered truly improved. This woman, who had been highly self-critical all her life, could now feel genuinely good about dealing well with a stressful situation. In particular, she had been desperately insecure about her capabilities as a mother and arranged it so that she was never alone with her children. Now, she reported feeling more confident in her abilities and was able to function independently in the role of mother. Not only was she able to perform the necessary maternal functions, but she felt good about herself and took pleasure in motherhood.

Emotional Changes

THERAPIST: It really seems to me that the internal blocks—those unresolved feelings and conflicts from the past—have largely been resolved and now you're freed up. You are involved and effective—no longer anxious and withdrawn.

PATIENT: I think that's right. I feel liberated from the past. It is really incredible. I'm tearing up.

THERAPIST: Tell me about that—you obviously have a lot of feeling.

PATIENT: As I drove here, I thought I don't feel haunted by it anymore. The past is there—it's my history and it has shaped me, but it doesn't haunt me. Now when things happen currently, I don't hark back to those feelings of helplessness and hopelessness. It's just about now and something I can handle. It's very different. It's amazing.

THERAPIST: So you feel at peace. I remember this being a primary goal. In the first session, you said, "I just want to be free". As we talk about this, you get tearful. Could we look at that?

PATIENT: It's an emotional thing to feel something I've carried around for so long, even when it wasn't acute, to have it not there is amazing.

THERAPIST: I wonder if you were so used to it, you habituated to it and didn't realize what a heavy weight it was. Only now that it's lifted, do you realize how heavy it was. It's sad. I also sense some feeling toward me. It is wonderful that you're doing so well, but then it means saying good-bye.

PATIENT: Yeah. It's sad, but I like to think you're still there if I should need you.

The termination phase presents another opportunity to face feelings around loss. Is it a problem that the patient wants to hold onto the idea that the therapist is still alive and available? In this case, I think not. This woman lost both her parents at an early age and adapted by becoming highly self-sufficient. Her ability to trust and rely on the therapist seemed a sign of health and one to be supported rather than undermined.

She fulfilled all the criteria for termination of an analysis as outlined by Nacht (1965):

1 An absence of suffering.

2 Modification of the structural and dynamic whole of the personality (changes in ego functioning).

3 The removal or minimizing of internal obstacles to health, happiness, and achievement.

4 The ability to live in harmony with oneself and with others.

5 Increased capacity to adjust to externally provoked frustrations.

That these results were obtained after only 25 sessions in this case, and in 10–12 sessions respectively in the previous two cases described, provides powerful support for the efficacy of this method of treatment. Short-term therapy does not require a compromise when it comes to goals. In fact, Alexander and French (1946) reported that many of the best therapeutic outcomes achieved in short term dynamic psychotherapy, as opposed to long-term treatment. One can have far-reaching goals and achieve them within a brief time, given the right combination of patient, therapist, and technique. Even though the cases described in this chapter thus far were complex and involved a good deal of traumatic loss, the termination process was smooth. With the Gentleman Scorned, the negative transference feelings, while strong, were identified immediately and worked through in speedy fashion. The two women just described had primarily positive feelings toward the therapist throughout treatment, which were maintained even in the face of separation.

In the following clinical vignettes, you'll notice how the therapist directly addresses the mixed feelings about termination and encourages the kind of "affect-laden" interaction Mann feels is optimal for the resolution of feelings around separation and loss.

Clinical Examples

The Detached Observer

This was a complex case in which rage toward both parents, as well as guilt about the same, needed to be experienced and integrated with love. Massive grief about the effects of repeated separations from his mother, and the sudden loss of her through death when he was 17, was another crucial phase of treatment. As rage, guilt, and grief were processed, his symptoms lifted and he experienced joy and desire for closeness, especially with women. Then, conflicts regarding intimacy, closeness, and sexuality emerged and were addressed. Finally, he was ready to terminate treatment. This had been a long (58 sessions) and very meaningful treatment for both patient and therapist. Saying good-bye was bittersweet.

THERAPIST: How are you feeling as you come in for the last time?

PATIENT: I'm incredibly proud of what I've done here and grateful for all your help, but it's also sad. I wanted to be able to tell you how I feel about you but it's hard (starting to get choked up).

THERAPIST: It stirs up a lot of feelings toward me that you want to be able to express.

PATIENT: I don't' know if it's wanting to tell you that stirs up the feelings or the other way around.

THERAPIST: Well why don't we just look at them.

PATIENT: Yeah. I thought about it this morning. I just thought how, when I first came to see you, how desperate I was. I just called the first person in the phone book and didn't get a referral or shop around or anything. I was thinking how lucky I was to get you. I mean, I could have gotten anybody and if I got somebody that didn't—who wasn't as good as you and couldn't deal with me the way have, how miserable I would have been (crying). I just feel really glad to have you.

THERAPIST: That touches me deeply.

PATIENT: It's nice.

THERAPIST: It's a gift I feel you've given me to let me know that, because what could be more important than being able to touch someone's life. And you have given me that opportunity.

PATIENT: Yeah.

THERAPIST: I don't know if I've told you that, in many ways, I feel the same. I feel lucky too. It's not just for you but for me too that I'm glad you didn't get somebody else.

PATIENT: Yeah.

THERAPIST: I have felt really touched by you.

PATIENT: I think I believe that. I thought about that too—that this has been a two-way street and I could tell that I've had an effect and meant something to you.

This very moving exchange revealed deep levels of change in the way this man related to himself and others. Most important was his ability to experience the therapeutic relationship as mutual and reciprocal. In the past, he was unable to have an emotional connection with or impact on his mother (or his father, for that matter). His mother was highly disturbed and used to tell him he was useless. His father told him that wanting to get close to his mother caused her symptoms and distress. This notion was generalized to others, who he "protected" by keeping his distance. As a result, he had never felt close to anyone. So, for him to feel and sense that he mattered and had had a positive impact on the therapist was completely new.

He went on to say that when he first entered therapy, he hoped he would leave feeling like a different person. Even though he went through massive changes, he reported feeling more like himself than ever. Furthermore, he really liked himself and believed he was worthy of good things. He was connecting deeply with his sisters, nieces, and nephews, as well as friends, had graduated from college, and had built a house for himself, with all the required adaptations. He had parlayed a meager $250,000 insurance settlement into a million-dollar portfolio by trading stocks himself. He was making a big difference in the lives of others, something that continued to expand and will be reported in his follow-up interview.

The Masochistic Artist: Termination

PATIENT: I'm feeling really good these days. It's wonderful. I feel calm and happy and productive. I feel this tremendous sense of relief—I'm on a better track.

The patient opened this session with a statement about her subjective sense of happiness and went on to detail all the changes in her life. These included the improved sense of well-being described in her opening statement, mutually gratifying personal relationships, an ability to assert herself in professional arenas, and a new productivity in her work.

Patient Raises Possibility of Termination

PATIENT: I saw a friend yesterday who's ending therapy, and I thought, "Maybe I could do that".

THERAPIST: So you've been thinking about ending.

PATIENT: Only recently—in the past two weeks or so.

THERAPIST: Look at what you've told me today. The obvious question is "Why would you need to come here anymore?" You're better.

PATIENT: Yeah! One thing that's always impressed me about you is that you've been so encouraging. You just don't slowly sort of begin to deal with your life—you get better. You actually get better, and you are able to leave some of this shit behind and be a person—a better person—someone capable of getting pleasure from life. That has always been a big draw for me to you—this hopefulness—that I won't be stuck in this mire forever and that there's a possibility for real growth.

Feelings of Hope and Confidence

Although critics of Davanloo's methods (Strupp & Binder, 1984) voice concern over how harsh and demanding the treatment may seem, patients frequently report the kinds of feelings this woman expressed. Positive and hopeful feelings are engendered by the therapist's active involvement and expectation for change and improvement. Particularly at termination, patients report feeling proud of themselves for working so hard and accomplishing what they set out to do (Flegenheimer, 1982). Sometimes this kind of positive response is evident earlier in the treatment process. I recall one patient who said, in response to my challenging her defenses against closeness, "I know you probably expect me to be angry, but I feel moved and deeply grateful that you care enough to dig a little. No one has ever made this kind of effort to get to know me beyond the surface".

This is what Davanloo (1990) meant when he referred to the complex nature of the transference feelings evoked by this intensive method of treatment. Patients feel hopeful and even excited about facing what they have avoided, while feeling increasingly confident in their own abilities to deal effectively with life.

Our expectations are powerfully communicated to our patients, so we must examine them carefully (Frank, 1961; Stotland, 1969). If we expect patients to be fragile and require a great deal of time to deal more effectively with life, in all likelihood, that is what will occur. In contrast, if we expect patients to work at their highest level of ability, challenge them to stretch, and are equally willing to work hard and deal with difficult material as it arises, they will often feel heartened and rise to the occasion, as the Masochistic Artist demonstrated.

Accepting the Good

In the case of the Masochistic Artist, love had become equated with pain and suffering. The patient had a history of difficulty in accepting good things. During the phase of working through, there was accumulating evidence that she was beginning to take good care of herself (eating well, allowing herself to rest, buying a couch, and making a comfortable home, etc.), but her ability to allow others to care for her in affectionate and loving ways was untested. This juncture in the treatment process proved an ideal time to test this out in the transference. I was very impressed with, as well as moved by, the changes this woman was reporting. In addition to all the changes she was discussing, there were very noticeable changes that are not reflected in the transcripts. These included a change in her appearance, speech, and manner of relating to the therapist. She behaved in a relaxed and confident, yet direct and engaging manner. I felt it was important to reflect and confirm these changes and to assess her ability to accept positive feedback. It should go without saying that any such comment on the therapist's part must be genuinely felt, as it was in this case.

The Sharing of Feelings of Termination

THERAPIST: So what's it like to hear me reflect on all the changes and to tell you how different it feels to be with you?

PATIENT: I feel kind of teary. It's emotional. It's important to me because I believe in you and what we've done together. I feel this is something we've done together. It's very moving and touching to me.

This response, both in word and tone, suggested that the patient was quite receptive to positive interactions. She was able to feel touched and to express that directly. She was able to receive positive feedback and offer it in return by emphasizing the joint nature of our venture. This kind of spontaneous interaction was a clear reflection of her newly developed capacity to form mutual and reciprocal relationships. Further material revealed these kinds of changes in her current relationships outside therapy.

Improvement in Intimate Relationships

A focus on the relationship, as it develops, is of central importance. Malan and Osimo (1992) have reported that the quality of intimate relationships has proven the most difficult change to effect in patients. Could this be an artifact of the treatment regimen in which the focus is too exclusively intrapsychic in focus? Davanloo's focus has shifted over time. Originally, he focused almost exclusively on intrapsychic phenomena. Gradually, he began to focus on patients' defenses against emotional closeness and highlighed the impact their intrapsychic functioning had on interpersonal relationships. In most cases, it is the difficulty in establishing and maintaining satisfying relationships that brings people into treatment. Sharpening our focus on the quality of relating, including work on the development of the therapeutic relationship, may facilitate substantial and enduring change in this critical area of functioning. In addition, careful monitoring of changes as they occur in the patient's current relationships should reinforce changes within sessions.

Internalization of the Therapist and the Therapeutic Process

PATIENT: I was just thinking I wanted to tell you how important it's been for me to be able to come here. I've been moving and getting things in order and it's all going so well. I'm enjoying my life and my friends.

It has to do with what has happened here in therapy. It's been very important to me.

THERAPIST: It sounds like it's not just therapy that has been important but that you have a lot of feeling toward me.

PATIENT: I do. It's more like a friendship than I thought it would be. Initially, it was like I was talking out loud to myself in the room, but I've become increasingly aware of and empathic with you. I really feel we've done this together. I will miss you. Even though I know we're not friends, there's an importance to the feelings I have for you.

THERAPIST: There's a depth of feeling. There are tender feelings and a sense of closeness. So, for us to say good-bye is painful too.

PATIENT: I miss you, but I carry your words around with me. A lot of this has been internalized. It's missing being here with you, but it doesn't feel like the process will end—it will continue inside me.

Once again, readiness for termination can only be assessed in terms of our goals. In ISTDP, as in psychoanalysis, the goals go beyond symptom removal to include alterations in ego functioning. According to Alexander and French (1946), this is accomplished by "inducing emotional discharge in order to facilitate insight and exposing the ego to those unresolved emotional constellations which it has to learn to master" (p. vii). This therapeutic work has as its aim an increase in "the patient's ability to find gratification for his subjective needs in ways acceptable to both himself and the world he lives in" (Alexander & French, 1946, p. 26). In the case being presented, this has been accomplished. The patient dealt with her traumatic past and all the intense and previously terrifying feelings she experienced in reaction to recalled events. Freed from the compulsion to repeat her past, she was able to discover new and gratifying means for working productively and for loving and being loved.

In addition to alterations in ego functioning, particularly the observing, anticipatory, and integrative capabilities, the nature and quality of parental introjects had also changed during the therapeutic process. The patient's newfound ability to care for herself, and to allow others to care for her in a nurturing way, indicated a change in the nature and quality of her parental introjects. The patient stated that she had internalized both the therapist's voice and the analytic process. She was now able to do for herself what the therapist had done for her. This is what makes loss bearable; a sentiment uttered by the patient. She noted that internalization of the therapist rendered separation possible without a feeling of traumatic loss. Patients frequently say things like "I don't feel like I'm losing you because I have you inside of me". This process of internalization seems to parallel that which occurs in normal development and allows a child to separate without undue anxiety. One evening, following a brief separation from my seven-year-old son I asked, "Did you miss me?" "Not really", he said, "You see, I have this picture of you in my mind—standing in front of the house". This internalized image of me and our home offered my son a sense of security that enabled him to separate without distress. This is the kind of process we seek to facilitate therapeutically in our patients.

How this occurs remains a matter of debate (Wachtel, 1993). Luborsky and Mark (1991) have suggested that "internalization is a gradual process by which external interactions between the person and others are taken in and replaced by internal representations of these interactions (Crits-Christoph & Barber, 1991, p. 116). More specifically, Ellman (1991) has suggested that it's the "analyst's equanimity in the face of conflict" that needs to be internalized so that the patient can face post-treatment conflicts with a similar attitude.

The Man with an Explosive Temper: Part 2

Several authors (Horner, 1984; Novick, 1982; Sterba, 1934) have emphasized the importance of the patient's ability to perform self-analysis as an indicator of preparedness for termination and a safeguard against future deterioration. In the case of the Man with the Explosive Temper (see Chapter 7), there was evidence of both symptom removal and the replacement of pathological defenses with adaptive alternatives. The patient's relationships were becoming closer, richer, and more reciprocal. In the following vignette, he told the therapist about a recent incident in which strong feelings were evoked. Following the experience, he was able to understand the personal meaning it had for him. This was particularly important in this case because he came for treatment, stating that strong feelings seemed to come out of the blue and he'd have no idea what triggered them. Evidence of self-understanding in which emotional and cognitive insights were integrated suggested a readiness to end treatment and carry on the work by himself.

Evidence of Capacity for Self-Understanding

PATIENT: My wife and I went to the theater to celebrate our anniversary. We have a new and deeper closeness now. We saw a dramatic production of *Phantom of the Opera*. I had read the book and knew that the manager of the opera house was the Phantom's father. The Phantom had been hiding because he was deformed by something his mother drank in an attempt to abort him. His father doesn't tell him who he is until he's been shot by the police, but the Phantom said he'd always known. I thought of you because I saw a connection between the play and my own father and me. I was really crying. I was so sad because this was me and my story. I identified with the Phantom—being wounded by

> rejection. He took so long to realize he was my father. His death won't be as painful as the loss of that bond.

Much of the therapeutic work in this case involved freeing the patient to experience the intense and conflicted feelings toward his brutal and sadistic father. Prior to treatment, his characteristic methods for defending against these feelings had left him in a state of detached confusion, punctuated with sudden and unintelligible emotional outbursts. This pattern was adversely affecting all his interactions, at work as well as at home. Now that he was able to experience and understand his emotions, he could use all his capacities to decide on an appropriate way to deal with them. This increased his personal confidence, as well as improving his relationships with others. He was especially grateful that the deep understanding he had developed of himself had expanded his capacity for genuine compassion for others resulting in newfound closeness with family members. In addition, his ability to understand his emotional reactions provided a reliable safeguard against repetitions of the past.

Defensive Withdrawal Replaced with Relatedness

PATIENT: This is it, huh?

THERAPIST: How are you feeling about that?

PATIENT: I had an interesting experience on Sunday. I am a convert and was asked to speak about the program for adults interested in joining the church. I did it on Sunday and I broke down. I got through the talk, but I cried. I felt embarrassed, but after the Mass I received an outpouring of warmth from others.

THERAPIST: What about it was so moving?

PATIENT: Memories of my grandfather, whom I talked about. I wasn't able to get to his funeral and I feel awful about that. He was more of a father to me than my own father. We would pitch horseshoes, fish together, ride in his pickup. I was the first grandchild, and I spent a lot of time with him. These new relationships with priests and other men in the class reminded me of him. That's when I cried. When I left the podium, I got a standing ovation. My family came over and surrounded me with love and support. Others came over with tears in their eyes, all choked up. Even strangers came up to me and said how moving it was. It felt so good to have these people respond.

This last vignette, along with the previous sessions in which the patient revealed a newfound ability to love his wife and children, demonstrates the kind of change in the quality of relating that Menninger (1958) has described. He wrote that "above everything else in life he wants to love and be loved and realizes that he can give love and get love and also that he can hate effectively when necessary" (p. 158).

Relations with others assume a real specificity. He was able to love those of his choosing while staying away from or confronting those who posed a threat. Both were essential in this case, as the patient had previously been unable to protect himself from violence. In fact, during the course of treatment, his home was vandalized. He was able to take firm and appropriate steps to apprehend the offenders and to protect himself, his family, and his home from violence.

The Cold Blooded Businessman

This cold, detached, rather narcissistic man, who had a long history of using women for his own temporary pleasure and then tossing them aside, became suicidally depressed when he was no longer able to seduce them. In our work together, we discovered a deep reservoir of rage toward women that had its origin in the relationship with his hostile and demanding mother. He had fused rage with sexual feelings and split women into two categories—the Madonna and the whore. He put his wife on a pedestal but was unable to function sexually with her, while acting out sexually with women with whom he had no emotional attachment. As the feelings of rage, pain, and longing were experienced, initially in the transference (and then linked to the past), he was able to integrate sexual and loving feelings. The relationship with his wife and all other women, including his daughters, were vastly improved.

In our last session, he freely expressed gratitude toward me for working so hard on his behalf and supporting him in the healing process. At the end, he handed me a gift—a copy of *To Kill A Mockingbird.* He had marked a passage he wanted me to read. It was the passage in which Calpernia, the family's maid, and Scout were on the balcony of the courthouse, watching her father, Atticus Fitch, walk by at the end of the trial. Calpernia said, "Stand up Jeanne Lousie (her proper name), your father's passing". This statement of profound respect was what he was trying to communicate to me. He neither idealized nor devalued me, but respected me—quite an achievement.

The Lonely Businessman

After only ten sessions, this man's anxiety and depression had been replaced with confidence and hope. He was able to proceed with divorce, and eventually met a partner with whom he shared a profound level of closeness. They remained together for 17 years, until his death. In addition to his newfound ability to love without restraint, he was able to pursue his professional life with assurance. He published four books and attained a very senior position in the federal government, commensurate with his education, experience, and capacity. As with many of the patients cited here, his creativity also blossomed; as the energy he had used to suppress his feelings was lifted, he published a volume of poetry and became an avid photographer.

He credited our therapy with these deep and lasting changes, as he had engaged in previous therapies that had no therapeutic impact. In particular, he cited the ability to get through his defensive barrier to release buried feelings and memories, which, as an adult, he was able to tolerate, experience, and integrate.

Return of Symptoms at Termination

In the analytic literature, one frequently finds reference to the phenomenon in which old symptoms return as termination is approached. This is certainly not a universal phenomenon and only occurs in a small percentage of patients treated with ISTDP. Should this kind of regression occur, it is an indication that specific feelings and defenses regarding separation and loss need to be worked through (Trujillo & Winston, 1985). This was the case with the Man with Primary Impotence (see Chapter 6). This highly dependent man had experienced a great deal of gratification from the intense and sexualized relationship with his mother. In treatment, he became increasingly aware of the underlying rage toward his mother for holding onto him and using him in ways that interfered with his optimal development. Still, as termination approached, old fears about being alone, along with the anger and pain associated with loss emerged. The re-appearance of passive-dependent defenses accompanied this upheaval. In addition to current feelings regarding the impending loss of the therapist, termination revived feelings about losses from the past that had not yet been mourned.

Evidence of Regression as Termination Approaches

The patient came into the session described in the following vignette saying he could feel himself reverting to procrastination as a way to avoid ending the therapy and facing all the feelings associated with the loss. This insight was crucial and directed the session toward the emotions that were being avoided.

PATIENT: I felt anxious coming here today because I haven't been working. I feel like a kid who doesn't have his homework done. I'm reacting to the pressure to get moving—I procrastinate.

THERAPIST: You cling to this old pattern of interaction in which you play the naughty boy and then I am either the harsh mother who scolds or the indulgent one.

PATIENT: And on and on. I like the times when I feel motivated and I move. The only way to do it is to do it.

THERAPIST: Let's look at what gets in your way.

PATIENT: I'm getting stuck in my head but there's pain inside. I'm sad and frustrated about the thought of ending. I told my friend about what I've been doing here. He said he felt sad about the things I had told him, but I couldn't really open up to him emotionally. I tried. I made the decision to tell him about these things but emotionally I didn't open up. I'm scared of overwhelming sadness.

THERAPIST: You have to pass through the pain to be free to open to others. It can be frightening, and the temptation is to pull back but . . .

PATIENT: It's like swimming. It's cold at first, but if you plunge in, it's great.

The patient proved to be highly motivated and demonstrated a good deal of intellectual insight into the meaning of his current difficulties with procrastination. In fact, he had enough insight to understand that awareness alone was insufficient to produce lasting change. The problem was an emotional one. The mechanisms he had developed during childhood to avoid painful and frightening feelings were interfered with the development and maintenance of close relationships in adulthood. He spelled this out quite clearly when discussing a current friendship. Toward the end of this sequence, he seemed to be encouraging himself to approach rather than avoid these painful feelings by using the swimming metaphor. The same struggle he had elaborated on in his current relationship with a friend needed to be outlined in the transference.

Feelings and Defenses in the Transference

THERAPIST: Here too, do you notice that each time the sadness starts to well up, you avoid my eyes and look at the floor? You keep a distance from me to avoid these feelings.

PATIENT: I look at you and it starts to hurt. I want to look you in the eye and tell you, but I'm avoiding it. There's a lot of tension but some excitement too. There's a part of me that isn't helpless with you anymore. I feel a strength from my center. It's charged—there's something strong inside.

Comparing New and Old Ways of Dealing with Loss

As we approached the grief-laden feelings he feared, the patient reported feeling strong and capable. At this point in treatment, he became aware of the positive consequences of using new, adaptive means of dealing with feelings, as well as the negative consequences of reverting to outmoded defenses. Processing how it feels to interact in this new way is essential in consolidating the changes. Often patients regress to avoid new feelings and experiences, not just to flee those from the past. In this case, to be a strong, capable man means facing the loss of the therapist.

Processing the Effect of New Changes

THERAPIST: What is it like to feel like a strong man with me?

PATIENT: I've been thinking about saying good-bye to you. Then I heard about someone who saw you for two years, and I thought "That gives me an out". I think I'm afraid to say good-bye. Then I also think she got more time than me.

THERAPIST: Feeling scared to leave and avoiding and procrastinating came after you found out about this other patient?

PATIENT: Yeah, and I thought she's pushing me out and now I'm clinging.

THERAPIST: What is your feeling toward me then?

PATIENT: I don't know why I'm afraid every time I think of leaving. I want to leave with a good feeling but it's painful. I don't know what a good parting is—I've never had it.

THERAPIST: Parting while retaining the good feeling. This certainly never happened with your mother.

Two things seem to be going on here. On the one hand, the patient is trying to do things differently, while resisting a regressive pull in the face of an impending loss. An additional factor has emerged regarding competitive feelings reminiscent of rivalries with siblings. Defending against these feelings, which had not been previously worked through, added fuel to his defensive clinging. Both issues needed to be addressed. The patient's ensuing associations indicated that the rivalrous feelings were most prominent. Avoiding this material could seriously interfere with his goal of ending treatment in a positive manner.

Competition and Sibling Rivalry

PATIENT: I used to have this dream where I would smash my sister's head, and she'd be tied to a cross. Dead—with stuff leaking out of her head, and some other member of the family would come and say, "Let's go", but I couldn't let go. I couldn't believe what I had done. There was terrible pain and a longing to change what had happened. How could I live with this? I feel it's bad. I'm wrong to leave (crying). I feel so responsible. It's my fault. My mother and sister were in such a bad way. How can I leave them behind and have a good life?

Talking about ending the therapy, and finding out that another patient had been involved in a longer-term therapy, revived competitive feelings toward siblings that had not come up in the therapy previously. This concurrence of events provided the opportunity to rework these feelings and to understand his tendency to cling to his mother in the past and to the therapist in the present as manifestations of maladaptive defenses against feelings of competitiveness with rivals. By having a special closeness with his mother, he felt he could "beat" his siblings.

When he became conscious of this, the cost attendant to this strategy began to outweigh the gains. He now felt he had won by losing. Not only did he end up saddled with a demanding, histrionic mother, but his relationships with his siblings suffered. Following this session, he began to reach out to his siblings in an attempt to develop a new sense of closeness with them as adults. In addition, he recognized how this pattern of competitiveness was repeated with peers with detrimental effects.

Finding a New and Adaptive Way to Say Good-Bye

Another important aspect of the work required at termination involves finding new ways to say good-bye. In the present case, simply putting an end to his tendency to procrastinate by working dutifully to the end of treatment would constitute progress but not substantive change.

Procrastination and regression need to be replaced by something adaptive. He made it very clear to the therapist that he had a specific goal in ending treatment—to say good-bye while maintaining the positive feelings he genuinely felt toward the therapist. This was something he had never been able to accomplish in the past. His goal could not be achieved by passing over the negative, competitive feelings and the guilt they engendered, but only by facing them directly. This material provided another opportunity to do so.

Special Consideration with Victims of Trauma

Nearly all the patients being described in this chapter experienced significant trauma in their childhood, whether the result of a mother's manic-depressive illness, a brother's psychotic decompensation, or brutal beatings by a sadistic father. According to Judith Herman (1992), who has devoted herself to the treatment of psychological trauma, termination should begin when "the survivor no longer feels possessed by her traumatic past", but, having dealt with it directly, feels free. This was expressed by the Manic-Depressive's Daughter when she said she no longer felt haunted by the past. As the patient is able to face the trauma and mourn for the "old self", a new self begins to develop. The damaged, victimized self begins to be transformed by a process of integration with the survivor self who has courageously faced the horrors of the past (Herman, 1992).

Mother's Little Angel reported feeling proud of herself for having faced all the trauma in her past and said she felt stronger and like a new and improved version of her old self.

In accordance with Malan's dictum that each pathological defense be replaced by something adaptive, Herman (1992) suggests that the replacement of a sense of helplessness and isolation with a feeling of empowerment and reconnection is a crucial factor in the recovery of patients who have been traumatized. "Having come to terms with the traumatic past, the survivor faces the task of creating a future" (p. 196). For health to be restored, it is necessary but insufficient to deal with the past. The patient must develop a revised sense of self which should include:

1 A reduction in physiological reactivity.

2 The ability to bear emotions associated with trauma.

3 Authority over memories such that they are neither repressed nor intrusive.

4 Memories of trauma that form a coherent narrative integrated with feeling.

5 A sense of self that is no longer damaged.

6 Close and trusting relationships with those who warrant it.

7 A system of belief and meaning that includes the experience of the trauma.

The Man with an Explosive Temper seemed to exemplify these changes. In addition to dealing with the past, this man found a new and enriched means for relating to his family and the community at large. Toward the end of treatment, his internal changes produced far-reaching changes in his functioning. He was able to use his own experience to understand, on a deep emotional and personal level, the struggles of others. By sharing his experiences with others, he was able to transform hurting into healing—perhaps the ultimate sign of recovery.

The treatment process did not simply stop the past from repeating itself by removing the negative, damaging cycle of explosive anger and fear, but facilitated a transformation in which real growth and reparative connections replaced hostile interactions.

Termination is dealt with in a straightforward fashion in ISTDP and requires little in the way of special techniques. Rather, the same tenacity in breaking through defensive avoidance and the same encouragement to face all the mixed feelings evoked by the loss of the therapist—which have characterized the treatment from the start—continue until the end. Termination is not considered traumatic. Losses are a part of life, and it is the way they are dealt with that is the focus of intervention. Allowing patients the freedom to end in new ways aids in the consolidation of positive feelings about the self and others. While loss cannot be prevented, regret about feelings unexpressed or actions not taken can be addressed and prevented. In addition to finding new ways to say good-bye to the therapist, termination provides another opportunity to mourn past losses.

Summary

Ideally, therapy ends when the patient's goals have been achieved. Furthermore, we want to obtain evidence that all symptoms and pathological defenses have been removed and replaced with healthy alternatives. In some cases, therapy will be ended prematurely due to unforeseen circumstances like the loss of a job or moving to a different state. In these cases, summarizing what has been achieved thus far, anticipating challenges in the future, and dealing with all the mixed feelings about leaving in the middle of treatment must be addressed.

When therapy is focused and short-term, termination tends to be uncomplicated and marked by a sense of pride and gratitude. When the treatment has been complex and challenging, resulting in profound levels of healing and transformation, both therapist and patient are changed. Termination is yet another opportunity to face and experience all the mixed feelings about loss. Since the therapist and therapeutic process often become internalized, positive feelings tend to predominate in the end.

It is also notable that ISTDP appears to be effective in cases that typically don't respond to psychotherapy, including personality disorders, treatment resistant depression, chronic pain, medically unexplained symptoms, and neurological symptoms including pseudo seizures, movement disorders, and fugue states (Abbass, 2015; Abbass, et al., 2008; Abbass, et al., 2012; Solbaken & Abbass, 2015; Town, et al., 2020). Furthermore, the effect sizes of ISTDP well outstrips medication and CBT (Shedler, 2010; 2017).

So, why isn't this method practiced more widely? As Alexander and French (1946) opined long ago, it takes clinicians far more time, energy, and dedication to develop the knowledge and skill required to facilitate deep and lasting change in a short period of time than administering "treatment as usual". To do this kind of work, the therapist must develop deep domain-specific knowledge, hone complex therapeutic skills, and be willing to devote a great deal of time and energy to supervision and training well beyond that offered in their degree programs. There is also evidence that the best therapists have superior meta-cognitive skills, such as working memory, and have high levels of emotional intelligence (Wampold, 2015).

Summary and Conclusions

In this chapter, the critical factors involved in termination phase of therapy were explored. The importance of achieving therapeutic goals, addressing the emotional complexities surrounding the end of treatment, and incorporating follow-up sessions to assess patient progress over time was emphasized.

Note

1. From "Breaking the Silence." Music and lyrics by Loreena McKennitt.

9 FOLLOW-UP

Sadly, studies have established the fact that over 50% of those seeking psychotherapeutic help receive no benefit (Abbass, 2015). For those who engage and improve, relapse often follows (Steinhart, et al., 2014). This is the case for psychopharmacology, as well as psychotherapy. Relapse rates for electroconvulsive shock treatment are greater than 50% (Jelovac, et al., 2013). In contrast, empirical studies on the long-term effectiveness of Intensive Short-Term Dynamic Psychotherapy (ISTDP) (Abbass & Katzman, 2013; Abbass, 2015; Driessen, et al, 2015; Shedler, 2017 Wiborg & Dahl, 1996) have achieved promising results. These data are especially significant since research has found that initial dropout rates in ISTDP are quite low (Abbass, 2015). This means that more patients engage and receive benefits from treatment, as well as retaining them. Additional clinical data can be obtained by therapists who conduct follow-up interviews with their completed cases. In the tradition of Malan and Davanloo, the author typically conducts one-, five-, and ten-year follow-ups and has follow-up data on some patients that span 20 and even 30 years. Much can be learned from in-depth interviews of these patients.

The Crucial Significance of Follow-Up

We are all indebted to Dr. Malan, one of the first clinicians to systematically study the effectiveness of brief dynamic psychotherapy. This work included detailed follow-up interviews years after psychotherapy had been terminated. Such data are essential in determining whether our interventions are truly curative.

DOI: 10.4324/9781003542131-9

The Tavistock group developed a rating scale to categorize patient response to treatment both at termination and follow-up (Malan, 1963). The criteria for success were as follows: 0 indicated no change; a score of 1 represented some symptomatic improvement but no evidence of greater coping skills in the area of the core conflict; a score of 2 reflected meaningful symptomatic improvement plus evidence of new coping strategies for dealing adaptively in previously conflictual situations; and a score of 3 indicated broad change beyond the specific conflictual area to reflect greater coping in relationships with both men and women and better performance at work. Malan's (1976) data suggest that those who were scored "improved" (a score of 2 or more) at termination maintained or exceeded this level of functioning at three- to five-year follow-up. In fact, 50% of those who scored a 2 at termination, moved up to 3 at follow-up.

It is also important to note that Malan (1979), in disagreement with Mann (1973; 1991), found that awareness of follow-up interviews in no way diluted feelings about termination or interfered with the process. It seems that the feelings evoked at termination are so robust, it is unnecessary to try to preserve them by adhering to a rigid structure in which there is no contact after treatment ends.

Davanloo (1978) reported that of 130 patients deemed suitable for ISTDP, 115 were successfully treated in an average of 20 sessions. These positive results were maintained in follow-up interviews conducted between two and seven years post-treatment. Davanloo engaged patients in an active reassessment of the process at follow-up. Both patient and therapist watched videotaped segments of treatment sessions. Davanloo invited feedback from patients and elicited their reflections about what they had found helpful. Of significance was a frequently reported perception that patients had improved as the result of their own hard work, rather than being passively cured by the therapist. This increased their sense of confidence and mastery—so essential for long-term resilience. They tended to report feeling "free" or "like a new person", attesting to the dramatic changes that had taken place.

Clinical Evidence of Further Improvement at Follow-Up

The Woman with Headaches

This 36-year-old woman suffered from crushing headaches since the age of eight, when she was first hospitalized for this condition. She came for therapy at the age of 36 because she was engaged to be married but couldn't go through with it. She loved her fiancé but every time a date was set for the wedding she would freeze with anxiety and literally be reduced to a fetal position, unable to get out of bed for days.

Her symptoms were severe and long standing, interfering with her most basic ability to function when acute. Many previous attempts at therapy were unsuccessful. She suffered brutal attacks by her father and had no protection from her mother, who was frequently ill and in the hospital. The therapist she consulted prior to engaging in ISTDP dissolved into tears when hearing about her past history. The patient clicked into caretaking mode and made no progress. Others steered clear of these painful memories altogether, offering strategies for how to cope with current life challenges. In her ISTDP treatment, she was supported to face the rage and grief that she had suppressed all her life. In a pivotal session, recounted in Chapter 4, she was able to experience the full brunt of murderous rage toward her father. Of note, she had seen him two weeks prior and had suffered with a severe headache ever since. Following our work on liberating these feelings, and the impulses that accompanied them, her headache went away.

These severe and long-standing symptoms were removed and replaced with healthy alternatives in only 20 sessions. This result confirms Malan's findings that neither history nor diagnosis predicts who will be able to respond to short-term dynamic psychotherapy. The method must be applied, with responses to intervention used to determine suitability.

The follow-up session recounted here took place five years after termination.

THERAPIST: What about the headaches?

PATIENT: You know, I haven't had one of those headaches since that session in which I really felt the rage toward my father.

THERAPIST: That's amazing. All that was getting turned back on you. Once you faced that it was his head you wanted to smash and his eyes you wanted to pierce, the need to do that to yourself lifted.

PATIENT: Yes, I guess that's how we can explain it. I just know I feel better than I've ever felt in my life.

THERAPIST: The other major reason you came to see me was because of the terror that would strike whenever you set a date to marry.

PATIENT: Yes! Well, let me tell you about that. When we ended therapy, I had set another date, but we hadn't yet gotten married. On the day of our wedding, I remember being really nervous. I was standing in the back of the church, but then I looked up and saw Bob, and all that anxiety melted away. It was as if the aisle was a bridge, from my old life to a new one. I never imagined I could be so happy.

THERAPIST: I can feel tears coming to my eyes as you tell me this—it's so touching.

PATIENT: It gets even better. You know how I was terrified to have children, in case I had a boy. There is such a long line of angry, violent men in my family, and I didn't know what I would do with a boy. Well, I got pregnant pretty fast and, wouldn't you know, my first was a boy. I call him my sunshine. He is nothing like my father or brothers and is just like Bob. He is so sweet and loving. Then I had a girl, so we feel complete and so happy.

THERAPIST: I am so glad to hear that.

PATIENT: I should tell you about my parents too. My mother died three years ago. I was with her at the end. I know there were times when you wanted me to get angry with her for not protecting me, but I never felt that way. She was so sick for so long and, despite it all, was a loving presence for us all. It felt so good to be able to be there for her. She died in my arms, and it was so peaceful. And I feel peaceful too.

Even though it was suggested that she would have to be angry with her mother for not protecting her, she had no awareness of any such anger. Furthermore, there was no evidence that she was avoiding anger by using pathological defenses or getting symptomatic. Again, it is response to intervention that guides the process, not our assumptions.

THERAPIST: Well, that's what's important. It sounds incredibly important that you could be there for and with her. How is it with your dad?

PATIENT: I see him how he is. There are no illusions and no hope that he will change or be different. I used to go home to see my mother and had to tolerate him. After she died, I decided I wasn't going to shut him out all together or avoid family gathering so I wouldn't have to see him. I am polite but keep my distance—and I would never leave my children alone with him.

THERAPIST: So you are a protective mother.

PATIENT: I really am.

THERAPIST: What do you think helped you get here? These changes are really huge—not only in the elimination of debilitating symptoms like headaches and freezing into a fugue state—but being happy, joyful, and close with your husband and children.

PATIENT: I was so afraid I might repeat that family pattern. I had to face what happened and all my feelings about it so I could resolve it and leave it in the past. You helped me face it and weren't overwhelmed by it yourself, like those other therapists. I trusted you that you wouldn't back away, and you didn't. I think that's what finally clicked when I was in the back of the church. I literally felt myself leaving that all behind and starting a new life.

THERAPIST: Just as you saw yourself leaving the kitchen and going into the living room, where the sun was shining.

PATIENT: Oh, you're right. How did you remember?

THERAPIST: How could I forget?

When we go to hell and back with patients, we are changed by the experience. If we are present and engaged, we will be deeply affected by these shared experiences. Given that level of involvement, forgetting is not a possibility. Just as patients carry me with them, I carry in my heart all those who have allowed me in deeply enough to make a difference. That kind of involvement is felt by the patient and is an important factor in therapeutic success. They have the felt sense that we are in this together. And, ultimately, that is what makes the unbearable bearable.

The Cold Blooded Businessman

Shortly after ending treatment, the patient decided to retire and move back to his wife's hometown. Following treatment, he had become very close to his relatives. In fact, his wife came to see me after his treatment ended to tell me about the profound changes she had witnessed and express her appreciation. While he had been detached from his own children as they were growing up, she reported that, currently, he was the first one to be down on the floor playing with his grandchildren. His individual healing became a healing force in the whole family system.

Ten years later, I received a letter from him in which he detailed further improvements. His relationships continued to deepen and existed at the very center of his life. Freed from the demands of work, he pursued his passion for music. Together with his wife, they had become important figures in the community, involved in philanthropy and charitable work. He was, in many ways, unrecognizable from the man who initially came to see me. These kinds of profound transformations are possible and have been documented here. While this does not always transpire, and not all patients require such extensive transformation, it speaks to what is possible. It also demonstrates how "to change one person is to change the world" (Fromm Reichman, 1950). One of the most important findings from these follow-up sessions is how frequently patients who are healed become a healing force in their families and communities.

The Woman on an Emotional Roller Coaster

This lifelong people pleaser was thrown into a crisis when she received a cancer diagnosis at the age of 42. She responded by alternatively repressing her feelings and becoming depressed, and acting out her anger in destructive ways. In only eight sessions, she was able to access and process the long-buried feelings of rage, guilt, and grief from her childhood and 25-year marriage. This was experienced as liberating, healing, and growth-producing. She was able to divorce her husband amicably and become an available and responsive mother to her children. Twenty years later, I received a letter from her.

> "Dear Dr Coughlin,
>
> I don't know if you remember me, but you saw me for a brief, but intensive course of therapy about 20 years ago. I have had a recurrence of the cancer that was supposed to have killed me long ago. It has metastasized and I know the end is near. Thanks to our work together, and the changes that wrought, I can die in peace.
>
> You helped me face the rage toward my mother and husband that I had long repressed. As a result, I was able to reconcile with my mother and divorce amicably from my husband. Before I came to see you, I was so depressed that I couldn't take care of my children. Subsequently I have been available and responsive to them. They are grown now, and we have a very strong bond.
>
> While I have participated in some cancer support groups over the years, I have never felt the need to get back into therapy. I think we really got to the heart of the matter. As a result, I have been able to build a happy, productive life with meaningful work and wonderful friends. Most importantly, I married a wonderful man, and we have created a truth-filled, passionate, and joyful relationship. I was finally able to be authentic in a relationship with a man, to really open up and reveal myself. That includes my sexual feelings and desires. If you recall, I never had an orgasm with my first husband. Now, sex is fun, passionate, and orgasmic!
>
> I wanted to let you know about the lasting impact of the work we did together and to thank you from the bottom of my heart."

This woman had developed a passive, dependent character as the result of repressing all her feelings and desires, while focusing on trying to please others. The cancer diagnosis triggered a crisis, as she suddenly realized she had abandoned herself and never shown up authentically in relationships. Research has repeatedly demonstrated that being in a crisis bodes well for deep and rapid change, if the therapist can help the patient face what they have been avoiding (Malan, 1978a).

This case supports those findings.

The Masochistic Artist

One Year Follow-Up

THERAPIST: Well, how are you?

PATIENT: I'm great. It's been a particularly good time for me since about last September. We ended in July, and I spent the summer with my husband. I realized I was playing something out that I just couldn't do anymore, but I needed to try it and to do it without you. I had to try being with him from this new position of self-awareness and resourcefulness that I have attained. The marriage seemed immutable. There was no openness. He continued to see me in a very fixed way and saw himself as the injured party. He wouldn't move. The message was that I would have to make amends. I could feel myself being eroded, and I just couldn't do it. So, by the end of the summer, it was clear the marriage was over. When he left, I felt such relief. There were feelings of loss—anger and sadness—but I felt like myself. Life has become rich. Things really took off after that and it's been steady ever since. I'm optimistic about myself and the world.

THERAPIST: This is very interesting, because you seemed to know all of this at the end of treatment. Still, you're saying it was important to test it out in reality. I remember you saying that you wanted to be with your husband now that you no longer had a need to be used and abused. You wondered if you had pulled this from him, and if you no longer needed him to be an oppressor, he might be free to change. It does take two to tango. You seemed to know that your changes would create change in the relationship. Either you could grow together or it would be over.

Post-Termination Transference Reactions

THERAPIST: Now the part you didn't seem aware of, and you didn't mention until today, was something going on between you and me—because you say you had to do it without me.

PATIENT: I didn't realize it until the Fall, after my husband left. I had this dynamic in my life where people would offer suggestions, and I was very susceptible to that. I had to make sure I wasn't just reacting to others' expectations but was exerting my own feelings.

THERAPIST: You wanted to be certain you weren't submitting to what you thought I wanted you to do. There was such intrusiveness in the past it was difficult to tell where the other left off and you began.

PATIENT: This is interesting in my friendships too. I notice how I tended to mirror their expectations and suppress my own. Now that I'm separated and getting divorced, I see how others play out their fantasies and fears on me. I'm much clearer when someone is projecting their concerns onto me and I can address it directly. Like with my friend . . . (gives concrete example).

The changes noted at termination in this woman's ability to form and maintain relationships that were positive, rather than sado-masochistic, were solidified over time. She was aware of her own dynamics and sensitive to unconscious forces in herself and others. In addition, she reported discussing these things freely with friends, all indicating significant growth. That enormous changes had occurred cannot be disputed. What factors were responsible for these changes? Following Davanloo's lead, I invite the patient to explore this with me.

Feedback from Patients on Factors Responsible for Change

PATIENT: So there's a whole new level of intimacy in my friendships.

THERAPIST: It really sounds like you feel released from this bondage. Obviously, this was a successful treatment. What do you think was responsible for the change?

PATIENT: Something very basic. Feeling someone being so sympathetic and empathic with a pain I was suffering. It sounds so simple, and, in a way, it is, but when you spend all your time and emotional energy denying that or feeling you're not entitled to it—because I really internalized my mother's voice. So I think that feeling I'm entitled to the pain, it's there, and I can bear it, made me understand how the avoidance of that pain set up this whole pattern of defensiveness. The other thing was your being very challenging and tough about bringing it back to the original source of pain and asking me how I actually feel it, cutting through the layers so I could really experience it. I don't know what else to say. It just makes it more difficult to return to denial. The layers get discarded.

The patient made it clear that her therapy provided two essential ingredients that enabled her to change. The first was a feeling of *empathic connection with the therapist*, and the second was *the rigorous examination of feelings*, both present and past. This feedback confirms the hypotheses formulated by Malan and Davanloo regarding both the specific (focus on the triangles) and nonspecific (empathy) factors responsible for the powerful results obtained with ISTDP.

PATIENT: Now if I start in on self-loathing, I just stop it because I see it as very destructive, and it's really not me.

This statement revealed how the patient's conscious ego had assumed control. The harsh and punitive superego, which had been dominating her functioning in all areas previously, now had a back seat. If it tried to assert itself, she recognized it as destructive and put a stop to it.

PATIENT: There are immediate rewards too, so it's not just an abstraction. There's more pleasure in life, more intimacy—so it's very reinforcing.

Here the patient confirmed one of the central hypotheses proposed by Wachtel (1993) regarding the cyclical nature of changes in the intrapsychic and interpersonal spheres of functioning. Internal changes beget external changes that are noticed and, in this case, reinforced by others. With her husband, these changes were not welcomed. Rather than revert to previous pathological accommodations to him, she left the marriage and selected those who supported her growth.

PATIENT: I've been dating some, and I think I see things much more clearly. I speak up for myself and don't just go along with the man. I'm also done with guilt. I say, "This is what I want and you'll have to decide if that's ok with you".

As Malan and Osimo (1992) reported in their follow-up studies, the change from passivity to active self-assertion is one of the most consistent findings in patients who respond to this form of treatment.

THERAPIST: So you take care of yourself but don't assume responsibility for others. You are clear about your needs and expectations and expect others to do the same.

The nature and extent of the changes reported (and observed) reflected profound character change rather than symptoms removal alone. What had gone wrong, kept going right, in large part because the changes in her way of being and interacting with others.

Ten-Year Follow-Up

THERAPIST: So nice to see you! Tell me about your life.

PATIENT: It's great. It's really great. A lot of wonderful things have happened. First of all, I met a wonderful man and we are married. It's like a miracle. We are so happy.

THERAPIST: Tell me.

PATIENT: I met him about 15 years ago and we knew each other casually. At the time, he was with someone, and I was married, but we always liked each other. He is a professor and has a studio in NYC. Mutual friends there had a dinner party, and we connected again. Turns out he always had a little crush on me, and I had a little crush on him. He's a real sweetheart. I just adore him. And we didn't have it easy from the start. We were both working things through, but because of all this motivation, hard work, and love, we are really happy together. I feel so lucky. Now I can't believe I was married to this other person!

THERAPIST: The contrast!

PATIENT: When we first got together, I thought, "He's too nice for me".

THERAPIST: Now this is what we have to look at. This is the cure right here, because that need to be punished . . .

PATIENT: Right. He is really good to me. I mean, he doesn't spoil me. He loves me because I'm a responsible person. He is too. We are very much alike. He's good looking in this athletic sort of way that I really like. He's smart and, look, we are really well matched—temperamentally well matched too.

THERAPIST: And both highly functional—not like with your former husband.

PATIENT: Right. The possibility of being in a really good relationship has an aspect of healing to it. Like, you don't change who you are but, if you find someone who is functional and motivated, you can trust enough so they can help heal you. I feel like I've done that for him too.

THERAPIST: So it's really mutual and reciprocal.

PATIENT: It's really wonderful. There are times when I was fantasizing about who I would find. I imagined it would be some perfect person, whatever that means. But I'm with a real person. He's not perfect, nor am I, but we love each other. I told a friend of mine a while ago, "I can't believe I'll ever be unhappy again". Of course, I have been unhappy about other things, but it's just such an important part of my life, and it enables me to do other things.

THERAPIST: That's so different—to have a relationship that is nourishing and energizing instead of so draining.

PATIENT: It's a terrible thing. I know I'll never want that again. I don't want that with anyone—not friends or colleagues. Actually, I am the Director at _____ now and I am very clear about what I want and expect, and I won't compromise or let myself be treated poorly. Of course, I consider the needs of others and am diplomatic, but I will never let myself be treated that way again.

THERAPIST: You no longer sacrifice yourself for others or allow yourself to be used.

PATIENT: I don't do that at all. It's like I'm a healthy person now (laughs joyfully)!

THERAPIST: You are indeed. And how is sex? I have to ask you that!

PATIENT: It's wonderful. We have this very strong mutual desire for each other and with each other. It feels like I'm more physically present than I've ever been. First of all, we have sex all the time, which is really great. I keep thinking, this can't last—but it has. It's so natural. I love his body, and he delights in mine. It feels like I love this whole person—his body and his being, so it's really wonderful. That tendency to play out being dominated just doesn't happen.

THERAPIST: It's integrated—how you feel with who you are. You are no longer play acting to please others but full yourself. What is your idea about how you got here?

PATIENT: All your help and support, first of all. I really trusted you, as I had never been able to trust anyone before.

THERAPIST: So how did that happen?

PATIENT: You were just so open and responsive to everything I said. You could even look at the ways in which the pressure you put on me to open up at the start could be experienced as the demands of my mother. That was huge. You clearly had no interest in repeating that, which was such a relief.

THERAPIST: And not wanting you to continue to comply in any way.

PATIENT: Absolutely. It was so important to be able to share all those intense and shameful feelings with you. It's strange, after feeling all that rage toward my mother, I ended up experiencing deep love and compassion for her. Ironically, it was almost the opposite with my father. He was no Boy Scout, as it turns out, but he played the good guy while utterly failing to protect me from my mother. It also became clear that he was projecting his sexual desires onto me. All this got played out with my first husband. I felt like I was permanently damaged and could never be loved, so I did whatever I could to be accepted. In a way, love had always been suffused with pain for me. No more—it is completely different now and I could never go back to that. Thank you so much. Talking through this with you is very moving.

THERAPIST: It is for me too. I am so happy for you and so glad we had the chance to do this together.

Data from this ten-year follow-up fulfil Malan's criterion for character change and, ultimately, cure; i.e., that all of the patient's presenting complaints and pathological defenses were replaced with healthy alternatives. Not only was she refusing to allow herself to be used and abused, but she had become a leader who held others accountable. Furthermore, she had co-created a deeply loving and respectful relationship with her husband. In the past, she could only come to orgasm when imagining being raped and tortured. Now she experienced a passionate and loving relationship with her husband that included joyful sensuality and robust sexual pleasure that was mutual and reciprocal.

Response to Subsequent Difficulties

As Freud suggested back in 1937, we can only tell if our interventions are curative if patients can face new difficulties without regressing. Both the Good Girl and the Manic-Depressive's Daughter began their follow-up interviews by saying that things in their lives could still be stressful at times, but they were handling the problems in their lives in new and more adaptive ways. In fact, the example provided by the Good Girl demonstrates a remarkable level of emotional maturity and both strength and resilience in the face of challenges.

The Manic-Depressive's Daughter: Part 3

THERAPIST: So how are you?

PATIENT: Well, I'm actually ok, which is surprising since we've had a very difficult time of it. My younger son was found to have some serious medical problems. I feel certain that if I had not done the work with you previously, I would have gone under with this one. But now I deal with it, and my husband and I deal with it together.

THERAPIST: How do you account for this—that the previous work prepared you to deal with this crisis with some sense of equilibrium?

PATIENT: Because it's just about now, it's not about the past, and because I have a closer relationship to my husband and some basic confidence in my ability to be a good mother. If I didn't have all that, this crisis would have sent me over the edge.

We cannot guarantee our patients will have lives free of pain and trauma. In fact, Wolberg (1965) has suggested that we prepare patients for the inevitability of struggles in life. Can our treatment have a prophylactic effect, insulating our patients from future symptoms when such upheavals occur? These cases suggest that it can. By enhancing the ego functioning of our patients, we help prepare them to weather these storms in adaptive fashion.

Follow-up interviews provide patient and therapist with the opportunity to review the process of therapy, to access the extent of change, and to note new or recurring problems. My experience has paralleled that reported by Malan and Davanloo, suggesting that the changes occurring during ISTDP are generally maintained and strengthened over time.

The Good Girl

This vignette, from a ten-year follow-up interview, revealed the extent of healing and change in this woman, both physically and emotionally. Furthermore, the information shared suggested tremendous resilience and a newfound and sustained ability to weather loss and challenge with grace, rather than returning to suffering and symptoms. Most therapies, including cognitive behavioral therapy (CBT), have a large relapse rates (Lorimer, et al., 2021; Steinhart, et al., 2014). To date, ISTDP is the only treatment that demonstrates continued growth and healing after therapy ends. The following is a dramatic example of this phenomenon.

PATIENT: Hello! It's so good to see you.

THERAPIST: And you. How are you these days?

PATIENT: I am just so happy. Life is really good.

THERAPIST: The last time I saw you, your sister had just died (killed suddenly in a traffic accident) and there was a brief revival of symptoms (a kind of survivor's guilt, in which she felt she shouldn't be happy and was depriving herself of pleasure).

PATIENT: That's no more . . . that's not a problem anymore. In fact, I have a real sense of peace about it. No matter how it comes up, I always end up with a feeling of peace.

THERAPIST: So, not only are you no longer punishing yourself, but you end up with a feeling of peace about your sister.

PATIENT: I also realize, in a deep way, that even though she is dead, my relationship with her goes on for the rest of my time on Earth. I can have all kinds of feelings come up now about her—I can love her, hate her—and, if she had lived, it would have been a very rich relationship.

This statement speaks to the ways in which healthy mourning leads to a feeling of peace and a largely positive memory of the deceased. As the patient said, their relationship continued within her. All was not lost.

Next, we explored her initial presenting complaint—an inability to form a relationship with a man that was "full blown and sustained". She reported having fallen deeply in love and marrying several years prior.

PATIENT: I feel very safe with him. I remember sitting in this chair and talking about how I had been humiliated for my physical kluziness. No, that would never happen with him—even though he is poetry in motion. I mean just watching this man twirl pots and pans is pure delight, but I never worry about being humiliated. I mean, I don't like to be ridiculed.

THERAPIST: Well, who does? But in the past, you tended to swallow your anger toward those who humiliated you—primarily your brother—and attack yourself. Now you don't do that to yourself, and you haven't repeated it by marrying someone like that.

PATIENT: Oh no, not at all.

THERAPIST: And is the relationship safe enough for conflict, as that is also something you tended to avoid at great cost.

PATIENT: Yes, I have gotten. I got very angry at him. (She went on to detail a particular incident in which she found out he lied about drinking, something he had previously sworn off of.) He lied to me.

THERAPIST: How did you deal with that?

PATIENT: At first, I was so angry I left the house. I was outraged. When I calmed down, I came back and spoke to him about it. I said, "This is a betrayal. I love you, but I won't have this in my life. You must decide. If you want to be with me, you've got to quit drinking. I will support you in every way possible, but I won't do it for you".

THERAPIST: You were clear you were not going to engage in any kind of destructiveness.

PATIENT: That's right. And I could have gotten on the phone and arranged things but that was not for me to be doing. I said, "You have a choice to make. I was clear what my conditions and requirements are. You can do what you like but this is where I stand. And, from my part, once he chooses, I will support him. He went into therapy on his own.

The patient revealed that her husband has a medical condition that could shorten his life. Since loss was such a prominent issue for her previously, I inquired about her response to this.

PATIENT: I feel sad, but I don't focus on it.

THERAPIST: And you don't distance in the face of it.

PATIENT: No, you never know what's going to happen. I think there is a lot of be said for loving and being loved—and having an optimistic temperament, which he does. (Research from the Grant study supports her view on this.) Every day I am grateful. The way I really feel is, I've had enough loss, and I celebrate what I have.

THERAPIST: The important thing is that you have the closeness now.

PATIENT: Oh yes, every single day, because, you know people say to me, even though it's been five years, "Oh, you're like newlyweds", but still, every day, I feel so happy. If I wake in the middle of the night, it just feels so beautiful and I come into the office saying, "I'm so happy". I treasure him and I feel treasured, so I feel that, in spite of the problems I told you about, I am so happy. My life has been changed. I love him and I feel loved by him.

This patient's ability to weather losses without becoming symptomatic, or employing pathological defenses, was striking. Furthermore, she was able to love fully, even in the face of inevitable loss.

Finally, I inquired about her physical health, as a severe case of ulcerative colitis had adversely affected her life. In fact, she came to therapy when her physician urged her to consider radical surgery to address the disease. In our work together, a link between the suppression of rage and guilt and her symptoms had been discovered. Her symptoms were eliminated by the end of treatment, but only follow-up would reveal whether this improvement was permanent

PATIENT: I must tell you, symptomatically, I feel fabulous! Ah, I don't, it just doesn't go to my gut anymore, I mean . . .

THERAPIST: So there's a feeling of vitality. You don't feel sick anymore.

PATIENT: Oh, I feel great.

THERAPIST: Really well. Energetic?

PATIENT: I'm energetic. I don't know where that anxiety goes anymore—well, it doesn't go somatically. I guess I just get it out now, directly. Now, most of the time I just feel relaxed and I savor, just savor, feeling so good—it's like an animal pleasure. Just to feel.

THERAPIST: Just savoring the feeling of being alive.

The Mind–Body Connection

Yearly colonoscopies revealed scarring from past bouts of acute ulcerative colitis, but no active disease. As noted by Lindemann (1944), sudden, traumatic, or early loss was found in the history of 85% of all patients with ulcerative colitis. In this case, the patient's father died when she was 14, and her first bout of ulcerative colitis occurred after her fiancé broke their engagement. Not only had her sister died suddenly, but her father-in-law and stepfather had also died since our treatment had ended. Even when faced with significant losses, there were no subsequent flare-ups in her symptoms or disease. She was able to grieve and, in each case, hold onto the positive memories of the deceased. At 15-year follow-up she reported that her much adored brother died of Amyotrophic Lateral Sclerosis (ALS), an especially cruel disease. Once again, she was able to deal with all of her mixed feelings toward her brother and did not become symptomatic. If that's not cure, I don't know what is.

In addition to massive changes in anxiety, depression, and relational capacity, the Woman on the Emotional Roller Coaster, the Woman with Headaches, and the Good Girl experienced profound levels of physical healing as well. The Woman on an Emotional Roller Coaster was given two to three years to live when we began treatment, but lived another 20 years post treatment. The Good Girl was spared life-altering surgery, and the ulcerative colitis never recurred, even when close family members died suddenly and tragically. The Woman with Headaches, who had been profoundly affected by headaches that required multiple hospitalizations, never had another crushing headache after our work together. This suggests that repressed emotions were a significant factor in the development of these physical symptoms and that the de-repression of same lead to physical as well as emotional healing.

From Conflict to Creativity

Another striking phenomenon observed at follow-up is a shift in patients from having their energy bound in conflict to being freed up for creativity. While she had the title of a novel in mind for ten years, it was only after the pivotal session in which the Good Girl faced her rage toward me and her mother that she was able to write the novel. The Man Divided integrated his life instead of keeping it divided by creating a whole new business that bridged the previous divide between his winter and summer homes. Furthermore, he stopped the pattern of affairs and was able to bring himself into his marriage wholeheartedly. As a result, the marriage had grown and deepened over time. In the case of the Detached Observer, his own healing prompted him to become a healing force in his family and community. Material from this ten-year follow-up interview revealed the extent of his creativity and contribution.

The Detached Observer—Ten-Year Follow-Up

THERAPIST: Hi. How are you? You look great. (He rolled in a slick racing chair.)

PATIENT: Actually, I am. I had some injuries a while back, which was a drag, but other than that, I am doing really well.

THERAPIST: What happened?

PATIENT: Well, you remember that, because I had been an athlete, people were always saying I should get involved in wheelchair racing. That never interested me. For me, it was always about a ball—football, basketball, baseball. Well, several years ago I was at a tennis match and saw a demonstration of wheelchair tennis. I thought, "That's for me", so I started playing. Most of the guys are paraplegics. Since I am a quad, I had to be strapped into the chair to play. I was playing pretty intensely and ended up on the national tour. I started breaking my ribs and eventually had to stop.

THERAPIST: Wait. That sounds amazing. You played on the national tour?

PATIENT: Yeah, I won the US Open two years ago and ended up being ranked #1. It was amazing, but it's so frustrating not be able to get back on the court.

THERAPIST: OK, but do you feel wonderful about what you were able to accomplish?

PATIENT: Oh yeah, like I say, before that injury came, I was feeling great and was ready to rock and roll. I was going to Europe on tournaments and had a great time.

THERAPIST: So you were enjoying, not just the competitive tennis, but the people and the adventure?

PATIENT: Honestly, it's mostly the competition. The people are great, and I have made some good friends, but that's not the crux of it with tennis. I love to get on the court and play. When I think about it, I wonder why I love knocking that ball around so much, but I get so much enjoyment out of it. At times I try to deny it, but when I get out there, I say, there's that feeling! Opportunities for tennis have grown tremendously in the five years I played in both recognition and money. There's still work to be done in that area, which I wouldn't mind getting involved in. Actually, with a friend back here, together we have created camps to get disabled kids involved in sports. We have the first disabled flag football league for disabled kids and have 200 kids involved in that. We are also doing tennis and have developed camps in four different locations and are trying to get funding. That's been really satisfying.

When this young man first came to see me, he was utterly withdrawn and isolated. Even as a star athlete in high school, he shied away from girls and avoided socializing. He reported that, as a child, he would look out at the night sky and wonder if he was living on the wrong planet. That revealed the extent to which he felt he didn't belong in his family, his community, and even the planet. Post-treatment, he was deeply involved with others at all levels, both personally as well as on the community level. His impact on the lives of others was significant and gave his life meaning.

THERAPIST: Wow—to be able to do something you just love and offer that to kids who would never have that opportunity otherwise.

PATIENT: We have kids who are both mentally and physically handicapped. Just to see them go crazy when they get the ball over the net is really satisfying.

THERAPIST: That's so meaningful. So, it's more than just getting out on the court and playing yourself. You can see a future past when you might be competitive, which will happen for every athlete. To get into coaching and mentoring.

PATIENT: Yeah, I haven't thought about more formal education like graduate school. Remember, I thought about that because I got interested in investing. I've done really well with my own investments, so I don't have to work for money. I can do what I love and contribute to others. In addition to the sports, I also got into astronomy. I bought a really high-powered telescope and set it up at the library so I can share it with others. I do some teaching there, which is cool.

THERAPIST: That's really touching, to go from feeling like you belonged on another planet to studying the universe and sharing it with others. Amazing.

PATIENT: It's a rich life.

THERAPIST: And what about relationships and romance?

PATIENT: With the injuries, romance was put on the back burner. I had a relationship with a woman on the tour, but we lived far apart and that eventually ended. I recently started dating a woman who saw an article about me in the newspaper. She asked a friend of mine if he could introduce her to me, so I've seen her a couple of times.

THERAPIST: How is that going?

PATIENT: Too early to say. She's a nice woman and I'll see her again to see what develops, but I don't get worked up about that anymore.

THERAPIST: What do you mean? Are you detached?

PATIENT: No, not at all, but you remember I used to get so anxious about approaching a woman that I would freeze. Now I am relaxed about it. I am comfortable with who I am and trust that things will work out. It's a huge change.

THERAPIST: Yes, indeed. How do you think that happened? Despite some hurdles, you are thriving. You no longer roll over and give up. You have created meaningful work and your relationships have improved.

PATIENT: Yeah, I'm really close to my sister and her family. I'm especially close to my nephews. Not long ago, one of them had to write an essay about his hero. I asked him who he wrote about, and he said, "YOU!" I tear up even now, telling you about it.

THERAPIST: I am getting choked up too. That is so beautiful.

PATIENT: Even with my father, the relationship has completely changed. As you know, I bought a place down south for the winter. He drove down with me this year. When he got back, it was January and really cold. His pipes froze and burst so I told him to come stay with me and he did, for three months. Plus, he has some physical problems, and it felt good to be able to do that.

THERAPIST: You don't feel all that conflict and animosity anymore?

PATIENT: No, no. It's a much better relationship with him. I can care for him now as he ages. It's better than ever.

THERAPIST: When you think back on the factors that helped you work through all that and create this rich and rewarding life, what do you remember?

PATIENT: Just being able to let out all those feeling—all the anger and grief and disappointment. It was a huge brick—a huge brick. To be able to face it and get it out and have it understood by you was huge. I felt a huge weight off me.

THERAPIST: And to resolve those competitive issues with your dad so you can both be close to him and go find your own woman.

PATIENT: For sure. I feel my life has changed completely. I am so grateful.

THERAPIST: Me too!

In this case, anxiety and depression were removed and replaced with vitality. His previous inhibitions with women had been overdetermined. In addition to a highly fraught relationship with his erratic and emotionally disturbed mother, the relationship with his father was harsh and demanding. He insisted on separating his son from his mother and even accused him of causing her psychiatric symptoms. What's more, his father coached him in sports and was clearly ambivalent about his son's athletic prowess and success. Instead of supporting and encouraging him, his father taunted him, threw the football in his face, and sought to undermine his confidence. A blatant Oedipal conflict was unearthed in the later phase of treatment—the resolution of which was vital in releasing him to pursue the women he desired and to be successful in his own right. This resolution also freed him up to have a caring relationship with his father in the present.

At 25-year follow-up, all gains were sustained. Further growth and development was reported. In fact, he had become a successful filmmaker. The extent of transformational change in this case, from a meager existence inside four walls, to a fully engaged human being who had healed himself and was a gift to all who encounter him, was astonishing and speaks to the power of this work. When defenses and resistances are relinquished in favor of facing and experiencing one's true feelings (which was quite a battle in this case), the patient's innate capacity to heal is unleashed, enabling development that had been arrested to take off.

When he first came to see me, his symptoms and presenting complaints fit the criteria for schizoid personality disorder, a diagnosis that carries with it a dire prognosis. But descriptive diagnoses like the *Diagnostic and Statistical Manual of Mental Disorders, Fifth Edition* (*DSMV*) tell us nothing about the cause of these disturbances or what therapeutic intervention is likely to be helpful. In fact, personality disorders are often a description of the patient's characteristic defenses. In this case, once his "schizoid" defenses of detachment and withdrawal were confronted and removed, his true self emerged. In fact, this man was quite sensitive and felt deeply. As defenses were abandoned and he was supported to experience, tolerate, and integrate all his feelings, needs, and desires, he healed and became capable of profound levels of connection with others. In so doing, he contributed significantly to the welfare of others and made a deep impression on many. So, he was not innately "schizoid", but developed schizoid defenses to guard and protect the true self from further harm. We only get to see and know another when they are in an open, unguarded state. Sometimes, when the masks are discarded and the walls are removed, I will say, "Hello. It's nice to meet you", as I am only then meeting the real person. We must not confuse and conflate patient's defenses with who they are at their core.

Man with Primary Impotence

At ten-year follow-up this man had completely changed his life. This case is an example of the research finding that patients who complete a course of ISTDP do better and better over time with no additional treatment (Abbass, et al, 2012; Driessen, et al, 2015; Town, et al, 2020) . Even though he had many therapies before our work together, he continued to re-enact traumatic experiences by working in an emergency room and engaging with women who were either completely inappropriate or erratic, unpredictable, and even abusive. Following ISTDP treatment, in which he faced and experienced all his intense mixed feelings toward significant others (rather than acting them out), his whole life changed. He shifted from emergency medicine to primary care, where he could form ongoing relationships with patients and have a predictable schedule. He met and married a lovely woman whom he both desired and respected. Together, they had four children and lived in a quiet country setting, so different from the dangerous and chaotic city where he grew up. Not only did he stop repeating the pattern of chaos and abuse, but he had also created an atmosphere of love, stability, and connection for himself and his family.

Summary

Follow-up studies on the long-term efficacy of psychotherapy are rare. Those that have been conducted suggest there is a significant relapse problem over time, even with CBT. In contrast, research indicates that relapse rates for patients receiving ISTDP is quite low (less than 10%). In addition, these studies have found that these patients continued to improve over time, with no further intervention. No other treatment method that I know of has demonstrated this kind of long-term effectiveness. Not only has ISTDP been shown to be clinically effective, but cost effective as well, saving $3 for every dollar spent on treatment (Abbass, 2015). In fact, that same level of cost savings were reported over three years post-treatment (Abbass & Katzman, 2013).

It is also notable that ISTDP appears to be effective in cases that typically don't respond to psychotherapy, including personality disorders, treatment resistant depression, chronic pain, medically unexplained symptoms, and neurological symptoms including pseudo seizures, movement disorders, and fugue states. Furthermore, the effect sizes of ISTDP well outstrips medication and CBT (Shedler, 2019).

So, why isn't this method practiced more widely? As Alexander and French (1946) opined long ago, it takes clinicians far more time, energy, and dedication to develop the knowledge and skill required to facilitate deep and lasting change in a short period of time than administering "treatment as usual". To do this kind of work, the therapist must develop deep domain-specific knowledge, hone complex therapeutic skills, and be willing to devote a great deal of time to supervision and training well beyond their degree program requirements. There is also evidence that the best therapists have superior meta-cognitive skills, such as working memory and pattern recognition. They also display high levels of emotional intelligence, allowing them to establish therapeutic alliances with difficult patients (Wampold, 2015). Davanloo (personal communication, 1991) suggested that ISTDP is to traditional psychotherapy what surgery is to general practice. Just as becoming a surgeon demands a great deal more time, study, and experience beyond their medical training, so it is for those who hope to master ISTDP. Therapists training in this model must be willing to develop a great deal of personal strength and self knowledge, as it is an intensive treatment in which strong feelings are aroused and often directed toward the provider.

In this chapter, the author has discussed the impact of ISTDP on patients, highlighting the resilience and growth individuals often experience, even after therapy has ended.

Follow-up interviews in ISTDP reveal that changes experienced during therapy often lead to sustained improvement over time, showcasing the therapy's lasting benefits compared to other methods. Overall, the chapter has emphasized the potential for long-term healing and growth through ISTDP.

Beyond the findings of empirical findings reviewed here, the detailed case studies included here offer a great deal of information on the factors associated with deep and lasting change. Most of those in our field are occupied with helping patients manage symptoms. In ISTDP the goal is to discover the conflicts responsible for symptoms so they can be resolved at the source. These cases have demonstrated that symptoms can be permanently removed AND replaced with healthy alternatives. In addition, the quality of growth in the patient's sense of self, and their ability to form genuine relationships with others. is self evident.

The almost universal report of energy that had been bound in conflict getting freed up for creativity is another fascinating finding of these follow up interviews. These patients have created new businesses and non-profit organizations, started to write plays, novels, and music, and often become a healing force in their families and communities.

Conducting regular follow up interviews provides therapists with an opportunity to review their work and assess its long-term effectiveness. This is also a way to review strengths and weakness, by tracking who benefits and who doesn't. A therapist might discover that she is quite effective with depressives, but not at all with patients who have a narcissistic character structure. That can inform further action—either deciding not to treat the kinds of patients with whom she has had little success, or seeking additional training and supervision targeted at improving skills with that particular population.

By routinely engaging in follow-up interviews, patterns emerge. In my own work, I received the same kind of feedback over and over again. When I ask what the important factors were in helping the patient heal, these are the most common responses:

"You were tough and focused, but compassionate at the same time".

"You were brave and courageous, never flinching, no matter what I threw at you".

"You were really solid and reliable—always on time and highly responsive to everything I said".

"Helping me get to the feelings I have avoided was key".

"Getting to that anger was huge. I was terrified of anger and didn't know what to do with it".

"You helped me put the pieces together and understand myself and others in a whole new way".

"You are highly skilled and obviously know what you're doing. Even though the work was really hard, I knew I was in good hands".

"I could sense your dedication and passion for helping people. It's not just what you did, but who you are that mattered".

"I always felt safe in this room".

Conclusions

In this chapter, the importance of achieving therapeutic goals, addressing the emotional complexities surrounding the end of treatment, and incorporating follow-up sessions to assess patient progress over time was emphasized.

Clinical examples were used to illustrate how ISTDP can lead to sustained improvement over time, with no further intervention. This underscores the finding that successful treatment results in the removal of symptoms, as well as fostering long-term growth and resilience in the patients who receive it.

Follow-up sessions are necessary in order to:

1. Assess long-term effectiveness.

2. Address remaining or emerging issues of concern.

3. Reinforce and celebrate positive change.

4. Therapist reflection and assessment of clinical effectiveness.

In summary, follow-up sessions are a vital component of the therapeutic process, ensuring that the work accomplished during therapy translates into long-term change and continual growth.

REFERENCES

Aafjes-Doorn, K., MacDonald, J., Stein, M., Cooper, A., & Tucker, S. (2014). Experiential dynamic therapy: A preliminary investigation into the effectiveness and process of the extended initial interview. *Journal of Clinical Psychology*, 00, 97–108.

Abbass, A. (2015). *Reaching through Resistance*. Kansas City, MO: Seven Leaves Press.

Abbass, A., Joffres, M., & Ogrodniczuk, J. (2008). A Naturalistic Study of the ISTDP Trial Therapy. *Brief Treatment and Crisis Intervention*, 8, 164–170.

Abbass, A. & Katzman, J. W (2013). The Cost-effectiveness of Intensive Short-term Dynamic Psychotherapy. *Psychiatric Annals*, 43 (11), 496–501.

Abbass, A., Kisley, S., & Town, J. (2018). Cost-effectiveness of the ISTDP Trial Therapy. *Psychotherapy and Psychosomatics*, 87 (4), 255–256.

Abbass, A., Sheldon, AM, Gyra, J., & Kalpin, A. (2008). ISTDP for DSM-IV Personality Disorders. *Journal of Nervous and Mental Disorders*, 196 (3), 211–216.

Abbass, A., Town, J., & Driessen, E. (2012). ISTDP: A systematic review and meta-analysis. *Harvard Review of Psychiatry*, 20 (2), 97–108.

Abbass, A., Town, J., Ogrodniczuk, J., Joffres, M., & Lillengren, P. (2017). ISTDP Trial Therapy: Effectiveness and role of "unlocking the unconscious". *Journal of Nervous and Mental Disorders*, 205, 453–457.

Alexander, F. & French, T. M. (1946). *Psychoanalytic therapy principles and application*. Lincoln: University of Nebraska Press.

Aronson, E. (1968). The theory of cognitive dissonance: A current perspective. In L. Berkowitz (Ed.), *Advances in experimental social psychology* (Vol. *4*). New York: Academic Press.

Balint, M. (1957). *The doctor, his patient and the illness*. New York: International Universities Press.

Bandura, A. (1986). *Social foundations of thought and action*. Englewood Cliffs, NJ: Prentice-Hall.

Bandura, A. (1989). Human agency in social cognitive theory. *American Psychologist, 44*, 1175–1181.

Bauer, G. P. & Kobos, J. C. (1987). *Brief therapy: Short-term dynamic interventions*. Northvale, NJ: Aronson.

Beck, A. T. (1976). *Cognitive therapy and the emotional disorders*. New York: International Universities Press.

Been, H. & Sklar, I. (1985). Transference in short-term dynamic psychotherapy. In A. Winston (Ed.), *Short-term dynamic psychotherapy*. Washington, DC: American Psychiatric Press.

Bettelheim, B. (1983). Preface and afterword. In M. Cardinal, *The words to say it*, pp. x–xii, 297–308. Cambridge, MA: VanVactor & Goodheart.

Bower, G. (1981). Mood and memory. *American Psychologist, 36*, 129–148.

Bowlby, J. (1970). *Attachment and loss* (Vol. *1*). New York: Basic Books.

Bowlby, J. (1973). *Separation: Anxiety and anger*. London: Tavistock.

Bowlby, J. (1980). *Loss: Sadness and depression*. London: Tavistock.

Brenner, C. (1976). *Psychoanalytic technique and psychic conflict.* New York: International Universities Press.

Breuer, J. & Freud, S. (1895). Studies in hysteria. In J. Strachey (Ed.), *The standard edition of the complete psychological works of Sigmund Freud* (Vol. *2*). London: Hogarth Press.

Bucci, W. (1985). Dual coding: A cognitive model for psychoanalytic research. *Journal of the American Psychoanalytic Association, 33*, 571–607.

Cardinal, M. (1983). *The words to say it.* P. Goodheart (Trans.). Cambridge, MA: VanVactor & Goodheart.

Carveth, D. (2006). Self-punishment as guilt evasion. *Canadian Journal of Psychoanalysis*, 14, 176–198.

Coughlin, P. (2022). *Facilitating the Process of Working through in Psychotherapy: Mastering the Middle Game.* New York: Routledge.

Coughlin, P. (2016). *Maximizing Effectiveness in Dynamic Psychotherapy.* New York: Routledge.

Coughlin, P. and Malan, D. (2018). *Lives Transformed.* New York: Routledge.

Crits-Christoph, P. & Barber, J. P. (Eds.). (1991). *Handbook of short-term dynamic psychotherapy.* New York: Basic Books.

Davanloo, H. (1978). *Principles and techniques of short-term dynamic psychotherapy.* New York: Spectrum.

Davanloo, H. (1979). Techniques of short-term dynamic psychotherapy. *Psychiatric Clinics of North America, 2*, 11–21.

Davanloo, H. (1980). *Short-term dynamic psychotherapy.* New York: Aronson.

Davanloo, H. (1986a). *Intensive short-term dynamic psychotherapy with highly resistant patients: I. Handling resistance* (pp. 1–28).

Davanloo, H. (1986b). *Intensive short-term dynamic psychotherapy with highly resistant patients: II. The course of an interview after the initial breakthrough* (pp. 29–46).

Davanloo, H. (1987a). *Intensive short-term dynamic psychotherapy with highly resistant depressed patients: I. Restructuring ego's regressive defenses* (pp. 47–80).

Davanloo, H. (1987b). *Intensive short-term dynamic psychotherapy with highly resistant depressed patients: II. The royal road to the dynamic unconscious* (pp. 81–100).

Davanloo, H. (1987c). The unconscious therapeutic alliance. In P. Buirski (Ed). *Frontiers of dynamic psychotherapy.* New York: Bunner/Mazel.

Davanloo, H. (1988). *The technique of unlocking the unconscious: I* (pp. 101–124).

Davanloo, H. (1990). *Unlocking the unconscious.* New York: Wiley.

Davanloo, H. (1990–1991). *Core Training in Montreal, Canada.*

Davis, D. (1988). Transformation of pathological mourning into acute grief with intensive short-term dynamic psychotherapy. *International Journal of Short-Term Psychotherapy, 3*, 79–97.

Della Selva, P. C. (1991). The emergence and working through of preverbal trauma in short-term dynamic psychotherapy. *International Journal of Short-Term Psychotherapy, 6*, 195–216.

Della Selva, P. C. (1992). Achieving character change in IS-TDP: How the experience of affect leads to the consolidation of the self. *International Journal of Short-Term Psychotherapy, 7*, 73–87.

Della Selva, P. C. (1993). The significance of attachment theory for the practice of intensive short-term dynamic psychotherapy. *International Journal of Short-Term Psychotherapy, 8*, 189–206.

Dewald, P. A. (1972). *The psychoanalytic process.* New York: McGraw-Hill.

Dickman, S. & Sechrest, L. (1985). Research on memory and clinical practice. In G. Strieker & R. H. Keisner (Eds.), *From research to clinical practice* (pp. 15–44). New York: Plenum.

Dubs, H. H. (Trans) (1928). *The Works of Hsunze.* London: Arthur Probsthain Publisher.

Duncan, I. (1927, 1955). *My life.* New York: Liveright.

Driessen, E., Gegelmaier, L. M., Abbass, A, Barber, J. P., & Dekker, J. J. M. (2015). The efficacy of Short term Dynamic Psychotherapy for depression: A meta-analysis and update. *Clinical Psychology Review*, 42, 1–15.

Ecker, B., Ticic, R., & Hulley, L. (2012). *Unlocking the emotional brain.* New York: Routledge.

Ellman, S. J. (1991). *Freud's technique papers: A contemporary perspective*. Northvale, NJ: Aronson.
Emde, R. N. (1989). The infant's relationship experience. In A. J. Sameroff & R. N. Emde (Eds.), *Relationship disturbances in early childhood: A developmental approach* (pp. 33–51). New York: Basic Books.
Engel, G. (1961). Is grief a disease? *Psychosomatic Medicine, 23*, 18–22.
Epstein, S. (1994). Integration of the cognitive and the psychodynamic unconscious. *American Psychologist, 49*, 709–724.
Esquivel, L. (1989). *Like water for chocolate*. New York: Doubleday.
Fairbairn, W. R. D. (1954). *An object-relations theory of the personality*. New York: Basic Books.
Ferenczi, S. (1924). *Further contributions to the theory and technique of psychoanalysis*. New York: Brunner/Mazel.
Ferenczi, S. & Rank, O. (1925). *The development of psychoanalysis*. New York: Nervous and Mental Disease Publishing Company.
Firestein, S. (1978). *Termination in psychoanalysis*. New York: International Universities Press.
Fisher, S. & Greenberg, R. (1977). *The scientific credibility of Freud's theories and therapy*. New York: Basic Books.
Flegenheimer, W. V. (1982). *Techniques of brief psychotherapy*. Northvale, NJ: Aronson.
Fosha, D. (1988). Restructuring in the treatment of depressive disorders with Davanloo's intensive short-term dynamic psychotherapy. *International Journal of Short-Term Psychotherapy, 3*, 189–212.
Frank, G. (1961). *Persuasion and healing*. Baltimore: Johns Hopkins Press.
Frederickson, J. (2013). *Co-creating Change: Effective Dynamic Therapy Techniques*. Kensington, MD: Seven Leaves Press.
Freud, A. (1937/1966). *The ego and the mechanisms of defense* (rev. ed.). Madison, CT: International Universities Press.
Freud, S. All references are to *The standard edition of the complete psychological works of Sigmund Freud* (Volumes *1–24*.). London: Hogarth Press, 1953–1974 (SE).
Freud, S. (1894). The neuro-psychoses of defense. *SE 3*: 45–61.
Freud, S. (1895). Studies of hysteria. *SE 2*: 255–305.
Freud, S. (1900). The interpretation of dreams. *SE 4/5*.
Freud, S. (1914). Remembering, repeating and working-through. *SE 12*: 147–156.
Freud, S. (1917). Mourning and melancholia. *SE 14*: 243–258.
Freud, S. (1920). Beyond the pleasure principle. *SE 18*: 3–64.
Freud, S. (1923). The ego and the id. *SE 19*: 1–66.
Freud, S. (1924). The economic problem of masochism. *SE 19*: 155–170.
Freud, S. (1926). Inhibitions, symptoms and anxiety. *SE 20*: 75–175.
Freud, S. (1930). Civilization and its discontents. *SE 21*: 59–145.
Freud, S. (1937). Analysis terminable and interminable. *SE 23*: 209–253.
Freud, S. (1949). An outline of psycho-analysis. *SE 23*: 139–207.
Freud, S. (1950). Extracts from the Fleiss Papers. *SE 1*: 173–280.
Friedman, S. B., Chodoff, P., Mason, J. W., & Hamberg, D. A. (1963). Behavioral observations on parents anticipating the death of a child. *Pediatrics, 32*, 610–625.
Friedman, S. B., Mason, J. W., & Hamburg, D. A. (1963). Urinary 17-hydroxycorticosteroid levels of parents of children with neoplastic disease. *Psychosomatic Medicine, 25*, 364–376.
Fromm, E. (1947). *Man for himself: An inquiry into the Psychology of Ethics*. New York: Rhinehart & CO, Inc.
Fromm-Reichman, F. (1950). *Principles of intensive psychotherapy*. Chicago: University of Chicago Press.
Geiselman, R. E., Fisher, R. P., MacKinnon, D. P., & Holland, H. L. (1985). Eyewitness memory enhancement in the police interview: Cognitive retrieval mnemonics versus hypnosis. *Journal of Applied Psychology, 70*, 401–412.
Gibran, K. (1923). *The Prophet*. New York: Knopf.

Gill, M. (1982). *The analysis of transference.* Volume *I.* New York: International Universities Press.

Glover, E. (1958). *The technique of psychoanalysis.* New York: International Universities Press.

Goin, M. K., Burgoyne, R. W., & Goin, J. M. (1979). Timeless attachment to a dead relative. *American Journal of Psychiatry, 7,* 988–989.

Greenberg, J. R. & Mitchell, S. A. (1983). *Object relations in psychoanalytic theory.* Cambridge: Harvard University Press.

Greenson, R. (1967). *The technique and practice of psychoanalysis.* New York: International Universities Press.

Haan, N. (1977). *Coping and defending.* New York: Academic Press.

Herman, J. L. (1992). *Trauma and recovery.* New York: Basic Books.

Henry, W., Sims, J. H., & Spicey, S. L. (1968). Mental health professionals in Chicago: Some preliminary observations on origins and practice. In J. M. Shlien (Ed.), *Research in psychotherapy.* Washington, DC: American Psychiatry Association.

Hollan, S. D., Evans, M. D., & DeRubeis, R. J. (1990). Cognitive mediation of relapse prevention following treatment for depression: Implications of differential risk. In R. E. Ingram (Ed.), *Psychological aspects of depression* (pp. 117–136). New York: Plenum.

Horner, A. (1984). *Object relations and the developing ego in therapy.* New York: Aronson.

Horowitz, M. J. (1979). *States of mind.* New York: Plenum.

Jacobs, S. & Ostfeld, A. (1977). An epidemiological review of the mortality of bereavement. *Psychosomatic Medicine, 39,* 344–357.

Janoff-Bulman, R. (1992). *Shattered assumptions.* New York: Free Press.

Janov, A. (1970). *Primal scream: Primal therapy, the cure for neurosis.* New York: Putnam.

Jelova, A., Kolshus, E., & McLoughlin, D. M. (2013). Relapse following successful ECT therapy for major depression: a meta-analysis. *Neuropsychopharmacology,* 38, 2467–2474.

Johansson, R., Eriksson, K., Aberg, K., Town, J., Abbass, A. (2024). ISTDP for depression: Treatment effectiveness and effects of unlocking. https://doi.org/10.21203/rs.3.rs-5404572/v1

Johnsen, T. J. & Friborg, O. (2015). The effects of Cognitive Behavior Therapy as an Anit-depressive treatment is falling: A meta-analysis. *Psychological Bulletin,* 141 (4), 747–768.

Kernberg, O. (1975). *Borderline conditions and pathological narcissism.* New York: Aronson.

Kernberg, O. (1976). *Object relations theory and clinical psychoanalysis.* New York: Aronson.

Kübler-Ross, E. (1969). *Death and dying.* London: Tavistock.

Laikin, M., Winston, A., & McCullough, L. (1991). Intensive short-term dynamic psychotherapy. In P. Crits-Christoph & J. B. Barber (Eds.), *Handbook of short-term dynamic psychotherapy* (pp. 80–109). New York: Basic Books.

Leichsenrig, F., Luyten, P., Hilsenrother, J. J., Abbass, A., & Barber, J. P. (2015). Psychodynamic therapy meets evidence-based medicine: A systematic review using updated criteria. *The Lancet Psychiatry,* 2(7), 648–660.

Lewin, K. (1951). *Field theory in social science.* New York: Harper & Row.

Lewis, C. S. (1961). *A grief observed.* New York: Bantam.

Lindemann, E. (1944). Symptomatology and management of acute grief. *American Journal of Psychiatry, 101,* 141–148.

Lindemann, E. (1945). Psychiatric aspects of the conservative treatment of ulcerative colitis. *Archives of Neurology and Psychiatry, 53,* 322–325.

Lindemann, E. (1979). *Beyond grief.* Northvale, NJ: Aronson.

Loewald, H. W. (1976). Perspectives on memory. In M. M. Gill & P. S. Holtzman (Eds.), *Psychology vs. metapsychology: Psychoanalytic essays in memory of George S. Klein* (pp. 298–325). New York: International Universities Press.

Loftus, E. F. (1993). The reality of repressed memories. *American Psychologist, 48,* 518–537.

Lorimer, B., Kellett, S., Nye, A., & Delgadillo, J. (2021). Predictors of relapse and recurrence following DBT for anxiety-related disorders: A systematic review. *Cognitive Behavior Therapy,* 50, 1–18.

Luborsky, L. & Mark, D. (1991). Short-term supportive-expressive psychoanalytic psychotherapy. In P. Crits-Christoph & J. P. Barber (Eds.), *Handbook of short-term dynamic psychotherapy* (pp. 110–136). New York: Basic Books.

Malan, D. H. (1963). *A study of brief psychotherapy*. New York: Plenum Press.

Malan, D. H. (1976a). *The frontier of brief psychotherapy*. New York: Plenum Press.

Malan, D. H. (1976b). *Toward the validation of dynamic psychotherapy*. New York: Plenum Press.

Malan, D. H. (1978a). Exploring the limits of brief psychotherapy. In H. Davanloo (Ed.), *Basic principles and techniques in short-term dynamic psychotherapy* (pp. 43–67). New York: Spectrum Publications.

Malan, D. H. (1978b). Evaluation criteria for selection of patients. In H. Davanloo (Ed.), *Basic principles and techniques in short-term dynamic psychotherapy* (pp. 85–97). New York: Spectrum Publications.

Malan, D. H. (1979). *Individual psychotherapy and the science of psychodynamics*. London: Butterworth.

Malan, D. H. (1980). The most important development in psychotherapy since the discovery of the unconscious. In H. Davanloo (Ed.), *Short-term dynamic psychotherapy* (pp. 13–23). Northvale, NJ: Aronson.

Malan, D. H. (1986). Beyond interpretation: Part I and II. *International Journal of Short-Term Psychotherapy, 1(2)*, 59–82, 83–106.

Malan, D. & Osimo, F. (1992). *Psychodynamics, training, and outcome in brief psychotherapy*. London: Butterworth.

Mann, J. (1973). *Time-limited psychotherapy*. Cambridge: Harvard University Press.

Mann, J. (1991). Time-limited psychotherapy. In P. Crits-Christoph & J. P. Barber (Eds.), *Handbook of short-term dynamic psychotherapy* (pp. 17–43). New York: Basic Books.

McCloskey, M. & Zaragoza, M. (1985). Misleading postevent information and memory for events: Arguments and evidence against memory impairment hypotheses. *Journal of Experimental Psychology: General, 114*, 1–16.

Menninger, K. (1958). *Theory of psychoanalytic technique*. New York: Basic Books.

Miller, A. (1986). *Thou shalt not be aware: Society's betrayal of the child*. New York: Meridian.

Moffat, J. (Ed.). (1986). *In the midst of winter: Selections from the literature on mourning*. New York: Random House.

Munroe, R. (1955). *Schools of psychoanalytic thought*. New York: Dryden Press.

Nacht, R. (1965). Criteria and technique for the termination of analysis. *International Journal of Psychoanalysis, 46*, 107–116.

Novick, J. (1982). Termination: Themes and issues. *Psychoanalytic inquiry, 2*, 329–366.

Parkes, C. M. (1970). The psychosomatic effects of bereavement. In O. W. Hill (Ed.), *Modern trends in psychosomatic medicine*. London: Butterworth.

Parkes, C. M. (1975). Unexpected and untimely bereavement. *In Bereavement: Its psychosocial aspects*. New York: Columbia University Press.

Parkes, C. M., Benjamin, B., & Fitzgerald, R. G. (1969). Broken heart: A statistical study of increased mortality among widowers. *British Medical Journal, 1*, 740–743.

Peppers, L. G. & Knoff, R. J. (1980). *Motherhood and mourning*. New York: Praeger.

Pine, F. (1985). *Developmental theory and clinical process*. New Haven, CT: Yale University Press.

Ranko, S. & Mazer, H. (1980, 1983). *Semrad: The heart of a therapist*. Northvale, NJ: Aronson.

Raphael, L. (1983). *Bereavement*. Northvale, NJ: Aronson.

Reich, W. (1933). *Character analysis*, 3rd ed. New York: Touchstone.

Reich, W. (1987). Character resistances. In D. S. Milman & G. D. Goldman (Eds.), *Techniques of working with resistance* (pp. 41–116). Northvale, NJ: Aronson.

Reitav, J. (1991). The treatment of character pathology with Davanloo's intensive short-term dynamic psychotherapy, Part I: Management of resistance. *International Journal of Short-Term Psychotherapy, 6*, 3–25.

Schnarch, D. M. (1991). *Constructing the sexual crucible: An integration of sexual and marital therapy.* New York: Norton.
Schoenewolf, G. (1990). *Turning points in analytic therapy.* New York: Aronson.
Seward, G. H. (1962–1963). The relation between psychoanalytic school and value problems in therapy. *American Journal of Psychoanalysis,* 22–23, 138–152.
Shainess, N. (1986). *Sweet suffering: Woman as victim.* New York: Bobbs-Merrill.
Shand, A. F. (1920). *The foundations of character,* 2nd ed. London: Macmillan.
Shedler, J. (2010). The efficacy of psychodynamic psychotherapy. *American Psychologist,* 65, 98–109.
Shedler, J. (2012). The efficacy of psychodynamic psychotherapy. In R. A. Levy, J. S. Ablon, & H. Rochele (Eds.). *Psychodynamic Psychotherapy: Evidence-based practice and practice-based evidence* (pp. 9–25). Totawa, NJ: Humana Press.
Shedler, J. (2017). Where is the evidence of "evidence-based psychotherapy"? *Journal of Psychological Therapies in Primary Care,* 4, 47–59.
Sifneos, P. (1972). *Short-term psychotherapy and emotional crisis.* Cambridge, MA: Harvard University Press.
Sifneos, P. (1979). *Short-term dynamic psychotherapy.* New York: Plenum.
Singer-Kaplan, H. (1974). *The new sex therapy.* New York: Brunner/Mazel.
Sklansky, M. A., Isaacs, R. S., Levitor, E. S., & Haggard, E. A. (1966). Verbal interactional levels of meaning in psychotherapy. *Archives of General Psychiatry, 14,* 158–170.
Solbaken, O. A. & Abbass, A. (2015). ISTDP residential treatment program for patients with treatment resistant disorders. *Journal of Affective Disorders,* 1 (181), 67–77.
Stark, M. (1994). *Working with resistance.* New York: Aronson.
Sterba, R. F. (1934). The fate of the ego in analytic therapy. *International Journal of Psychoanalysis, 15,* 117–126.
Steinhart, C., Hofman, M., Kruse. J., & Leichsenrig, F. (2014). Relapse rates after psychotherapy for depression – Stable long-term effects: A meta-analysis. *Journal of Affective Disorders,* 168, 107–118.
Stern, D. (1985). *The interpersonal world of the infant: A view from psychoanalysis and developmental psychology.* New York: Basic Books.
Stotland, E. (1969). *The psychology of hope.* San Francisco: Jossey-Bass.
Strupp, H. H. & Binder, J. L. (1984). *Psychotherapy in a new key.* New York: Basic Books.
Suttie, I. (1937, 1988). *The origins of love and hate.* London: Free Association Books.
Swift, J. K. & Greenberg, R. P. (2012). Premature discontinuation of adult psychotherapy: A meta-analysis. *Journal of Consulting and Clinical Psychology,* 80, 547–559.
Teyber, E. (1992). *Interpersonal process in psychotherapy: A guide for clinical training.* Pacific Grove, CA: Brooks/Cole.
Town, J., Abbass, A., Stride, C., Nunes, A., Bernier, D., & Berrigan, P. (2020). Efficacy and cost effectiveness of ISTDP for treatment-resistant depression: 18 month follow-up of the Halifax Trial. *Journal of Affective Disorders,* 273, 194–202.
Town, J., Abbass, A., & Bernier, D. (2013). Effectiveness and cost-effectiveness of Davanloo's Intensive Short-term Dynamic Psychotherapy: Does unlocking the unconscious make a difference? *American Journal of Psychotherapy,* 67, 89–108.
Trevor, W. (1991). Reading Turgenev. In *Two lives* (pp. 1–222). New York: Penguin.
Trierweiler, S. J. & Donovan, C. M. (1994). Exploring the ecological foundations of memory in psychotherapy: Interpersonal affordance, perception, and recollection in real time. *Clinical Psychology Review, 14,* 301–326.
Trujillo, M. & McCullough, L. (1985). Research issues in short-term dynamic psychotherapies: An overview. In A. Winston (Ed.), *Clinical and research issues in intensive short-term dynamic psychotherapy.* Washington, DC: American Psychiatric Press.
Trujillo, M. & Winston, A. (1985). Termination. In A. Horner (Ed.), *Treating the neurotic patient in brief psychotherapy.* Northvale, NJ: Aronson.

Vaillant, G. (1993). *The wisdom of the ego*. Cambridge, MA: Harvard University Press.

van der Kolk, B. A. (1987). *Psychological trauma*. Washington, DC: American Psychiatric Press.

Wachtel, P. (1977). *Psychoanalysis and behavior therapy*. New York: Basic Books.

Wachtel, P. (1993). *Therapeutic communication*. New York: Guilford.

Wampold, B. E. (2015). *The Great Psychotherapy Debate: What makes psychotherapy work*, 2nd edition. New York: Routledge.

Wampold, B. E., Fluckiger, C., Del Re, A. C., Yulish, N. E., Frost, N. D., Pace, B. T., Goldberg, S. B., Miller, S. D., Baardseth, T. P., Lask, K. M., & Hillsenroth, M. J. (2016). *Psychotherapy Research*, 27, 14–32.

Weinberger, J. (1995). Common factors aren't so common: The common factors dilemma. *Clinical Psychology, 2(1)*, 45–69.

Weiss, J. (1993). *How psychotherapy works*. New York: Guilford.

Whisman, M. A. (1993). Mediators and moderators of change in cognitive therapy of depression. *Psychological Bulletin, 114*, 248–264.

White, W. A. (1937). The origins of love and hate by I. D. Suttie. *Psychoanalytic Review, 24*, 458–460.

Wiborg, I. M. & Dahl, A. A. (1996). Does brief dynamic psychotherapy reduce relapse rates of panic disorder? *JAMA Psychiatry*, 53, 689–694.

Winnicott, D. W. (1965). *The maturational process and the facilitating environment*. New York: International Universities Press.

Wolberg, L. R. (1965). The technique of short-term psychotherapy. In L. R. Wolberg (Ed.), *Short-term psychotherapy*. New York: Gruner Stratton.

Zeigarnik, B. (1927). *Psychologische Forschung*, 9, 1–85.

Zilbergeld, B. (1992). *The new male sexuality*. New York: Bantam.

INDEX

Abbass, Allan 119
abdomen, heavy feeling 111
acceptance (grief stage) 111
achievement, internal obstacles (removal/minimization) 208
active alcohol abuse 29
active intervention strategies, usage 174
activity, inhibition 109
acute distress 158
acute grief, somatic/psychological symptomatology 110
acute grief syndrome 111; characteristics 111
adaptive alternatives, usage 214
adaptive capacity, increase 166
adaptive functioning, prevention 171
adolescence, re-doing 80
adult ego, mastery opportunities 3
adulthood, self-defeating consequences 61–62
affair, occurrence (anxiety/guilt) 156
affect: access, deepening 100; activating, techniques 104–107; breakthrough 185; centrality 100–101; deepening, techniques 104–107; defense, handling 106; depressive affect, handling 83; detail, focus 104–105; direct experience, anxiety intensity (reduction) 78; feeling, handling 106; focus, maintenance 107; imagery, usage 105; importance 101; modulation, improvement 165; research support 102–103; specificity, focus 104–105; therapist empathy/encouragement, providing 107
affect, experience 7, 31; patient acquaintance 106–107; tolerance, increase 171
affective activation process 108
affective attunement, deficit 106
affective experience 101–102; components *7*
affective expression, freedom 166
affective information, usage 66
affective involvement, intensification 14
affect-laden experiences 120–121
affect-laden interaction 208
affect-laden unconscious communications, production 30
aggressive feelings 54; sexual, 148; feelings, fusion 138
aggressive impulses/sexual impulses, handling (therapeutic strategies) 148–155
alliance, resistance (contrast) 13
aloneness, fear 59, 178
Amyotrophic Lateral Sclerosis (ALS), death 238
analysis: process 169; termination criteria, fulfillment 208
"Analysis Terminable and Interminable" (Freud) 197
analysts: idiosyncratic interventions 4; radicalness 65
analytic focus 47
analytic treatment, ISTDP (contrast) 174

anger: acute grief syndrome characteristic 111; appearance 66–67; avoidance 33, 72, 183, 227; breakthrough 64; defenses 84–85; defenses, examination 33–34; direct experience 74; direction (Man with Sexual Difficulties, a) 125–126; direction (Woman with Panic Attacks, the) 130–131; experience 39, 56–57, 67; experience, freedom 89; feeling, evocation 45; feeling, trouble 42–43; focus 33–34; grief stage 111; growth 182–183; memories 159; motoric element 71; patient examination 43; physiological element 71; presence 63, 71, 80; self-defeating approach 83; swallowing, tendency 236
antidepressants, usage 46
anxiety: assessment 37; baseline, obtaining 11; channels *9*, 10; cognitive disruption, impact 10–11; de-coupling 168; disappearance 226–227; diversion 98; emotional reaction 80; excess 166–167; exploration 6, 68, 79; feelings/defenses, relationship (understanding) 166; flooding 89; Freud perception 4–5; increase 167; intensity, reduction 78; link, insight (increase) 78; modulation, improvement 165; muscles, involvement 10; operational definition 10–11; optimal range 77; overcoming 197; pathways 10; patient exploration 60; physiological manifestations, exploration 89; positive feelings, relationship 137–138; presence 60–61; provocation 149; second theory (Freud) 4–5, 52
anxiety-provoking events 2–3
anxiety-provoking feelings, examination 108
anxiety, reduction 166, 171; changes 166–167; methods 89; techniques 88–89; Woman with Panic Attacks, the 132–133
arms: pain, presence 48; tension 68
associations: outpouring 77; spontaneous flow 151
associations, de-repression (central dynamic sequence phase) 15; history-taking, de-repression 21–22; unconscious material, de-repression 21–22
attachment: figures 154–155; theories 137–138
attention: evidence 96; non-verbal communication, comparison 119
avoidance, disadvantages 141
avoidant stance, maintenance (consequences) 18–19

baby, death (mourning) 117–120
backing off, impact 20
back spasms, experience 160
bargaining (grief stage) 111
barrier, maintenance 69
Beck, Aaron 103
behavior: change, failure 194; compliance 85; transference pattern, interpretation 198
beliefs: de-repression 121–122; pathogenic beliefs, role 156
belief system, trauma experience (inclusion) 221
belligerence 49
bereaved: emotional upheaval, endurance 113; survival/adaptation 113
bereavement 110
boarding school, attendance 60, 61
bondage, release 231
boss, anger (direction) 125–126
breakdown, approach 124
Brief Symptom Inventory (BSI) 28
buried feelings, liberation 181
business failures 42

cancer diagnosis, internal crisis 80, 229
Cape Fear (movie) 157
Cardinal, Marie 154
catharsis 2, 185

central dynamic sequence 15–23, 27; defense analysis 17–19; feelings, breakthrough 19–21; initial phases, abandonment 45; inquiry 15–17; insights, interpretation/consolidation 15, 22–23; phases 15–23; unconscious material/history-taking, de-repression 21–22
change: achievement 13; cyclical nature 232; deep change, facilitation 104; evidence 199; factors, feedback 231–232; instance, focus 175; process, acceleration 65; resistance, problem 192–193
character: armor 12, 54; change, processing 164; pathology 12; resistance 54; structure 78
character defenses: addressing 45–46; ego attack 83–84; reliance, self-defeating consequences 194
characterological defenses 29
chest: heavy feeling 111; pains, presence 48; tension 68
children: dependence 5; separation 205
choice, freedom 154–155
choking, desire 90
clarification: process 60; requirement 39
clinical depression 41
clinical examples: Cold Blooded Businessman, the 216, 228; defense analysis 58–65; Detached Observer, the 67–74, 140, 208–210, 239–243; erotic feelings 140–141; Gentleman Scorned, a 40–45; Good Girl, the 235–239; grief 116–120; Lonely Businessman, the (grief response) 58–65, 216–222; Manic-Depressive's Daughter, the 30–36, 206–208, 235; Man in a Fog, the 116–120; Man with an Explosive Temper, the 182–191, 214–216; Man with Primary Impotence 147–148, 243; Man with Sexual Difficulties, a 125–129; Masochistic Artist, the 156–162, 177–182, 210–214, 230–235; Mother's Little Angel 204–206; positive feelings 140–141; termination 204–222; Woman on an Emotional Roller Coaster, the 79–91, 228–229; Woman with Headaches, the 92–99, 225–228; Woman with Panic Attacks, the 130–133
closeness: conflict 209; defenses, challenge 211; desire 209; feeling 86; issue 61; longing(s) 138, 139, 190; result 215; terror 62
Coconut Grover disaster, grief 110–111
coffin, dream 133–134
cognitive behavioral therapy (CBT): effectiveness, decrease 103; relapse rates 236
cognitive clarity, defenses 159–160
cognitive disruption, impact 10–11
cognitive information, usage 66
cognitive modes, affective modes (integration) 103–104
cognitive perceptual disruption 29
cognitive re-analysis 77, 185–186; feeling breakthrough, relationship 87; usage 83–84
cognitive understanding 169
Cold Blooded Businessman, the: clinical example 216; follow-up, improvement (clinical evidence) 228
coldness, feeling 184
collaborative atmosphere 23
communication: disguised means 161; recognition 203
competition: enjoyment 240; sibling rivalry 219–220
competitiveness, feelings 219–220
complex mixed feelings, rise/breakthrough (central dynamic sequence phase) 15
compliance, targeting 26
confidence, feelings 211
conflict: anxiety-laden area 33; emphasis 40; examination 38; identification/denial pattern 42; intensity 36, 43; shift 239
conflicted feelings, resolution 82
conflicting forces, impact 19–20
conflictual feelings, role 13
conscious ego, handling 2

consciousness: impulse/feeling pathway, re-directing 87; impulses, appearance 98–99; repressed material, appearance 197
conscious therapeutic alliance 107–108
contact: avoidance 67; resistance 147
control, loss (fear) 34
Control Mastery theory, development (Weiss) 170
cool, losing 126
coping, definition 168
corrective emotional experience 64, 145
creative functioning, capacity (increase) 172
creativity: blossoming 216–217; observation 239
crime, punishment 129
cumulative trauma, result 124
curiosity, evidence 96
Current figures-Past genetic figures (C-P) link 80–81, 123, 126; Manic-Depressive's Daughter 32–33; Man with Sexual Difficulties, a 126; pathological beliefs 123–124; Woman on an Emotional Roller Coaster, the 80–81
cyclical psychodynamics 188
cynicism, impact 196

Davanloo, Habib: defense analysis 116; defense work approach 54–55; innovations 22; intensive short-term psychotherapy 1; intrapsychic crisis, creation (advocacy) 164; pathological mourning studies 115; re-interpretative interventions, development 27; psychotherapy, approach 202; termination findings 201–202; treatment model 172; trial therapy process, development 25
death: loss, mourning 133; manner, impact 114; misery 22
deceased: identification, exaggeration 111; image, preoccupation (acute grief syndrome characteristic) 111; patient identification 134–135; relationship, impact 114
decompensation, absence 123–124
deep change, facilitation 104
deep signing 111
defense(s) *8*; acquaintance 55–65; assessment 9, 37, 38; breakdown 129; challenges 21; clarification 47–48; cognitive clarity 158–159; consequences, examination 57; contra-indication 77; cost-benefit analysis 61–62; cost, examination 55; cost, grief (relationship) 62; defense theory concept 52; distinction 48; ego, attacks 18, 63–64, 65–74; emotional closeness, defenses 183–184; emotional closeness, defenses (focus) 61; erection 72; feelings/anxiety, relationship (understanding) 166; focus 199; fortification 30; function, elucidation/clarification 55, 56–57; fusion 81; identification 18, 56; internalization defense, cost-benefit analysis 97–99; mix, patient experience 48–49; mobilization 63; operation 6, 7; operational definition 8–9; outward direction 53; positive feelings, relationship 137–138; regressive defenses, restructuring 76; release, pressure/challenge 18; reliance, decrease 172; reliance, decrease (evidence) 168–169; restructuring, technique 65, 77–78; theory, concepts 51–53; therapist identification 56; transference, relationship 119–120; types 8–9; usage 9; work 19; work, approach (Davanloo) 54–55; work, goals 66
defense against emotional closeness (DOEC) 12
defense analysis: responses 57–58; responses, anger (appearance) 66–67
defense analysis (central dynamic sequence phase) 15, 17–19; advances 53–55; clinical example 58–65; complex mixed feelings, rise/breakthrough 15, 19–21; defenses, identification/clarification 18–19; ego/defenses, attacks 18–19; feelings, complexity 21;

impulse, portraiting 20–21; patient release, pressure/challenges 18, 19; responses 57–58; transference, breakthrough 19–21
defense analysis (Davanloo) 116
defenses, handling 51, 106; techniques 55
defensive barriers, impact 12–13
defensive behaviors 168; awareness 18
defensive displacement, evidence 94
defensiveness: experience 63; pattern, setup 231
defensive processes, reliance (decrease) 166
defensive structure, alteration 165
defensive system, examination 53
defensive withdrawal: meaning/impact, awareness 185; relatedness replacement 215–216
defiance: defense 43; presence 41
dejection, feeling 109
denial: grief stage 111; regressive defense 33–34
dependency, tendency (observation) 194
depression: clinical depression 41; episodes 78; exploration 79–80; grief stage 111; history 30; meaning 15
depressive affect, handling 83
depressive mechanism, restructuring 82–83
depressives, restructuring (usage) 78–79
de-repression: central dynamic sequence phase 15; continuation 144–146; Man with an Explosive Temper, the 186; mother, death 132; phenomenon 101–102; post trauma, sudden de-repression 130; primal scene, de-repression 143–144; process 108, 137; research support 102–103
desire: emergence 140–141; evidence 96; feeling 150
despair, feeling 113
Detached Observer, the 77; clinical example 67–74, 208–210, 239–243; desire, emergence 140–141; detachment, consequences (examination) 68–69; detachment, defense (challenge) 69–70; fantasy 146–147; feeling, defense 141; follow-up, improvement (clinical evidence) 239–243; longing, emergence 140–141; loved, attached (tenacity) 133–135; memories, de-repression 73–74; needs/desires, reconciliation 153–154; pressure and challenge technique, usage 70; resistance, head-on collision 70–71; sadistic impulses, breakthrough 71–72; T-P link 73; transference, anger (presence) 71; transference, anxiety (exploration) 68
detachment: defense 184; presence 41, 147; schizoid defenses 242–243
developmental history, exploration 22
developmental material, revealing 204–205
Diagnostic and Statistical Manual of Mental Disorders, Fifth Edition (*DSMV*), usage 242–243
diarrhea, report 10
direct therapeutic intervention, aim 138
disablement 110
discrimination, deficit 106
disequilibrium 40
disordered mourning, occurrence 115
disorganization, feeling 113
displacement 8, 34; elements, removal 95; usage 92
dissociated state 132
dissociation 29; episodes 29
distance, maintenance 69
distancing 39; defenses, cost (examination) 62
distorted beliefs, examination 122–123
distress, physical state 10
disturbance areas, examination 15
doctors, fear 132–133
dog: hatred 73–74; murder (flashback) 186
"do or die" procedure 66
dreams: depiction 133; de-repression 22; work (Masochistic Artist, the) 158
drive theory, impact 191–192
Duncan, Isadora 116
dynamic concepts, operational definitions 7–14

dynamic diagnosis, obtaining 28–29
dynamic psychotherapy 165; accelerated form 198; effectiveness 224–225; ISTDP, distinctions 142–143; notion 193; practice 51; speed/effectiveness 108–109
dynamic unconscious, discovery 2
dysfunctional thoughts/beliefs, identification 103
dystonic defense 28–29, 33; assessment 9, 38
dystonic feelings 30–31; avoidance 56–57

ego: attacks 18–19, 63–64, 65–74; character defenses (attack) 83–84; clinical example 67–74; conscious ego, handling 2; defense theory concept 52; desensitization 22, 66; fragility 11, 168; function, observation 56, 105; functions, development (increase) 172
ego-adaptive capacity 9, 10, 172; building 87; evaluation 25; high level 60; increase 115; information, providing 16; patient functioning 191; patient level 237
ego functioning 78, 165; alterations 213–214; changes 208; high level 8, 10; increase 95–96; low level 11
Elavil, usage 46
electroconvulsive shock treatment, relapse rates 224
emotional activation 55; increase 166; prevention 104
emotional changes 207–208
emotional closeness 154–155; barriers, absence 28–29; defenses 38, 125, 183–184; defenses, focus 61
emotional contact, deflection/prevention 8
emotional detachment 93, 120
emotional experience: cognitive understanding 103; elements 7
emotional expression, freedom (increase) 169
emotional healing, de-repression 239
emotional involvement 20, 38, 102; intensification 91; prevention, resistance (impact) 76–77
emotional reactions, detachment 110
emotional upset, absence 159
emotional withdrawal, requirement 128
emotions: handling, ability 221; importance 101
empathic connection 231
empathic contact, maintenance 162
empathy, distinction 98–99
enemas, memory 180
energy, suffusion 94
enjoyment, derivation 180
enthusiasm, renewal 171
epiphenomenon 137
erectile failure 125
erection, loss 147
erotic feelings: anxiety/defense, presence 139; clinical example 140–141; handling 136
evaluator, contact 55
excessive anxiety 166–167
excitement, sense 41
experience, cognitive modes/affective modes (integration) 103–104
explosive anger/fear, cycle (damage) 221
exposure, importance 166–167
external constraints 52
externally provoked frustrations, adjustment capacity (increase) 208
external stimuli, approach 86
eye contact 49; avoidance 9, 68

factual inquiry 46
false self 12
family: dynamics, assumptions 158; gathering, avoidance 227
father: alcoholism 98; attacks, brutality 226; brutality, anger 188; death 238; displacement 153; fight 97; glaring 95; hatred 95; Man with an Explosive Temper, the, link 190; murder, desire 97, 189; pain, empathy 98–99; replacement, desires 143, 145–146; sexual abuse 189–190; Woman on an Emotional Roller Coaster, the, relationship 82

feelings: aggressive feelings 54; anxiety/defenses, relationship (cognitive understanding) 166; assessment 38; avoidance 32, 56–57, 60, 65, 218; breakthrough 19–21, 86–87; buried feelings, liberation 181; cognitive element 7, 8; complexity 21; components, absence (meaning) 7; confidence 211; conflict 215; conflictual feelings, role 13; dangers, assessment 160; defense 38, 141; de-repression 90–91, 132, 180–182; detachment 33; directed experience, gradual exposure 77; direct experience 87; distinction 48; erotic feelings, handling 136; examination 104; experience 39–40; experience, enhancement 20–21; exploration 31, 59; facing, motivation/capacity (increase) 78; fusion 81; handling, adaptive means 218; helplessness, feelings (mastery) 166; hope 211; inquiry 37; intensification 133; mix (patient experience) 48–49; motoric element 7; narrative coherence (integration), trauma memories (impact) 221; negative feelings 49, 54; negative transference feelings 108; numbing, feeling 112; Oedipal feelings 140; operational definition 7–8; pain 70; pathway, re-directing 87; patient experience 17–18; patient exploration 41; physiological element 7; repressed feelings, functional disorder symptoms (link) 92–94; resentment 127–128; rivalry 140; sadness, feelings 118–119; sexualized feelings, emergence 138–139; strength 5; therapeutic relationship, sexual feelings 138–140; transference, relationship 119–120; upsurge, experience 61, 95
"fishing for feelings" 106
flashbacks, occurrence 187–190
focused attention, requirement 173
focused interview, usage 104–105
follow-up 224; Cold Blooded Businessman 228; Detached Observer, the 239–243; Good Girl, the 235–239; growth, increase 201; importance (Freud emphasis) 177; improvement, clinical evidence 225–243; inquiries 177; Manic-Depressive's Daughter, the 235; Man with Primary Impotence 243; Masochistic Artist, the 230–235; session 65; significance 224–225; Woman on the Emotional Roller Coaster 228–229; Woman with Headaches, the 225–228
follow-up interviews 239; awareness 225
forbidden feelings/impulses, reduction/elimination 167
forgetting (regressive defense) 33–34
forgiveness, distinction 98–99
formal defenses 53; operational definition 8
freedom, feeling 177
freedom of choice, increase 154–155
freedom of emotional expression, increase 169
Freud, Anna 53
Freudian slip 151
Freud, Sigmund: "Analysis Terminable and Interminable" 197; follow-up, importance 177; grief, discussion 109–110; *Inhibitions, Symptoms and Anxiety* 5; *Interpretation of Dreams* 52; *Mourning and Melancholia* 109; "On the History of the Psychoanalytic Movement" 4; *Outline of Psychoanalysis, An* 121; second theory of anxiety 4–5, 52; "seizing the resistance by the throat" 174; working through, consideration 165
friendships, expectations (mirroring) 230–231
Fromm-Reichman, Freida 169, 175
frustration 184; growth 182–183
functional disorders (suffering), restructuring (usage) 92; clinical example 92–99
fury: feeling 130; mother, fury 148

gender-related behavior, shaping 156
genital sexual longing 146
Gentleman Scorned, a 204, 208; anger, examination 43; clinical example 40–45; feelings, exploration 41; resistance, examination 41–42; self-defeat, exploration 42–43; T-C-P interpretation 44–46; triangle of conflict 44
good, acceptance 211–212
good-bye (saying), difficulty 152, 220
Good Girl, the: clinical example 235–239; conflict, shift 239; creativity, observation 239; follow-up, improvement (clinical evidence) 235–239; mind-body connection 238–239
good things, acceptance 211
graded pressure and challenge technique: systematic desensitization, similarities 86; usage 86
grandmother: death/loss 123; matches theory 155; sickness 122
gratification, finding (ability) 213
grief: acute grief, somatic/psychological symptomatology 110; acute grief syndrome 111; bearing, inability 125; Bowlby, contribution 112–113; characteristic 112; clinical example 116–120; deceased, identification (exaggeration) 111; defense, mother (erotic attachment) usage 152–153; defenses, cost (relationship) 62; despair/disorganization, feeling 113; duration 112; emotion, awareness 106; experience, decompensation (absence) 123–124; experience, defenses 106; facing (Man with Sexual Difficulties, a) 127–129; findings (Kübler-Ross) 112–113; Freud discussion 109–110; mourning process, distortions (transformation) 111; numbing, feeling 112; occurrence 208–209; outpouring, complexity 109; process 109–113; reorganization, process 113; response (Lonely Businessman, the, clinical example) 58–65; sessions, results 122; sharing 119; sharing, prevention 117; syndrome, occurrence 111; treatment, implications 115–116; ulcerative colitis, appearance 111; unresolved grief, defenses 137; work (Lindemann) 110–111
grief, feelings: avoidance 90–91; evocation 44–45; pain 118
grief-laden feelings, experience (facilitation) 100
grief work 108–109; difficulty 133; focus 115
growth: change 171–172; sign 203
guilt: acute grief syndrome characteristic 111; de-coupling 168; experience, defenses 106; facing (Man with Sexual Difficulties, a) 127–129; feelings, avoidance 90–91; sense, pervasiveness 129; survivor's guilt 135

Haan, Norma 168
hand, fist configuration 20
happiness: continuation, belief 233; internal obstacles, removal/minimization 208
"head-on collision" 66, 70
health: confirmation 40; internal obstacles, removal/minimization 208
helplessness 70; character defense, clarification 47–48; experience 90; feelings 180, 207; feelings, mastery 166; sense, pervasiveness 171; usage 69
Herman, Judith 220
history-taking, de-repression 21–22
homosexual rape, memory 189–190
honesty 70
hope, feelings 178, 211
hopefulness 210
hopelessness: feelings 207; sense, increase 124
hospitalization: approach 124; requirement 92
hostility (acute grief syndrome characteristic) 111
human attachments, centrality 5

humor, usage 235
hurt, direct expression (importance) 54
husband: conflict 35; exit 230; fury 130–131; mistreatment 46; murder, imagining 131; physical abuse 46; stabbing, desire 131, 167; substitute, usage 205; Woman with Panic Attacks, the (anger) 130–131
hypnosis, usage 3

ideas, de-repression 121–122
imagery, usage 105
impulse control disorder, severity 29
impulses: assessment 38; control 35; control, evaluation 182–183; defense 38; direct experience, gradual exposure 77; direct feeling 87; instantaneous internalization 89; mobilization 7; operational definition 7–8; pain 78; pathway, re-directing 87; "portraiting the impulse" 20–21; sexual impulses/aggressive impulses, handling (therapeutic strategies) 148–155; strength 5
inhibitions, overcoming 197
Inhibitions, Symptoms and Anxiety (Freud) 5
innate aggressive drives 192
innate instincts, focus 52
inner guardedness 60
inquiry, patient involvement 45–46
insight-oriented psychotherapy 47
insights: consolidation, triangles of conflict (link) 199; discovery 102; interpretation/consolidation (central dynamic sequence phase) 15
insights interpretation/consolidation 15, 22–23; therapeutic contract, making 23; therapeutic tone, control 23
integration, role 169
intellectual functioning, capacity (increase) 172
intellectualization 8, 23, 59
intense affect: experience, functions 22; mobilization 104
intensive short-term dynamic psychotherapy (ISTDP): active intervention 174–175; analytic treatment, contrast 174; benefits, patient usage (assessment) 26; changes, occurrence 235; circular process 165–166; demands 76; development 51; dynamic psychotherapy, distinctions 142–143; ego-adaptive capacity/suitability data 30; focus 173; focused interview, usage 104–105; goals 108, 213; initiative 142; intention 23; label 4; long-term effectiveness, studies 224; patient defenses, identification/clarification/exhaustion 109; patients, active role (encouragement) 170; patient treatment 217; power/strength 173; practice, therapist (impact) 176; revisions, translation 121–122; strategies/techniques, incorporation 54–55; termination, presence 201; therapeutic goal 108; therapeutic process 136; therapist, focused interview 105; therapist, openness/honesty 14; trial therapy, comparison 27–28; working through 186
intensive short-term psychotherapy (Davanloo), theory/technique (integration) 1
interaction, modes 186
intercourse, attempt 147
internal crisis 40; creation 65–66
internal images, interpersonal experience (impact) 188
internalization: mechanism, undoing 95–96; process 214
internal obstacles, removal/minimization 208
interpersonal conflict, childhood patterns 103–104
interpersonal context, importance 6
interpersonal difficulties 47
interpersonal distance 120
interpersonal dynamics 188
interpersonal experience, effect 188
interpersonal reality 121
interpersonal relationships, rule 154

interpretation: links 22–23; usage 27, 52
Interpretation of Dreams (Freud) 52
intervention: occurrence 66; patient response 30
intimacy: conflict 209; isolation, contrast 154–155; issue 61
intimate relationships: formation/maintenance, ability (increase) 172; improvement 212
intrapsychic conflicts: concepts 51–52; conceptualization 7; genesis 33; genesis, intrapsychic conflicts (relationship) 66
intrapsychic crisis, creation 14; advocacy (Davanloo) 164
intrapsychic disequilibrium 40
intrapsychic phenomena 212
intrapsychic solution, interpersonal consequences 183
intrapsychic system, loosening 22
Inventory of Interpersonal Problems (IIP) 28
irritation: examination 183–184; experience, suppression 182–183
isolation, impact 196

jealousy, memories 159
joy: capacity, evidence 136; experience 209; tenacity 106

Kübler-Ross, Elizabeth 111, 113

learning, application 176
learning-theory based approaches 166–167
lethargy, experience 16
Lewis, C.S. 112
libidinal cathexis, withdrawal 109–0110
life: constriction 69; episodes, representations 187; misery, mother (impact) 36; self-critical aspect 207; self-defeat 70; shortening 237
life-affirming counterforce 154
life-events, recall (facilitation) 187
Like Water for Chocolate (Esquivel) 155
Lindeman, Erich (grief work) 110–111
living: harmony 208; process 168
Lonely Businessman, the (grief response) 65; anxiety, exploration 60; clinical example 58–64, 216–222; competition, sibling rivalry 219–220; emotional closeness, defenses (focus) 61; good-bye (saying), finding 220; loss, handling (comparison) 218; new changes, effect (processing) 219; T-P link 64–65; triangle of conflict, examination 59–60
Lonely Businessman, the (grief response), defenses: cost-benefit analysis 61–62; cost, grief (relationship) 62; ego, attack 63–64
Lonely Businessman, the (grief response), termination: approach, regression (evidence) 217–218; symptoms, return 217
Lonely Businessman, the (grief response), transference: anger, presence 63; anxiety, presence 60–61; feelings/defense, appearance 218
longer-term therapy, involvement 219–220
longing: direct expression, importance 54; emergence 140–141; feeling 150
loss: approach 124; handling, comparison 218; pain 124, 133, 200
lost object, patient replacement 205
love: display 215; torture, absence 182; trap, feeling 180
loved one: attachment, tenacity 133; loss, grief 9
lovemaking, satisfaction 159
love-making scene, description 144
loving feelings: avoidance, rationalization (attempt) 141; sexual feelings, integration 149–150

"Madonna and Whore" split, development 148, 216
maladaptive defenses, manifestations 219–220
manic behavior 81
Manic-Depressive's Daughter, the: anger, focus 33–34; changes, review 206–207; clinical example 30–36, 206–208,

235; control, loss (fear) 34; C-P link 32–33; emotional changes 207–208; evaluation, smoothness 36; follow-up, improvement (clinical evidence) 235; inquiry, return 35–36
manic-depressive mother 31
manic-depressiveness 83
Man in a Fog, the 125; clinical example 116–120; portrait, resumption 120; sadness, feelings 118–119; transference, feelings/defense 119–120
Mann, James 171, 178
Man with an Explosive Temper, the 221; affect, breakthrough 185; clinical example 182–191, 214–216; cognitive re-analysis 185–186; cyclical psychodynamics 188; defensive withdrawal, relatedness replacement 215–216; de-repression 186; emotional closeness, defenses 183–184; father, link 190; father-son relationship, P-C link (impact) 191; homosexual rape, memory 189–190; impulse control, evaluation 182–183; life-events, recall (facilitation) 187; self-understanding, capacity (evidence) 214–215; triangles, link 186
Man with Primary Impotence 171; clinical example 147–148, 243; follow-up, improvement (clinical evidence) 243
Man with Sexual Difficulties, a: anger (at boss) 125–126; clinical example 125–129; C-P link 126; guilt/grief, facing 127–129; rage, facing 126–127
marital separation 80; reason 58–59
marital therapist, usage 58
marriage: briefness 46; collapse 79; decision 92; enjoyment 232–233; failure 162; immutability 230; terror 226
masochism, roots 160–162
Masochistic Artist, the 168; change, factors (feedback) 231–232; clinical example 156–162, 177–182, 210–214, 230–235; cognitive clarity, defenses 158–159; confidence, feelings 211; difficulties, response 235; dream work 158; fantasy interpretation, creation 159–160; feeling, dangers (assessment) 160; feelings, de-repression 180–182; follow-up, improvement (clinical evidence) 230–235; good, acceptance 211–212; hope, dawning 178; hope, feelings 211; intimate relationships, improvement 212; masturbatory fantasies, exploration 157–158; mother rape, memories (de-repression) 180–182; post-termination transference reactions 230–231; re-playing, re-living (contrast) 162; self-care, development 178–179; sexual fantasies, usage 179–180; symptoms, changes 179–180; therapeutic process, internalization 212–214; therapist, internalization 212–214
Masochistic Artist, the, termination 210–214; feelings, sharing 212; possibility, patient idea 210
mastery: goal 121; sense, achievement 170–171
masturbatory fantasies 152; exploration 157–158
"matter-of-fact" tone, information communication style 117
meaning system, trauma experience (inclusion) 221
memories: approach, defenses 117; authority 221; evocation 187; fallibility 187; outpouring 77; pain 70; reconsolidation, research 102; retrieval 102, 105; return 132–133; slippage 33–34; surfacing 104
memories, de-repression 30–31, 121–122, 132; Detached Observer, the 73–74; Woman on an Emotional Roller Coaster, the 90–91
memories, de-repression (central dynamic sequence phase) 15, 66; history-taking, de-repression 21–22; unconscious material, de-repression 21–22
Menninger, triangle of insight (drawing) 6
mental illness, appearance 74

migraines, presence 48, 92
Miller, Alice 160, 171
mind-body connection 238–239
minimization 8
misalliance, impact 43
mistreatment 46; vulnerability 85
mixed feelings, experience 122, 196
mother: access 145–146; attachment 133; connection 63; coolness/aloofness 140; death, de-repression 132; desire 143; discussion, failure 127; disturbed character 209–210; erotic attachment 152–153; fantasy 151; feelings, intensity 74; fucking 150; fury 148; histrionic aspect 220; jealousy 152; manic-depressive mother 31; Man with Sexual Difficulties, a (rage) 126–127; murder, imagining 128–129, 171; nervous breakdown 122–123; physical abuse, imagining 127; physical exhaustion 206; rape, memories (de-repression) 180–182; relationship, reassessment 129; selfishness 152–153; sexual desire 151; touching, avoidance 141
Mother's Little Angel: clinical example 204–206; feeling 220; new self, emergence 206; task, accomplishment 206
motivation: display 30; increase 45
mourning: disordered mourning, occurrence 115; pain, avoidance 114; pathological course, translation (absence) 117; pathological mourning 113–115; phase, fixation 114; process, distortions (transformation) 111
Mourning and Melancholia (Freud) 109
muscles, tension 96
muscular weakness, feeling 111
mutual pleasure, fantasy 179
myopia 144

negative consequences, outlining 19
negative feelings 49, 54
negative memories, impact 196
negative response, occurrence (absence) 187
negative transference feelings 108
neurosis: core conflicts, nature (revealing) 22; origin 11; transference neurosis 140
neurotic fear, consideration 34
neurotic maladjustment 147
neurotic suffering: cure 100–101; origin 11
new changes, effect (processing) 219
newness, sense 41
new self, emergence 206
non-verbal communication 119
nonverbal tactical defenses 9
numbing, feeling 112

object-related attachment theory 146
object relations, theories 137–138
Oedipal conflict, appearance 242
Oedipal feelings 140
Oedipal myth 146
Oedipal victor 152
one-to-one connection 96
"one two punch" (Coughlin) 55–56
"On the History of the Psychoanalytic Movement" (Freud) 4
"on the spot" situation, experience 60–61
openness 70
others: distorted beliefs, examination 122–123; perceptual distortions 104
outcome: success, chance (optimization) 121; termination, importance 198–203
Outline of Psychoanalysis, An (Freud) 121
outpatient psychotherapy 16

pain: cause 191; contact 32; feeling, description 31; internal pain 59; presence 21; resistance 179; source 185
panic, episodes 78
parental introject: ouster 153–154; quality 213–214
parents, destructiveness 154
passivity: character defense, clarification 47–48; targeting 26
past: exploration, possibility 36; forgetting, ability 32
Past genetic figures-Current figures (P-C) link (father-son relationship) 191

pathogenic beliefs, role 153
pathogenic defenses, reliance 206
pathological beliefs: accuracy, assessment 124–125; C-P link 123–124; dispelling 120–124
pathological defenses: replacement 214; usage 237–238
pathological mourning 113–115; death, manner 114; deceased, relationship (nature) 114; distinction 110; premorbid personality adjustment, impact 114; presentation 116; studies (Davanloo) 115; susceptibility 114–115
pathological processes, repetition fear (absence) 197
patient: anger, focus 33–34; benefits, ability (assessment) 26; clinical example 30–36; contra-indications 29; control, loss (fear) 34; core conflict, origin 91; counteroffer 14; C-P link 32–33, 80–81, 123, 126; defensiveness, interpretation 3; defensive system, restructuring 3; evaluator, role 26; feedback, invitation 225; focus, development 27; fragility 53; functioning, issues 114; initial evaluation, purposes 26; insight, need 57; intervention response 30; intrapsychic workings, understanding 37; life, active role (assumption) 174; mobilization 66; pathological processes, repetition fear (absence) 197; psychopathology, usage *28*, 28–29; selection criteria 26–28; suffering, factors (determination) 26; symptoms, suffering (cessation) 197; therapist, collaborative effort 199; training 175
patient defenses: acquaintance 55–65; analysis, responses 57–58; consequences, examination 57; function, clarification 56–57; identification 56
patient difficulties, inquiry/survey (central dynamic sequence phase) 15–17; clarity, absence (challenge) 16; focus, maintenance 17; inquiries, specificity 15–16; survey, obtaining 16; work, patient willingness (securing) 17
patient (developmental history), exploration (central dynamic sequence phase) 15; developmental history, exploration 22; history-taking, de-repression 21–22; therapeutic value 22; unconscious material, de-repression 21–22
patient treatment: active role, assumption 174; suitability assessment 26–30; undermining, defenses cost (examination) 55
patronization 84
people, loss 183
personality, structural/dynamic whole (modification) 208
personal relationships, gratification 210
pessimism, experience 16
Phantom of the Opera 214
phenomenological inquiry, return 89
physical abuse 46
physical healing, de-repression 239
physical motion, description 73
physical pleasure, experience 182
physical symptoms, defense function 92
physical violence 235
physiological reactivity, reduction 221
"portraiting the impulse" 20–21
portraiting, usage 20–21, 105, 176–177
positive feedback, receiving 212
positive feelings: appearance (treatment, midphase) 139–140; clinical example 140–141; defense, presence 139; defenses 137–138; handling 136; nervousness 149
positive feelings, anxiety: impact 137–138; presence 139, 149
post trauma, sudden de-repression 130
post-traumatic stress disorder 114
pre-interpretative interventions, development (Davanloo) 27
premorbid personality adjustment, impact 114

pressure and challenge technique 65–66; Detached Observer, the, example 70; graded pressure and challenge technique, systematic desensitization (similarities) 86; graded pressure and challenge technique, usage 86
primal scene, de-repression 143–144
privacy, violation 155
procrastination: replacement 220; reversion 217
projection 29; regressive defense 88
psychic functioning, responsibility 52
psychic weaning 147
psychoanalytic inquiry, focus 52
psychoanalytic principles, adherence 54–55
psychoanalytic theory, tenets 2–3
psychodynamic(s): cyclical psychodynamics 188; theory, therapeutic implications 11–13
psychodynamic psychotherapy, essence 3
psychological growth 166
psychopathology: maintenance 153; spectrum *28*, 28–29, 38
psychosomatic complaints, exacerbations 78
psychotherapy: approach (Davanloo) 202; development 15; entering 17; goal 167; insight-oriented psychotherapy 47; process, initiation 11
punishment: fear 179–180; masochistic suffering, usage 161

rage: control, absence 92, 205; direct expression, importance 54; experience 33–34, 97, 182; expression, fantasy 21; facing 97, 126–127, 161; feeling 181; mechanism, blocking 95; murderous rage 126–127, 226; pattern 93–94; reservoir, access 35; sadistic rage, breakthrough 90; violence 86
rape: fantasies 157; flashback 189–190; imagining 234
rationalization 8, 23, 34
reaction formation 8
reactive sadism, defenses 137
ready-made negative transference, patient exploration 46–47
reciprocal interaction 188
regression: change 171–172; replacement 220
regressive defenses 106; operation 84–85; reliance, absence 13; reliance, decrease 78; restructuring 76; undoing 87; usage 33–34
regressive weepiness, experience 90
rejection: fear 150; meeting 62
relapse rates 236
relationships: closeness/trust 221; current relationship, triangle of conflict 84–85; development, satisfaction 135; gratification 193; improvement 241; intimate relationships, formation/maintenance ability (increase) 172; intimate relationships, improvement 212; safety 237; separation/loss/disappointment 124; triangle of conflict, usage 78
relief, feeling 177
reorganization, process 113
repetition compulsion 191–193
re-playing, re-living (contrast) 162
repressed feelings, functional disorder symptoms (link) 94
repressed impulses: link, insight (increase) 78; self-attack, link 90; targeted symptom, link 86
repressed material, appearance 197
repressed pain/sorrow, trigger 133
repression: balance, shift 30–31; defenses, reliance 78–79; label 2; undoing 101
repressive barrier, penetration 101
resentment: direct expression, importance 54; feeling 49; presence 152
resistance: alliance, contrast 13; continuation 72; defense theory concept 52–53; focus 199; head-on collision 70–71; increase, passivity increase (Freud reaction) 12; low level, demonstration 57–58; overcoming 52–53; patient examination 41–42
resourcefulness 230
restlessness (acute grief syndrome characteristic) 111

restructuring 77–78; clinical example 79–91; cognitive re-analysis 77; cyclical process 97; defense restructuring, technique 77–78; depressive mechanism, restructuring 82–83; elements 77; goals 87; process 95; usage (depressives) 78–79
re-working 100
rights, violation 155
romance, back burner 241

sadism: disguised act 92; reactive sadism, defenses 137
sadistic impulses: breakthrough 71–72; severity 98
sadistic rage, breakthrough 90
sadness: arrival 185; experience 16
sadness, feelings 99, 118–119, 152; depth 127
safe distance, keeping 62
sarcasm: defenses 43; usage 88
second theory of anxiety (Freud) 4–5, 52
"seizing the resistance by the throat" (Freud) 174
selection criteria (patient) 26–28
self: child sense 124; distorted beliefs, examination 122–123; false self 12; internalized images, modification 165; internalized models, revisions 188; living, harmony (ability) 208; perceptual distortions 104; sense, damage (cessation) 221
self-attack, repressed impulse (link) 90
self-awareness 230
self-care: deficit 179; development 178–179; emergence 179
self-contradiction, defense 43
self-defeat 70, 145; patient exploration 42–43; pattern 42
self-defeating consequences 18
self-defeating defenses 87; abandonment 65–66; ego attack 83; reliance, absence 13
self-defeating effects 130
self-defeating nature, examination 85
self-defense 180
self-image, loss (effects) 124–135
self-protection: deficit 179; inability 85
self-sacrificing 160
self-soothing, capacity 182
self-understanding, capacity (evidence) 214–215
self-validation, focus 177
separations, pain 124
sessions, change (attention) 174
sex: acting out 156; discussion 142
sexual arousal, feeling 150
sexual contact, response 145
sexual desire, absence 125
sexual dysfunction, history 147
sexual encounters 36
sexual fantasies 157–158; changes 179–180
sexual feelings: aggressive feelings, fusion 138, 148; avoidance, rationalization (attempt) 141; loving feelings, integration 149–150; memory 150; presence 151; projection 158–159; therapeutic relationship 138–140; usage, tactical defense 138
sexual impulses/aggressive impulses: freedom of choice, increase 154–155; handling, therapeutic strategies 148–155; mother, erotic attachment 152–153; parental introject, ouster 153–154; T-P link 150–151
sexuality, conflict 209
sexualized feelings, emergence 138–140
sexual longings: dangers 141–146; de-repression, continuation 144–146; emergence 149; primal scene, de-repression 143–144; transference, occurrence 142–143
sexual prowess, power/toughness (equivalence) 146
sexual relationship, satisfaction 129
short-term anxiety-provoking therapy 200
short-term dynamic psychotherapists, agreements 198
short-term dynamic psychotherapy (STDP): benefits, absence 13;

change, process 169; development 104; effectiveness 26–27, 174; research 103–104; therapeutic outcomes, achievement 208
short-term dynamic therapists, tools/techniques 104
short-term treatment, development (Sifneos) 26
sibling rivalry 219–220
silence, usage 69, 72
sisters, sexual molestation 139
sleep disturbance, report 10
“Sleep Watchers” (Picasso) 158
smooth muscle (anxiety channel/pathway) 10
social supports, role 113
somatic discharge 110
somatic distress (acute grief syndrome characteristic) 111
somatization 29
son: conflict 35; pathological mourning 123
specificity 15–16; assumption 216; focus 104–105; importance 203; need 202–203
splitting 29, 106
stabbing, imagining 90
state-dependent learning, reference 102
stillborn, disappearance 117
strangulation 88
striated muscle (anxiety channel/pathway) 10
substance abuse 29
suffering: absence 208; factors, determination 26; freedom 14; perpetuation, defenses cost (examination) 55; pleasure 161; punishment 153; symptoms, patient cessation 197
support: continuation 237; display 215
survivor’s guilt 135
symptomatic behavior, economy 169
symptomatic disturbances 29, 205
symptoms: changes 179–180; meaning 108; phenomenological experience, exploration 79; return 217
syntonic character defenses, ego attack 97
syntonic defense: assessment 9, 38; indication 68
systematic desensitization, graded pressure and challenge technique (similarities) 86

tactical defenses 138; operational definition 8–9
temper tantrums 94–95; verbal temper tantrums 182
tender feelings, expression 6
tenderness: longings 138; taboo 146–148; tenacity 106
tension: experience 63; impact 192; increase, description 93–94
termination 196; approach, regression (evidence) 217–218; clinical examples 204–222; consideration 197; criteria, fulfillment 208; expectations 202; findings (Davanloo) 201–202; findings (Mann) 200–201; findings (Sifneos) 199–200; importance, determination 198–203; Masochistic Artist, the 210–214; opportunity 207; planning, specificity/flexibility (need) 202–203; possibility, patient idea 210; post-termination transference reactions 230–231; preparedness, consideration 201; regression, tendency 170–171; research (Malan) 198–199; symptoms, return 217; therapist expectations, effect 202; uncomplicated termination 199, 204, 206
theory-guided technique, importance 4–6
therapeutic alliance: increase 45, 62; usage 34
therapeutic contract, making 23
therapeutic efforts (undermining), defiance (impact) 42
therapeutic goal 23; attention 108; interference 36
therapeutic interaction 89
therapeutic intervention: design 109; goals 77–78; resistance 2–3

therapeutic misalliance, result 19
therapeutic process: emotional involvement 103; intensification/acceleration 105; internalization 212–214; re-analysis 23
therapeutic relationship 121; sexual feelings 138–140
therapeutic stance 13–14
therapeutic strategies 148–155
therapeutic success 169, 228
therapeutic tone, control 23
therapeutic work, resistance 116
therapist: activity, high level (impact) 174; alliance, strength 96; closeness, feeling 86; empathy/encouragement, providing 107; expectations, effect 202; follow-up inquiries 177; internalization 212–214; longing, direct expression (importance) 54; longing, presence 140–141; mixed feelings 21; openness/honesty 14; rage, expression (fantasy) 21
therapy, learning-theory based approaches 166–167
throat, tightness 111
time-limited psychotherapy 200
To Kill A Mockingbird (copy, gift) 216
torture: chamber 157; desire 98; imagining 234
toxic affects (experience), ego (desensitization) 22, 66
transference: anger, presence 63; anxiety, exploration 68; anxiety, presence 60–61; breakthrough 19–21; distortion 67; examination 102; mixed feelings 14; negative transference feelings 108; neurosis 140; neurosis, possibility 142; occurrence 142–143; pattern of behavior, examination 199; relationship 72, 193; resistance 193; sexual longing, emergence 149; triangle of conflict, involvement 87–88
Transference-Current figures (T-C) links 49; importance 175
Transference-Current figures-Past genetic figures (T-C-P): interpretation (Gentleman Scorned, a) 44–46; interpretation, affective/cognitive information (usage) 66; making 66
Transference-Current figures-Past genetic figures (T-C-P) link 103; frequency 173; interpretive work focus 156; Lonely Businessman, the (grief response) 64–65; making 23, 45
transference feelings 21; complexity 67, 69–70, 76–77; defense 119–120; intensification 65–66; priority 45; surface appearance 71
Transference-Past genetic figures (T-P) link 150–151; Detached Observer, the, clinical example 73; Lonely Businessman, the, clinical example 64–65; sexual impulses/aggressive impulses, handling 150–151; Woman on an Emotional Roller Coaster, the 89–90
transformations, possibility 228
trauma: conscious ego, handling 2; cumulative trauma, result 124; definition 5; de-repression, post trauma (sudden de-repression) 130; emotions, handling (ability) 221; experience, inclusion 221; Masochistic Artist, the, clinical example 156–162; memories, impact 148, 221; memories, resurfacing 105, 178; recovery 221; re-living 162; response, gender differences 155–162; victims, special consideration 220–222
traumatic events 192
traumatic experiences 187, 243
traumatic interactions, re-enactment 161–162
traumatic loss 208
treatment: defense, focus 199; goals 172–173; implications 172–173; midphase, positive feelings 139–140; patient suitability, assessment 26–30; resistance, focus 199; sterility/disappointment 67; termination 203
Trevor, William 109
trial therapy 25; conducting 108; effectiveness, studies 28; Gentleman

Scorned, a, clinical example 40–45; Manic-Depressive's Daughter, the, clinical example 30–36; process, development (Davanloo) 25; treatment suitability, assessment 26–30; triangles, usage 37–39
triangle of conflict *6*; clarification/differentiation, extent (determination) 37; current relationship 84–85; defense restructuring, clarification/differentiation 77; elements, distinction (inability) 77; elements, linking 37; insight consolidation, link 199; interpretation 68; involvement 87–88; label 6; link 22–23, 173; patient examination 44, 58–59; trial therapy usage 37–39; triangle of the person, links (making) 22; triangle of the person, relationship 27; usage 78; Woman on an Emotional Roller Coaster, the 81; working 81
triangle of conflict, corners: assessment 37–38; differentiation 38–39; linking 39
triangle of insight, drawing (Menninger) 6
triangle of the person *6*; elements, linking 37; focus, switch 89; label 6; link 22–23; trial therapy usage 37–39; triangle of conflict, links (making) 22; triangle of conflict, relationship 27
triangle of the person, corners: assessment 37–38; differentiation 38–39; linking 39
triangles: link 186; "working the triangles" 18
triangle work (central dynamic sequence phase) 15
trust, problems 44
Two Lives (Trevor) 109

ulcerative colitis 238; appearance 111; suffering 110
uncertainty, cause 191
uncomplicated termination 199, 204, 206
unconscious: direct communication 21; genetic system, relationship *12*; material, de-repression 21–22; signal 19–20; unlocking 21–22, 58, 107, 184
unconscious feelings: approach 29; unlocking 150
unconscious forces, understanding 25
unconscious memories, unlocking 150
unconscious therapeutic alliance (UTA) 14, 107–108; increase 76–77
unresolved grief, defenses 137

vagina, fondling 151
vaginal area, approach 151
vagueness: response 16; targeting 26
Valentine's Day, recollection 191
verbal tactical defenses 9
verbal temper tantrums 182
victimization, identity (consolidation) 155–156
visualization 176–177

"walking wounded" (appearance) 117
well-being, confirmation 40
wheelchair tennis, participation 239
Woman on an Emotional Roller Coaster, the 238–239; anxiety, exploration 79; anxiety, reduction (techniques) 88–89; character defenses, ego (attack) 83; clinical example 79–91, 228–229; cognitive re-analysis, usage 83–84; C-P link 80–81; depression, exploration 79–80; depressive mechanism, restructuring 82–83; feelings, de-repressions 90–91; follow-up, improvement (clinical evidence) 228–229; graded pressure and challenge technique, systematic desensitization (similarities) 86; graded pressure and challenge technique, usage 86; memories, de-repression 90–91; restructuring, goals 87; T-P link 89–90; transference, triangle of conflict (involvement) 87–88; triangle of conflict 81; triangle of conflict, current relationship 84–85; triangle of conflict, father (relationship) 82

Woman with Headaches, the 238–239; clinical example 92–99, 225–228; follow-up, improvement (clinical evidence) 225–228; internalization defense, cost-benefit analysis 97–99; trigger, exploration 92–93
Woman with Headaches, the, symptoms: exploration 92–93; reemergence 95–96; repressed feelings, link 94–95
Woman with Panic Attacks, the 167; anger, direction 130–131; anxiety, reduction 132–133; clinical example 130–133; loved one, attachment (tenacity) 133; mother (death), de-repression 132; post trauma, sudden de-repression 131
Woman with Two Failed Marriages, the: clinical example 45–49; defenses, clarification 47–48; inquiry 45–46; ready-made negative transference, exploration 46–47; transference, feeling/defense mixture 48–49
women, relationships (sado-masochistic quality) 139
"working the triangles" 18
working through 164, 171; change (absence), insight (impact) 193–194; changes, display 166; clinical examples 177–191; essence 186; follow-up inquiries 177; phrase, defining 165; process 172–173; repetition compulsion 191–193; technical considerations 174–175; treatment, implications 172–173
working through, process 165–172; facilitation, active intervention strategies (usage) 174; integration, role 169

Xanax, usage 46

For Product Safety Concerns and Information please contact our EU representative GPSR@taylorandfrancis.com Taylor & Francis Verlag GmbH, Kaufingerstraße 24, 80331 München, Germany